Intraosseous Vascular Access

James H. Paxton

Editor

Intraosseous Vascular Access

A Guide for Healthcare Professionals

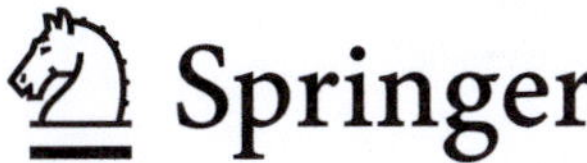

Editor
James H. Paxton
Department of Emergency Medicine
Wayne State University School of Medicine
Detroit, MI, USA

ISBN 978-3-031-61203-9   ISBN 978-3-031-61201-5   (eBook)
https://doi.org/10.1007/978-3-031-61201-5

This Springer imprint is published by the registered company Springer Nature Switzerland AG
The registered company address is: Gewerbestrasse 11, 6330 Cham, Switzerland

If disposing of this product, please recycle the paper.

Preface

My first exposure to intraosseous (IO) vascular access was as a trauma surgery resident working in a busy urban Level I trauma center. My mentor, Dr. Thomas Knuth, had a wealth of military experience and had become familiar with IO cannulation techniques during his military service. I was surprised by the lack of civilian experience with this technique but immediately grasped the value of this somewhat unorthodox approach to vascular access. Under Dr. Knuth's tutelage, I first studied a cohort of trauma patients in 2008, who received the proximal humerus approach to IO vascular access, and found that this technique was not only invaluable but also incredibly safe and effective. Over the last 15 years, I have seen the growth of this approach in the civilian world and have personally witnessed the potential of IO infusion to salvage the resuscitation of patients who cannot receive direct venous access rapidly enough to achieve clinical stabilization.

Although explorations of therapeutic IO cannulation have been underway for more than a century, much of the early research into this modality is squirreled away in obscure journals, some of which are no longer in print. Even recent data can be hard to find, leading to a somewhat disjointed view of this approach in many modern reviews on the topic. Our goal with this "primer" is to present the modern clinician with at least a scoping review of relevant knowledge in a cohesive and cogent manner. Despite the extensive growth of the IO approach in the prehospital and emergency medicine environments, consideration of the IO technique remains underutilized in the clinical arena. We believe that lack of familiarity and education with this modality is a key factor contributing to this phenomenon and hope to improve upon this situation through a targeted discussion on several fundamental aspects of the technique.

As an emergency medicine physician, I am haunted by the memory of patients who suffered intolerable delays in vascular access due to inaccessible peripheral veins. This is never a problem when IO cannulation is considered in the vascular access algorithm, but providers must be comfortable with IO cannulation and competent in the use of this technique for its potential to be fully realized. When we published our primer, "Emergent Vascular Access," in 2021, only a single chapter was dedicated to IO access. After publishing that "primer," it became obvious that an entire book was needed to describe the many nuances of the IO technique. This book is the result of that unanswered need for improved awareness of the risks and benefits of the IO approach to indirect venous access.

Modern patients can expect to live longer with chronic diseases than ever before due largely to recent diagnostic and therapeutic advances that prolong life by reducing the risk of emergent complications. But chronic diseases lead to recurrent hospitalizations and other acute care events, ultimately requiring repeated direct venous access attempts. Each direct venous access attempt (successful or failed) carries with it the potential for venous injury or other traumatic effects that can render future attempts at venous cannulation at that site more difficult or even impossible. Patients carry these scars of previous venous injury with them into future care events, eventually leading many patients with chronic illness toward a state of difficult venous access that may overwhelm the ability of providers to safely and efficiently establish therapeutic venous access during an emergency. Thus, as we get better at keeping people with chronic illness alive, we are likely to experience an increasing threat of difficult or impossible direct venous access. Alternative routes for providing fluids and medications to critically ill patients are needed to combat this threat, and I believe that indirect routes of venous access such as the IO approach will become increasingly important to future generations of clinicians and patients.

This book is dedicated to the emergency care provider who has attempted or at least considered the need for direct venous access but has found that direct methods for venous access are not adequate or feasible. Recognition that IO access is an available option is a crucial step toward improving the care of our emergency patients under austere conditions where direct venous access is not assured. It is our hope that a better understanding of this approach will yield better outcomes for patients with difficult venous access, both now and far into the future.

Detroit, MI, USA   James H. Paxton

Contents

1 A History of Intraosseous Vascular Access 1
Jacob Dougherty and James H. Paxton

2 Anatomy and Physiology of Intraosseous Infusion 43
Andrew Mizerowski and James H. Paxton

3 Indications and Contraindications 59
Jacob C. Lenning and James H. Paxton

4 Intraosseous Access Site Selection 93
Katherine Quibell and Julia Yip

5 Manual Intraosseous Devices 115
David Greiver, Sarah Chung, and James H. Paxton

6 Automatic and Semiautomatic Devices 131
Parker J. Marsh and James H. Paxton

7 Flow Rates with Intraosseous Catheterization 149
Nicholas Righi and James H. Paxton

8 Intraosseous Medication Administration 167
Paul Dobry, Stephanie B. Edwin, Renée M. Paxton, Tsz Hin Ng,
and Christopher A. Giuliano

9 Complications of Intraosseous Access 215
Stephanie Cox, Aleksandria Bartosiewicz, Erin Rieck,
Jacob Fanning, Amanda Pierce, Jonathon Verde, Sameer Jagani,
and James H. Paxton

10 Pain with Intraosseous Infusion 249
Bobak Ossareh, Aaron J. Wilke, and James H. Paxton

11 Decision-Making for Intraosseous Infusion 287
Zaid Mohsen and James H. Paxton

12 The Future of Intraosseous Vascular Access 301
James H. Paxton

Index 319

Contributors

Aleksandria Bartosiewicz Michigan State University College of Osteopathic Medicine, East Lansing, MI, USA

Sarah Chung Department of Emergency Medicine, Wayne State University School of Medicine, Detroit, MI, USA

Stephanie Cox Michigan State University College of Osteopathic Medicine, East Lansing, MI, USA

Paul Dobry Department of Pharmacy, Eugene Applebaum College of Pharmacy and Health Sciences, Wayne State University, Detroit, MI, USA

Jacob Dougherty Department of Emergency Medicine, Wayne State University School of Medicine, Detroit, MI, USA

Stephanie B. Edwin Department of Pharmacy, Ascension St John Hospital, Detroit, MI, USA

Jacob Fanning Michigan State University College of Osteopathic Medicine, East Lansing, MI, USA

Christopher A. Giuliano Department of Pharmacy, Eugene Applebaum College of Pharmacy and Health Sciences, Wayne State University, Detroit, MI, USA

David Greiver Department of Emergency Medicine, Wayne State University School of Medicine, Detroit, MI, USA

Sameer Jagani Michigan State University College of Osteopathic Medicine, East Lansing, MI, USA

Jacob C. Lenning Department of Emergency Medicine, Western Michigan University Homer Stryker M.D. School of Medicine, Kalamazoo, MI, USA

Parker J. Marsh Department of Emergency Medicine, Wayne State University School of Medicine, Detroit, MI, USA

Andrew Mizerowski Department of Emergency Medicine, Wayne State University School of Medicine, Detroit, MI, USA

Zaid Mohsen Department of Emergency Medicine, Wayne State University School of Medicine, Detroit, MI, USA

Tsz Hin Ng Department of Pharmacy, Ascension St John Hospital, Detroit, MI, USA

Bobak Ossareh Department of Emergency Medicine, Wayne State University School of Medicine, Detroit, MI, USA

James H. Paxton Department of Emergency Medicine, Wayne State University School of Medicine, Detroit, MI, USA

Renée M. Paxton Department of Pharmacy, Ascension St John Hospital, Detroit, MI, USA

Amanda Pierce Michigan State University College of Osteopathic Medicine, East Lansing, MI, USA

Katherine Quibell Western University of Health Sciences, Pomona, CA, USA

Erin Rieck Michigan State University College of Osteopathic Medicine, East Lansing, MI, USA

Nicholas Righi Department of Emergency Medicine, Wayne State University School of Medicine, Detroit, MI, USA

Jonathon Verde Michigan State University College of Osteopathic Medicine, East Lansing, MI, USA

Aaron J. Wilke Department of Emergency Medicine, Wayne State University School of Medicine, Detroit, MI, USA

Julia Yip Department of Emergency Medicine, Wayne State University School of Medicine, Detroit, MI, USA

A History of Intraosseous Vascular Access

Jacob Dougherty and James H. Paxton

History of Intraosseous Vascular Access

The earliest reference to studies of the intraosseous (IO) circulation can be traced back to **Franz Müller** (1871–1945), of Humboldt University (Berlin, Germany), at the turn of the twentieth century. In animal studies, Müller observed that blood taken directly from the nutrient vein of the canine tibia was identical in its composition to blood drawn from other parts of the animal [1]. Around the same time, the first bone marrow samples from living patients were obtained independently by two physician-scientists, Italian hematologist **Giuseppe Pianese** (1864–1933) at the Anatomical-Pathological Institute of Naples and German hematologist **Alfred Wolff-Eisner** (1877–1948) of Berlin, circa 1903, in an effort to diagnose parasitic infections [2, 3]. While none of these early scientists developed a technique for IO infusion, their groundbreaking work would stimulate interest across the globe in studying the bone marrow and its blood supply.

Building on Müller's research, **Cecil Kent Drinker** (1888–1956), a professor of physiology at Harvard University Medical School (Cambridge, Massachusetts), noted the extensive vascular network that existed within the canine tibia and suggested that substances injected into the tibial bone marrow could be taken up and distributed into the central circulation [4]. Although Drinker was an anatomist and physiologist, his early publications were among the first in the English-language literature to propose the potential therapeutic use of intraosseous infusion. Drinker published his report on maintaining circulation through the tibia of an anesthetized dog in 1916, including a proposed method for perfusing the bone marrow, as illustrated in Fig. 1.1 [4]. Drinker's technique involved exposure of the nutrient artery of

J. Dougherty (✉) · J. H. Paxton
Department of Emergency Medicine, Wayne State University School of Medicine, Detroit, MI, USA
e-mail: hl6843@wayne.edu; james.paxton@wayne.edu

J. H. Paxton (ed.), *Intraosseous Vascular Access*,
https://doi.org/10.1007/978-3-031-61201-5_1

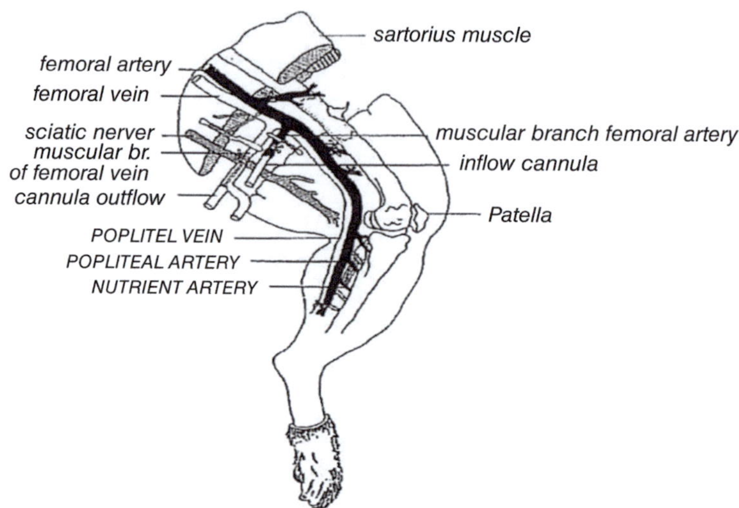

Fig. 1.1 Drinker's original sketch of his technique for studying intraosseous blood flow [5]

Fig. 1.2 Cecil K. Drinker *(Image courtesy of Harvard T.H. Chan School of Public Health. © 2023 The President and Fellows of Harvard College. All rights reserved.)* [6]

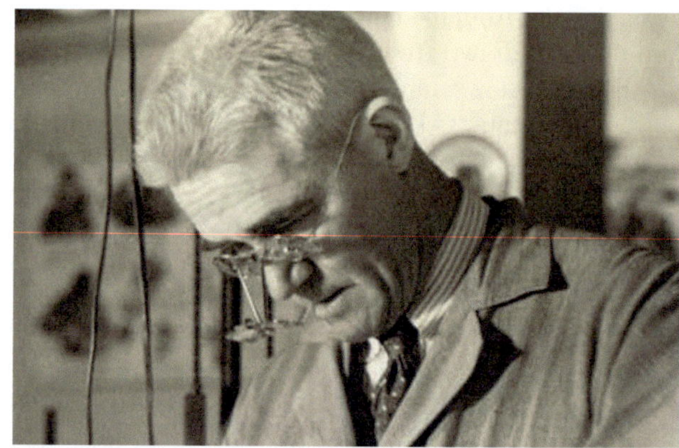

the tibia following ligation of the popliteal artery branches. Cannulation of the popliteal artery was performed, and study solution was then shunted through the cannula into the tibial nutrient artery, with the aid of a thigh tourniquet [5]. Drinker's experiments, in which he injected various substances into the live canine tibia to observe their movement and removal from the marrow, demonstrated that infused substances were subsequently distributed into the central circulation [5]. A photograph of Drinker examining his work can be seen in Fig. 1.2.

Perhaps inspired by the early work of Drinker and others, **Charles A. Doan** (1896–1990), a medical student at Johns Hopkins University (Baltimore, Maryland), similarly explored the role of bone marrow in the circulation of adult pigeons [7]. While attempting to deliver ink, mercury, and saline into the pigeon's circulation through intraosseous infusion, Doan found that infusion pressures near 130 mm were

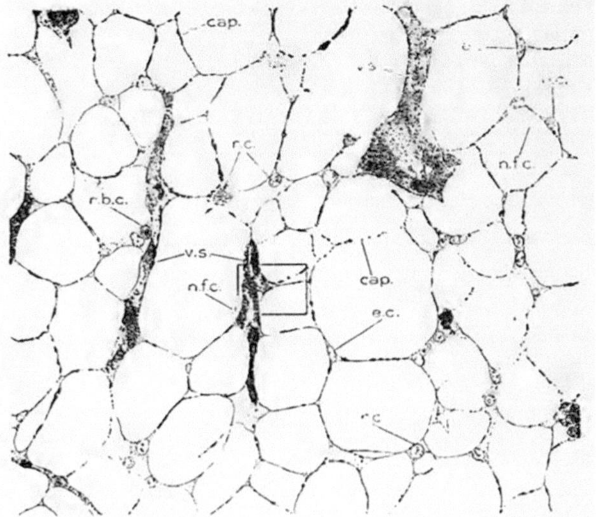

Fig. 1.3 Doan's original sketch of the intraosseous capillary system [7]

required, but pressures above that level led frequently to tissue injury. In his 1922 publication, Doan reported that a well-defined and extensive network of capillary beds existed to drain the marrow space of adult pigeons. Although much of the hematopoietically active marrow had been replaced with fatty tissue in adult subjects, he speculated that these channels were "functionally dormant" and might be activated to drain the marrow space in times of urgent need [7]. Doan's original sketch of the capillary is illustrated in Fig. 1.3, with endothelial cells (ECs), reticular cells (RCs), nuclei of fat cells (NFCs), red blood cells (RBCs), capillaries (CAPs), and venous sinusoids (VSs). The interstitial capillaries can be surrounding the nuclei of fat cells and communicate with the larger venous sinusoids, with carbon granules distributed via injection scattered throughout the capillaries. A photograph of Doan is provided in Fig. 1.4.

This pioneering work by Drinker and Doan laid the framework for subsequent experiments involving human subjects and clearly inspired other scientists to explore the use of intraosseous infusion for therapeutic purposes. German physician **Paul Carly Seyfarth** (1890–1950) of the University of Leipzig investigated the use of sternal trephination for the diagnosis of malaria [9] and brought this technique with him as director of the German Alexander Hospital in St. Petersburg (Russia) from 1922 to 1923. A Russian physician, **Mikhael Innokent'evich Arinkin** (1876–1948) of the nearby Military Medical Academy at Leningrad, adopted Seyfarth's technique using a spinal needle for the diagnosis of various hematological disorders as well as typhus and tuberculosis in 1922 [10].

Arnold R. Josefson (1870–1946), a Swedish internist and pathologist by training, had already become very well known for his work in the diagnosis and treatment of a variety of endocrinologic and hematological disorders. In the early 1930s, Josefson began to explore the possibility of infusing campolon (liver extract) into the sternum and manubrium of human patients as an alternative to intravenous injection in the treatment of pernicious anemia. His report of these experiments in

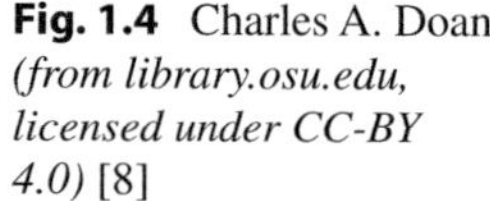

Fig. 1.4 Charles A. Doan *(from library.osu.edu, licensed under CC-BY 4.0)* [8]

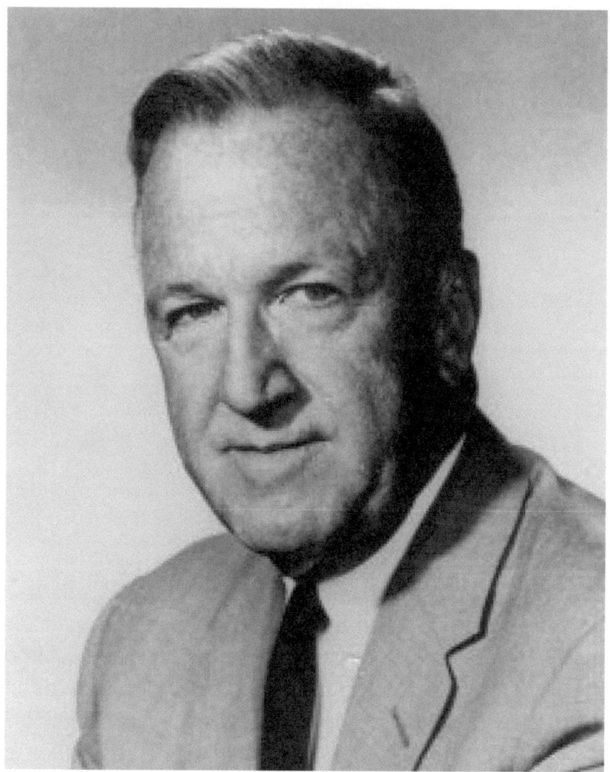

1934 included a claim that intraosseous infusion of this substance was equally effective as intravenous infusion and much simpler to perform. Josefson deemed the IO method superior as a result of less frequent injections being needed when compared to other common routes of infusion [11].

Although Josefson is generally considered to be the first clinician to treat a human patient with intraosseous infusion, his work built on the efforts of Seyfarth, Arinkin, and a host of other European hematologists who pioneered sternal and tibial IO access for diagnostic bone marrow sampling. Italian physician **Giovanni Ghedini** (1877–1959) at the University of Padua (Italy) published the first report of a bone marrow biopsy technique for use in live human subjects in 1908, building on the work of mid-nineteenth-century physicians **Charles-Philippe Robin** (1821–1885) and **Rudolf Albert von Kölliker** (1817–1905), who had described a similar approach for the sampling of cadaveric specimens [12]. Although Ghedini endorsed the tibial bone as a site for marrow sampling, the sternum was generally preferred by Seyfarth and most other investigators. Another early clinician who expanded upon Ghedini's work was the American physician **Francis Weld Peabody** (1881–1927) of Harvard Medical School (Boston, Massachusetts), whose research focused on bone marrow changes with pernicious anemia [12].

Within a few years of Josefson's report, other clinician-scientists began reporting on their own experiences with sternal IO infusion. By 1937, French scientists were

Fig. 1.5 Leandro M. Tocantins. *(Image courtesy of Thomas Jefferson University, Philadelphia. © 2023 Thomas Jefferson University. All rights reserved.)* [16]

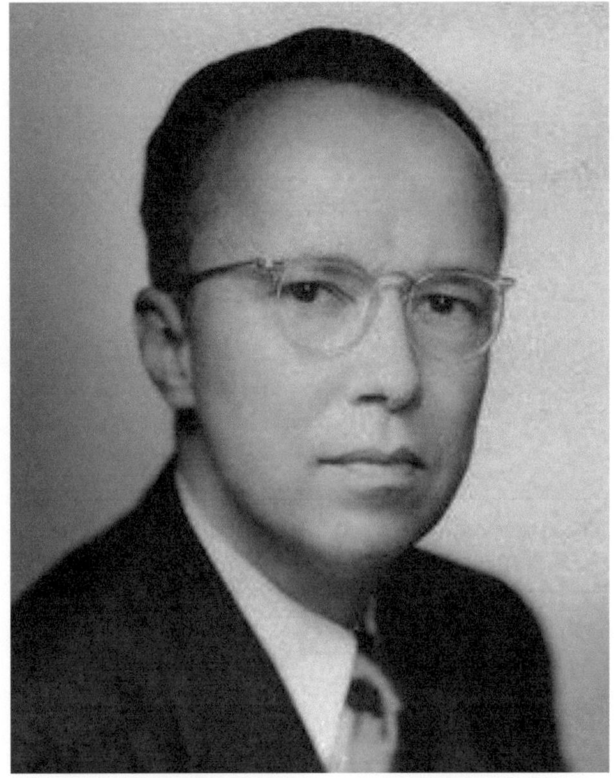

experimenting with IO infusion of drugs, bacteria, air emboli, and various radi-opaque substances in guinea pigs and human subjects [13–15]. In 1940, hematologist **Leandro M. Tocantins** (1901–1963) at the Jefferson Medical College and Hospital (Philadelphia, Pennsylvania) published his first of many reports on the use of sternal IO injection in the treatment of patients suffering from "acute failure of the peripheral circulation" (i.e., shock) (Fig. 1.5). Tocantins' subsequent work with **James F. O'Neill**, a surgeon at the Wake Forest Bowman Gray School of Medicine (Winston-Salem, North Carolina), and internist **Alison H. Price**, a recent graduate of Jefferson Medical College, emphasized the importance of this technique, describing the bone marrow as a superior route of infusion in the setting of hypotension and hypovolemia for both pediatric and adult subjects [17–20]. He found that blood, dextrose, and dye infused into the human sternum or rabbit tibia were absorbed just as quickly as with intravenous infusion, with emergent IO infusion of dextrose capable of rapidly correcting dangerous levels of hypoglycemia [21].

Tocantins' study of the sternal site for IO infusion revealed that the pediatric sternum (especially in infants) appeared to be relatively undeveloped and generally unsuitable for IO infusion. Figure 1.6 demonstrates the path of a solution following injection into the manubrium, with the solution rapidly traveling to the internal mammary veins.

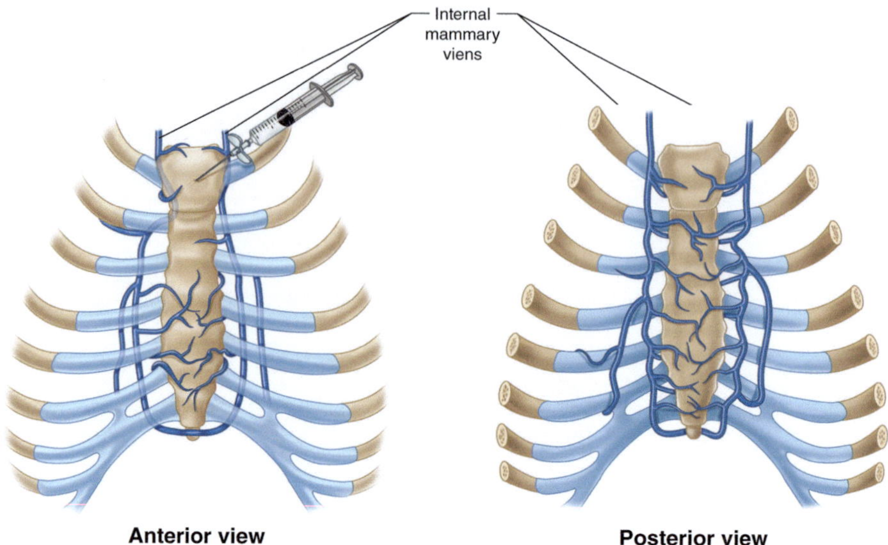

Fig. 1.6 Tocantins' sternal infusion approach, including relevant venous anatomy [18]

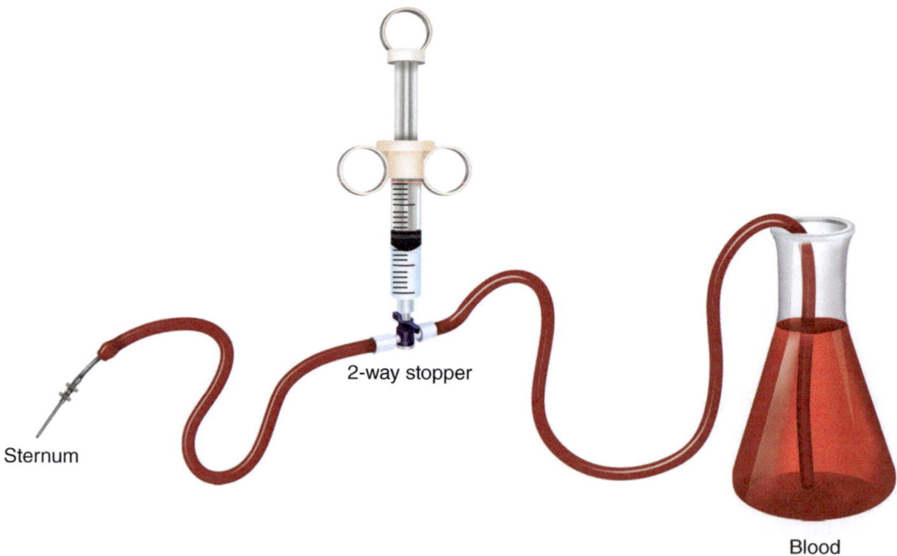

Fig. 1.7 Tocantins' push-pull system for IO infusion [18]

Tocantins' push-pull infusion system (Fig. 1.7) called for the infusate to be first placed into a flask, with tubing including a two-way stopcock placed between the flask and the needle. After closing the infusion tubing system to the sternum, the fluid was drawn from the flask into the syringe. The stopcock was then turned to close the flask tubing system, and the syringe contents were injected through the sternal tubing into the patient's sternum. This process could be repeated without requiring disconnection of the syringe from the infusion tubing, greatly improving the efficiency of high-volume IO fluid infusions [17, 18].

Tocantins was among the first clinician-investigators to propose the use of the proximal tibia (preferred) or distal femur (as a secondary site) for pediatric IO infusions, and he also reported satisfactory results with the proximal humerus site decades before this site was commonly used [19]. Tocantins was also one of the first to develop his own IO device, later known as the "Tocantins needle," which was manufactured by the George P. Pilling and Son company (Philadelphia, 1900–1960) [22]. This needle was described as a "needle with a wide wing top, having a ball guard which slides along the shaft to fix the needle after it is in place, another indwelling needle for marrow aspiration, a stylet, and a curved adapter" [22]. The Tocantins needle was manufactured in four different lengths.

Around the same time, several Spanish- and German-language reports were published extolling the virtues of intraosseous infusion [23–32]. During the late 1930s, German hematologist **Norbert Henning** (1896–1985) began studying the use of IO infusion at the University of Leipzig [25–27]. Although his multiple German-language publications were relatively unreferenced in American medical circles, Henning was a vocal advocate for the use of IO infusion as an alternative to intravenous infusion [27]. Henning also developed his own biopsy needle, which included a side hole for irrigation of the marrow space and graduated centimeter depth markings ringing the cannula [25, 28]. His studies of sternal blood flow revealed that substances injected into the sternum were transmitted to the central circulation via the internal thoracic and brachiocephalic veins with a speed and efficacy comparable to intravenous injection [26]. This led him to announce his findings at the annual meeting of the German Society of Internal Medicine in May 1940, several months before Tocantins published his groundbreaking article [26]. While Tocantins strongly discouraged the IO infusion of hypertonic saline and glucose-containing solutions due to the risk of extravasation with resultant soft tissue necrosis, Henning showed that these substances could also be safely administered, and he was a pioneer in the infusion of blood products through the IO route [29, 30]. Though largely neglected in the English-language IO literature, Henning's work undoubtedly influenced the use of IO technology by other European practitioners much as Tocantins influenced those in the United States and England. Two German surgeon-scientists, **Joseph Korth** (1907) at the University Clinic of Leipzig and **Werner Lamprecht** (1900–1970) of Osnabrück, developed their own eponymous IO catheters that were widely used within the German-speaking world during the 1940s [25, 31, 32].

Emanuel M. Papper (1915–2002), while an anesthesiology resident at Bellevue Hospital (New York, New York) during the early 1940s, built on Tocantins' work by demonstrating that an injection of macasol solution (containing a combination of magnesium and calcium salts) infused at the human sternum was absorbed only slightly less quickly than the same compound injected into the antecubital vein of seven adult subjects (Fig. 1.8) [34]. He discovered similar comparable results with a range of different infusates, reporting that some drugs appeared to be absorbed more quickly from the IO space than others [22]. In fact, 2% sodium cyanide appeared to

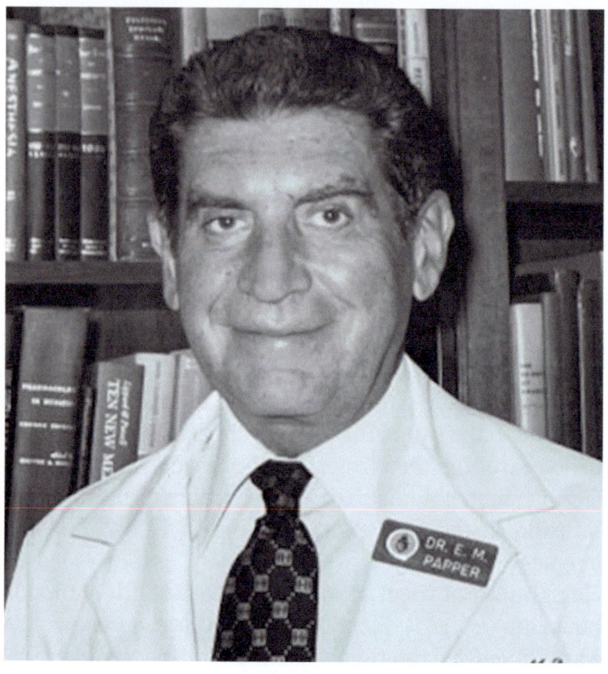

Fig. 1.8 Emanuel M. Papper. (*Image courtesy of the University of Miami Louis Calder Memorial Library collection. © 2023 University of Miami Louis Calder Memorial Library. All rights reserved.*) [33]

be absorbed more quickly from the sternal IO space than from peripheral veins [22]. Papper published his initial findings in 1942 (the same year that he finished residency), along with his mentor, **Emery A. Rovenstine** (1895–1960), then Chair of Anesthesiology at Bellevue. While he acknowledged the utility of the Tocantins needle, Papper suggested that a "wide-bore [Becton-Dickinson] Luer-Lok type (1.5 mm in diameter) sternal needle with accurately ground stylets" was more than adequate [22]. Papper's needle of choice featured a 3 cm long shaft (exclusive of the hub) for adults, with a short (4 mm) bevel and a sharp point and cutting edges [22].

Although intraosseous access had its origins in civilian medicine, the potential benefits of this approach on the battlefield were readily evident. Papper himself was a Major (1942–1946) in the Army Medical Corps and appears to have been a major advocate for the use of IO access to treat injured soldiers during the war. One very-high-profile case of IO infusion involved a Boeing B-29 Superfortress aircraft gunner from Detroit, Michigan, named **Romeo Rendina**. While flying a mission over Nagoya, Japan, on 18 February 1945, an explosive shell penetrated Rendina's aircraft and exploded in his lap. More than 100 shell fragments ripped through his right hand, right arm, and left leg, causing significant blood loss and necessitating immediate vascular access to treat hypovolemic shock [35]. After multiple failed peripheral IV attempts, crew members ultimately inserted a sternal IO device and infused 150 mL of plasma (and morphine) through the sternal IO catheter while Rendina was being transported to a military hospital. This successful resuscitation brought national attention to the use of the IO route for combat resuscitation and appears to be the first documented use of a sternal IO catheter by a medical first responder, although Rendina was only one of many soldiers who benefited from IO infusion during the war [35]. From 1939 to 1945, an estimated 4000 intraosseous infusions were performed on injured Allied soldiers and civilians in the military arena.

As Rendina's case demonstrated, wartime conditions made the establishment of direct peripheral venous access challenging and central venous access was not yet commonplace. British surgeon **Henry Hamilton Bailey** (1894–1961) described situations of extreme hypovolemia, poor lighting conditions ("blackout"), and the chaos of battle in his rationale for proposing IO access as first-line therapy for injured soldiers during wartime [36]. Bailey had served in the British Royal Navy during World War I and experienced these difficulties in caring for injured soldiers first-hand. At the time, stainless steel hypodermic needles were still being used for peripheral venous cannulation and were especially prone to dislodgement and/or iatrogenic vascular injury. Bailey reportedly used a trocar needle with winged handle designed by Whilen Brothers of England to treat patients during the London Blitz (1940–1941).

Penicillin was only just becoming available during the mid-1940s, and ineffective antiseptic methods for peripheral IV catheter placement contributed to a high rate of infection and thrombophlebitis [36]. These factors led to tremendous growth in the use of IO infusion therapy during the 1940s, as the IO route was considered to be a safer (or at least no more dangerous) route of infusion than peripheral IV infusion at the time.

British physician **Joseph Bramhall Ellison** (1898–1953) of the Grove Fever Hospital (London, England) had also served in World War I, and described the intraosseous technique as "utterly simple and the discomfort momentary" [37]. By 1944, Ellison had treated 40 "collapsed and dehydrated" infants with tibial IO infusion in his own civilian practice. As he put it, "no one who has fumbled with a Bateman's cannula and a vein like a bit of chewed cotton, no one who has seen the last available venous channel firmly clotted up, no one hard pressed for time, once having tried this new method is likely to revert to the old. The only snag (barring over-enthusiasm engendered by facility) is the difficulty at the present time of getting needles sharpened" [37]. The Hamilton Bailey-type infusion needle was also one of interest at this time. It was made with a gold cannula for enhanced sterility with a beveled tip to help guide needle insertion on one end and a bulb directly attached to rubber tubing on the other [38].

While Papper and some others advocated for the use of simple "serum needles" to cannulate the sternum, many practitioners preferred Tocantins' winged catheter [37, 39]. Sternal infusion, which had already been largely replaced by tibial infusion in infants and small children, remained a risky venture due to the risk of perforation through the sternum with subsequent infusion into the mediastinum [36, 40–42]. To counter this risk, Bailey developed a winged cannula (Fig. 1.9) intended to prevent the instrument from being advanced too far into the sternum [36].

The Bailey needle itself was a derivative version of the "Witts needle," first introduced to the medical literature circa 1936 by British hematologist **Leslie John Witts** (1898–1982) and first developed for bone marrow biopsy by unnamed clinicians practicing in Egypt [43]. The Witts needle featured a stylet (a) inserted into a needle (b) with an adjustable guard (c) to prevent overpenetration (Fig. 1.10).

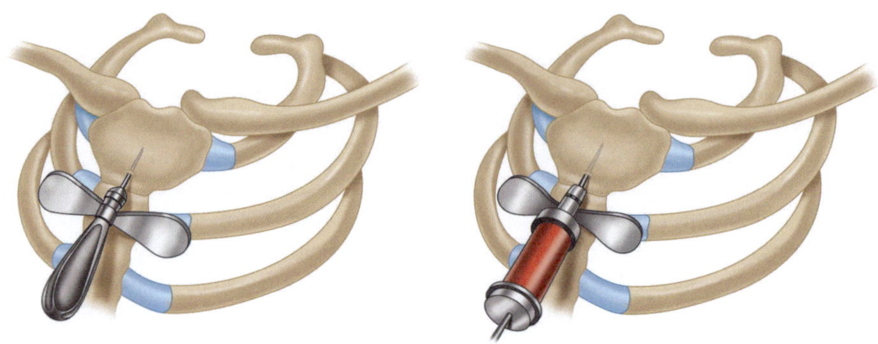

Fig. 1.9 Bailey's winged catheter design [36]

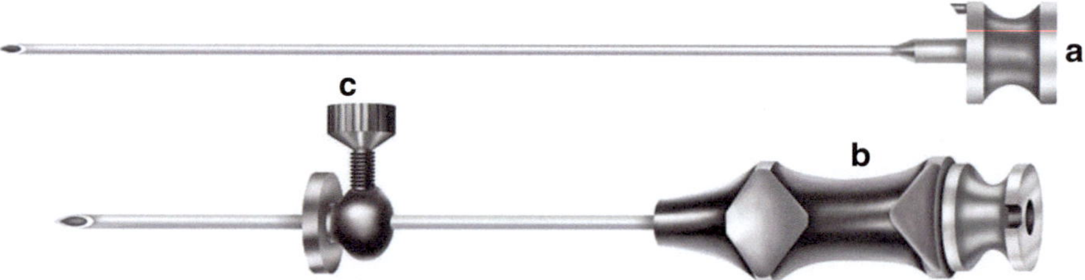

Fig. 1.10 Witts lumbar puncture needle, including internal stylet (**a**), infusion needle (**b**), and adjustable guard (**c**) [43]

The addition of wings to stabilize and guide insertion for IO catheters may have solved the problem of overinsertion with sternal placement, but some felt that these newer devices were inappropriate for use at the pediatric tibia due to their heft and size. In 1944, British pediatrician **Janet Dinah Gimson** (later Roscoe; 1914–2002) of the Hospital for Sick Children, Great Ormond Street (London, England), introduced a needle system (Fig. 1.11) specifically designed for tibial infusion among infants and small children that was lighter, smaller, and more versatile, with needle lengths of $\frac{1}{4}$, $\frac{3}{8}$, $\frac{1}{2}$, and $\frac{5}{8}$ inches. The needle was manufactured by Allen & Hanburys (London), a prominent pharmaceutical company and medical supply manufacturer, in their Bethnal Green factory. Gimson emphasized the need to insert the needle at a right-angle perpendicular to the bone's surface and to use a "strut" with a rubber strap wrapped around the infant's leg to better stabilize the device [44]. As shown in Fig. 1.11, the Gimson needle also featured a large handle to facilitate control over needle insertion.

Many other important IO researchers published their earliest results during the 1940s. Pharmacologist **David I. Macht** (1882–1961), who was working at the time for Hynson, Westcott, and Dunning pharmaceuticals (Baltimore, Maryland), reported on his work with IO epinephrine injection in 1942 [45]. Macht found that

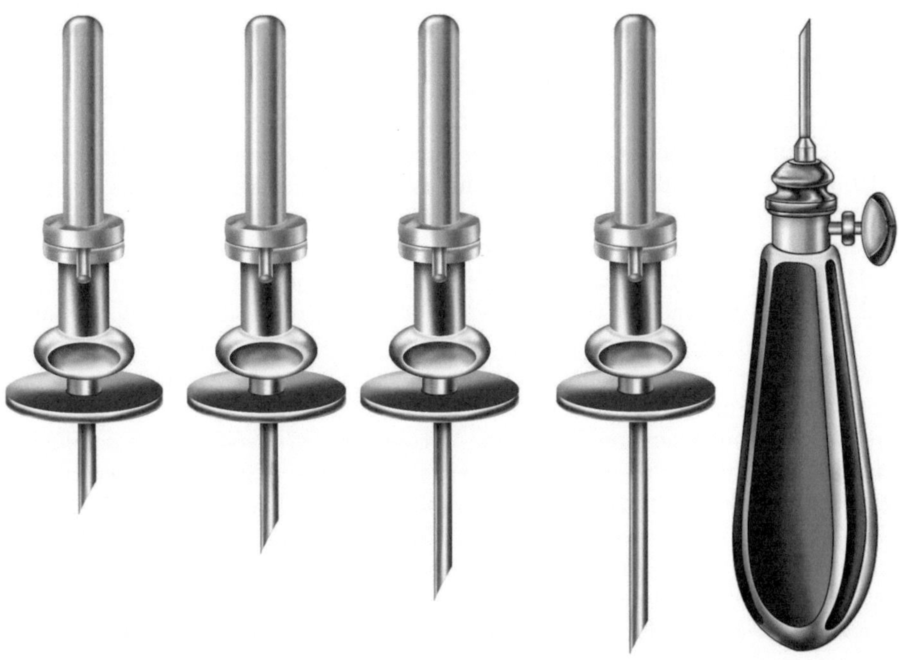

Fig. 1.11 The Gimson needle, demonstrating variable lengths of cannulae (*left*) and large attachable handle to stabilize insertion (*right*) [44]

aqueous solutions of epinephrine administered through the tibia of various animals (e.g., cats, dogs, rabbits, rats, guinea pigs) yielded results that were virtually indistinguishable from intravenous infusions, including a sharp rise in blood pressure followed by a rapid decline [45]. Suspensions of epinephrine in oil, on the other hand, yielded only a moderate increase in blood pressure (i.e., about half of that produced with aqueous solutions), although the effect was longer lasting - up to an hour in some cases [45]. His experiments with various vegetable oil diluents demonstrated the "depot" effect of medications suspended in oil within the IO medullary cavity, suggesting that the drug was being slowly released into the general circulation. While intravenous infusion of these oil suspensions was believed to be "fraught with great danger," he found that IO infusion of oil suspensions rarely resulted in any adverse events among those animals studied [45].

Maurice Morrison (1895–1983) and **AA Samwick** of the Jewish Hospital (Brooklyn, New York) reported a successful human bone marrow transfusion at the sternum for the treatment of idiopathic pernicious anemia in 1940 [46]. Meanwhile, dermatologists **Udo J. Wile** (1882–1963) and **Ira L. Schamberg** (1909–1980) at the University of Michigan (Ann Arbor, Michigan) investigated the effects of IO injection of mapharsen (arsenious oxide), a common treatment for syphilis, on rabbits [47, 48]. They found histological evidence of fat emboli in the pulmonary arterioles of five of the seven rabbits sacrificed in this experiment, with one presumed death due to embolism, although the other four rabbits showed no immediate or delayed clinical evidence of adverse effects [47]. The authors concluded that, "the more rapid the bone marrow infusion and the higher the pressure of the stream of fluid, the greater would be the likelihood of rupturing fat cells and forcing fat globules into the venous system" [47]. In fact, the one fatal embolism noted in this series occurred in the subject exposed to the most rapid infusion rate, approximately 10.9 mL/min (4.54 mL/kg/min). The authors did not entertain the notion that massive rapid infusion of mapharsen, an arsenic-containing substance, may have contributed to the single death in this series.

Heinrich "Henry" Turkel (1903–1992), an Austrian-born American physician and inventor, was another vocal advocate for the use of IO technology. He introduced the IO infusion of amino acids and other fluids at the sternum, ilium, femur, and tibia at the University of Michigan in 1935 and later at Wayne County General Hospital (Detroit, Michigan) in 1937. His collaborators at the University of Michigan included surgeon **Frederick A. Coller** (1887–1964) and hematologists **Frank H. Bethell** (1903–1959) and **Cyrus C. Sturgis** (1891–1966) [49]. Coller (Fig. 1.12) had earned the rank of Major in the US Armed Forces during World War I as a member of the American Ambulance Service and was a surgical consultant to the US military during World War II. As Chairman of the Department of Surgery at the University of Michigan (1930–1957) and President of the American College of Surgeons (1949), Coller was an influential figure in American medical circles

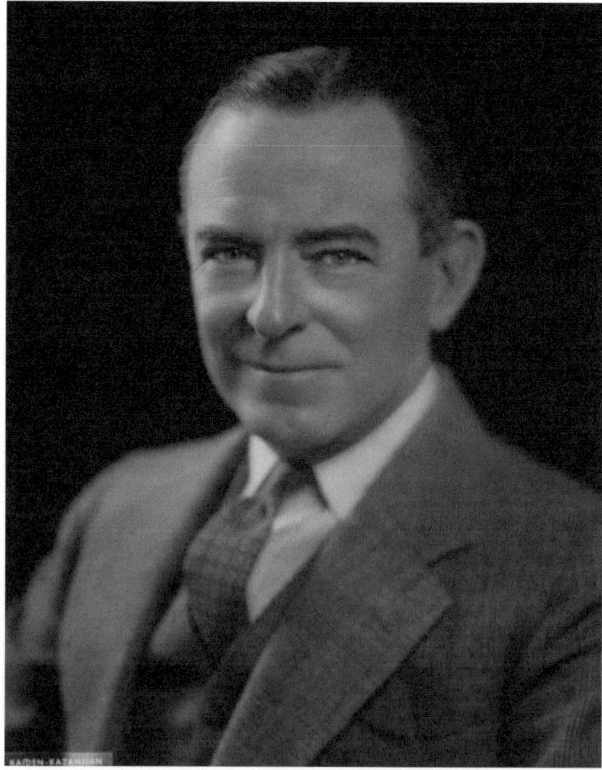

Fig. 1.12 Frederick A. Coller (1887–1964) *(Image courtesy of the Archives of the American College of Surgeons. All rights reserved.)* [50]

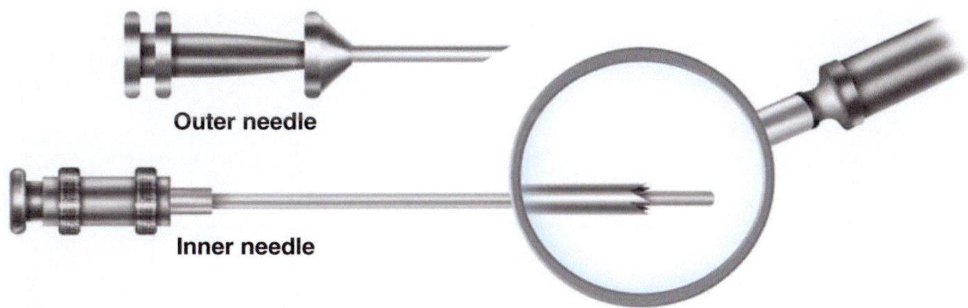

Fig. 1.13 The Turkel trephine instrument [52]

during the 1940s and 1950s. Turkel himself was a consultant to the Surgeon General's Office during the war. Consequently, these two men were instrumental in securing a place for IO catheters in every combat medic's tool kit during World War II.

Henry Turkel developed a novel trephination and IO infusion device that would come to be marketed by Turkel Trephine Instruments (Detroit, Michigan) and was ultimately adopted by the US National Research Council for use by the American military during and after World War II [49, 51]. Turkel claimed that his proprietary trephine (i.e., hole saw) catheter tip needle (Fig. 1.13), with the use of an internal stylet, had been proven safe for infusions up to 24 h in duration [49].

The Turkel Trephine Instruments for Biopsies and Marrow Infusions, Adult Sternal Infusion Set, was manufactured by Trephine Instruments (1302 Industrial Bank Building, Detroit, Michigan) and included a 14–17 gauge catheter with 20 mm length. This kit included right-angle connectors, which served to connect the IO cannula to the infusion tubing (Fig. 1.14).

The use of intraosseous vascular access among adults declined sharply after the end of World War II, but pediatric use would continue in many countries. Danish pediatrician **Svend Heinild** (1907–1994) at the Refsnaes Kysthospital (Refsnaes, Denmark) reported the largest case series to that time, with nearly 1000 pediatric infusions, in 1946. Most of his infusions were of crystalloid fluids for the treatment of acute gastroenteritis, with patients often receiving more than one infusion [53]. Heinild highlighted the safety of the approach in children, but did mention the risk of osteomyelitis as a potential complication [53].

Following the end of World War II, civilian reports of therapeutic intraosseous infusion within the English-speaking literature became more rare, although they continued to filter in from Dutch-, Russian-, German-, and Bulgarian-language journals [54–58]. The reasons for this declining interest in IO infusion remain unclear, although several factors likely contributed to the trend. While combat medics were uniformly taught IO insertion techniques (usually at the sternum), most of these medics resumed their nonmedical civilian jobs at the end of the war. Thus, most of the training and familiarity with IO infusion that these medics developed was ultimately lost to the medical community. The introduction of penicillin and other antibiotics may have also mitigated concerns about potential infectious risks associated with direct peripheral venous infusion, which seemed to be more prominent at the time when compared to the rare reports of osteomyelitis attributed to IO infusion.

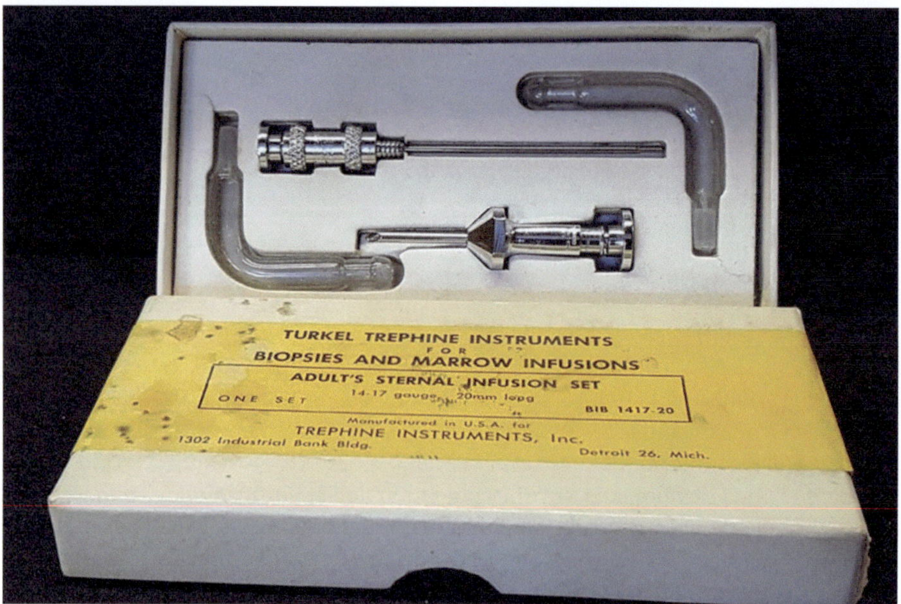

Fig. 1.14 Turkel Trephine Instruments for Biopsies and Marrow Infusions, Adult Sternal Infusion Set. (*Image provided by the authors*)

Newer materials and methods for intravenous infusion also became available during this time, likely drawing attention away from the use of IO devices. During the first half of the twentieth century, intravenous access was generally achieved with steel needles that were sterilized between uses by boiling them in water [59]. The sterilization process caused the needles to become dull or barbed after multiple uses, increasing the risk of venous injury and complicating their insertion. Once dulled, the needles had to be hand-sharpened with flint stones [59]. But the introduction of disposable intravenous needles dramatically improved the provider experience with IV insertion. The first disposable peripheral IV cannulae (made of polyethylene) were introduced by Becton-Dickinson in 1945, followed by the Rochester needle in 1950, and the first over-the-needle plastic winged catheter in 1963 [59]. Disposable needles proved to be much cheaper and easier to insert than multiuse steel cannulae, signaling the end of the steel needle era for intravenous access. As steel IO catheters featured many of the same disadvantages as steel IV catheters, these trends likely contributed to decreased interest in reusable IO devices as well.

Central venous catheters, designed to be inserted into the major veins of the thorax, also became more commonly used in the 1960s, often made of "modern" disposable materials (e.g., silicone rubber and polyurethane) that allowed for greater flexibility with insertion [59]. The Seldinger technique, named for the Swedish radiologist **Sven Ivar Seldinger** (1921–1998), was introduced in 1953 and was rapidly applied to central line placement, making central venous access an increasingly feasible alternative to IO or peripheral IV access in the unstable patient [60]. Each of these advances in direct venous access likely moved indirect (e.g., IO) venous access further and further down the vascular access algorithm for medical providers [61].

Occasional voices from outside of the United States were heard promoting the use of IO access during the late 1970s. One of the first clinicians to promote IO use in the English-language literature during the 1970s was **Manuel M. Valdes** at the Institute of Tropical Diseases (Mexico City, Mexico). Valdes routinely used intraosseous venography for phlebographic studies and noted that IO infusions of fluids and medications other than contrast agents appeared to be both safe and effective. In 1977, he reported a case series of 15 adult patients who received 2–42 L of fluid over a period of up to 30 days via either medial malleolar (12 cases) or lateral malleolar (3 cases) IO infusion using a standard 14-gauge Becton-Dickinson needle [62]. This publication by Valdes appears to have stimulated additional interest in the IO route during the late 1970s and early 1980s, including bovine studies of epinephrine injection at the distal tibia [63] and early studies on IO infusion for regional anesthesia during orthopedic surgery [64].

A resurgence of interest in IO cannulation came during the early 1980s, following a series of editorials published in the United States. The first of these editorials was from Henry Turkel, now retired and living near Detroit, Michigan. In his 1983 editorial published in *Southern Medical Journal*, Turkel commented on a local news story involving a 3-year-old child who was allegedly blinded and brain-damaged when her anesthesiologist was unable to establish an intravenous line for the infusion of general anesthesia in a timely manner [65]. Turkel lamented that the IO route was being "ignored in medical schools" and suggested that the use of an IO catheter to obtain earlier vascular access could have prevented these complications [65]. Turkel's claim that IO cannulation was not being widely taught in American medical schools was fairly accurate. In fact, the first American Heart Association (AHA) Advanced Cardiac Life Support (ACLS) guidelines (published in 1974) did not mention IO access at all, although these early guidelines did suggest the use of cutdowns or intracardiac injections of medication when peripheral veins were not immediately accessible [66, 67]. The first appearance of IO infusion in the ACLS guidelines would come in 1986, but only for use in pediatric emergencies [68, 69]. The first reference to IO access in the adult ACLS guidelines emerged in 1992, couched in the claim that, "intraosseous infusion of drugs is an excellent alternative when IV access is not readily available, particularly in pediatric patients" [70].

Robert A. Berg (b. 1950), a pediatric intensivist at Maricopa County General Hospital (Phoenix, Arizona), was the first to report in the English-language literature on the continuous IO infusion of dobutamine and dopamine following cardiac arrest (Fig. 1.15) [71]. The subject of this report was a 6-month-old infant who had already failed multiple intravenous catheterization attempts, including a femoral vein cutdown, but was able to receive bilateral proximal tibial IO cannulation using a standard 18-gauge hypodermic needle [71].

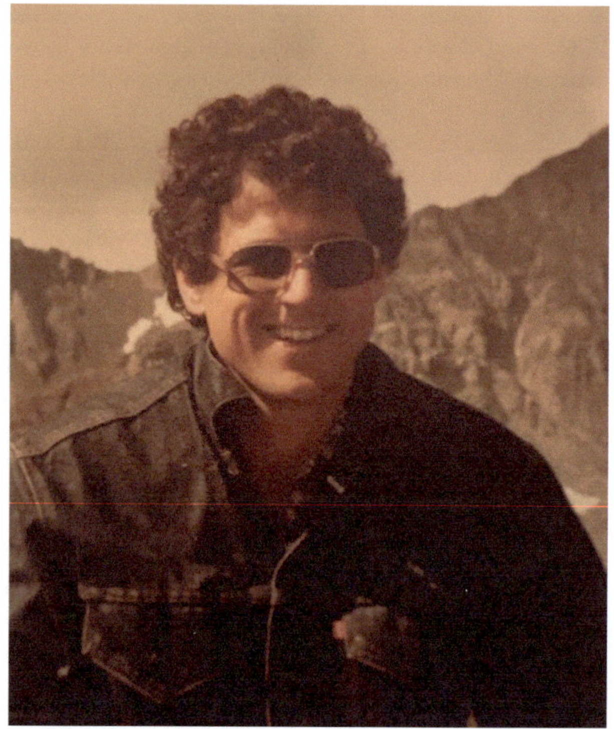

Fig. 1.15 Robert A. Berg. *(Image courtesy of Dr. Robert A. Berg. © 2023 Robert A. Berg. All rights reserved)*

As Berg recalled,

I actually learned how to place a needle in the proximal tibia IO space from Hem-Onc physicians to obtain specimens for diagnostic purposes, such as cancers and for karyotyping newborns (e.g., to diagnose Trisomies 21, 13 and 18 in newborns). Thus, I had learned that IO access could be used for resuscitation and I had developed the clinical skills of IO access for bone marrow diagnostic purposes. The case report was the first time that I [had] used this combination of historical knowledge and clinical skill experience to provide IO access for resuscitation. I had never seen anyone use it for resuscitation before I used it, and I was not aware of others using over the last couple decades (but that says more about what I knew than whether others were using it elsewhere).

I wrote the case report for *AJDC* (now renamed *JAMA-Pediatrics*) because the editor Vince Fulginiti (Chair of Pediatrics at U of Arizona in Tucson at the time) specifically wrote an editorial that year asking for case reports of experiences using clinically important interventions that had been part of medical care in the past but were not as well known in the early 1980s.

Apparently, that simple case report and accompanying editorial by Jim [Orlowski] led to increased interest over the next several years with both animal studies and clinical studies supporting its value. Perhaps most importantly, the first [American Heart Association Pediatric Advanced Life Support] course in 1987 and the associated first PALS textbook published in 1988 highlighted the importance of prompt vascular access for fluid resuscitation and drug administration during resuscitation. Under Priorities in Venous Access, the PALS textbook stated, 'In children under 3 years of age, an intraosseous cannula should be placed immediately and used for volume expansion and additional medications.' *(Communication between RA Berg and the authors, 2022, unreferenced)*.

An editorial accompanying Berg's report in the September 1984 issue of the *American Journal of Diseases of Children* (AJDC) written by pediatric intensivist **James P. Orlowski** (b. 1947) of the Cleveland Clinic (Cleveland, Ohio) further advocated for increased use of the IO route [72]. Orlowski had learned about the use of IO catheters on a medical missionary trip to India as a senior-year medical student at Case Western Reserve University (Cleveland, Ohio) in 1973. While there, he witnessed profoundly dehydrated patients being treated with IO infusions of fluids during a cholera epidemic. Returning to Cleveland, he began using IO infusion in his own practice. As Orlowski wrote:

> There is no more exasperating situation than the inability to establish intravenous (IV) access in a critically ill child. Yet this predicament confronts physicians. It is not uncommon for a child to come to an emergency room in severe shock, with no visible or palpable veins, or for the only venous access to a child to be lost in an emergency [72].

In a 2002 interview with Larry Miller, Orlowski reported that many of his colleagues considered the use of IO catheters to be "barbaric, or overly aggressive. The IO route had become a lost skill." Despite this resistance, Orlowski continued to teach manual IO catheter placement and infusion to his residents and colleagues. Over the next two decades, Orlowski would contribute significantly to the IO literature. In 1989, he reported a study of 21 canine subjects demonstrating that all of the dogs had "fat and bone marrow emboli" in their lungs following femoral IO infusion of ACLS drugs, regardless of which drugs were used [73]. However, none of the animals developed any clinical symptoms of fat embolism syndrome, suggesting that the emboli remained clinically insignificant [73]. That same year, he reported on the similarity of common laboratory studies (e.g., electrolytes, hemoglobin, lactate, liver function tests) from IO marrow samples when compared to arterial or venous samples [74]. In 1990, he reported that the pharmacokinetics of six common ACLS drugs (epinephrine, sodium bicarbonate, calcium chloride, hydroxyethyl starch, 50% dextrose, and lidocaine) in a canine cardiac arrest model did not appear to differ significantly whether the drugs were administered through a 14-gauge distal femoral IO, 16-gauge forepaw peripheral IV, or 16-gauge femoral central venous catheter [75]. In this series of experiments, Orlowski compared each drug's magnitude of peak effect, drug level, and duration of action among both normovolemic and hypovolemic subjects [75]. Although IO infusion of sodium bicarbonate or hydroxyethyl starch was associated with increased time to peak level and increased duration of effect when compared to the other routes, the differences that he found were not statistically significant with any drug [75].

Meanwhile, other authors were studying the potential role of IO access for cardiac arrest resuscitation. In 1992, **William H. Spivey** (1954–1993) and colleagues at the Medical College of Pennsylvania (Philadelphia, Pennsylvania) reported that 0.1 mg/kg rapid IO infusions of epinephrine (but not 0.01 mg/kg aliquots) were able to increase blood pressure in a swine model of cardiac arrest [76]. Other studies by Spivey and colleagues included IO infusion of anti-epileptic medications [77], sodium bicarbonate for cardiopulmonary arrest [78], and crystalloids and blood

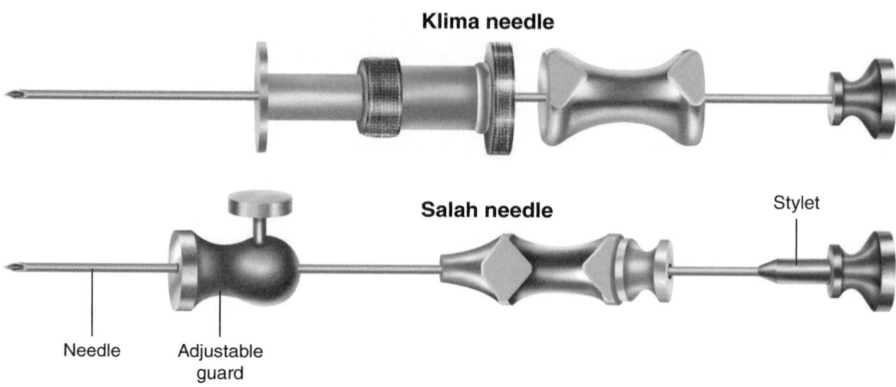

Fig. 1.16 Klima and Salah needles [83]

products using standard 13-gauge hypodermic needles [79]. Spivey would go on to serve as a scientific advisor to LifeQuest Medical (San Antonio, Texas) on the development of that company's Osteoport® device, before his sudden death on 20 February 1993.

Although many researchers and clinicians in the 1980s were still using standard hypodermic needles to access the intramedullary space, various specialized manually placed IO devices had been developed. The earliest IO devices were modeled on bone marrow biopsy needles and were generally developed by hematologists for use in bone marrow aspiration. Some of the earliest models included the Vim-Silverman needle with pronged bifid needle insert [80], the Favorite needle with a screwlike obturator [81], the Turkel needle [49, 52], and the grooved Reddy needle [82]. Despite a wide range of needles developed during the mid-twentieth century, the most popular for sternal IO biopsy appears to have been the Klima-Rosegger needle developed by **Rudolph Klima** (1896–1983) and **Hellfried Rosegger** (d. 1940) of the University of Vienna circa 1935 [83] and the Salah needle, both of which featured an adjustable guard to prevent overpenetration (Fig. 1.16).

In 1971, Iranian hematologist **Khosrow Jamshidi** (b. 1929) reported the development of a new bone marrow biopsy needle with a T-bar handle, tapered edge, and a cutting interior [84]. The Jamshidi™ needle (Fig. 1.17) was designed for iliac crest biopsies, featuring a much longer cannula than most previous devices used for sternal and tibial access. The Jamshidi needle design would inspire a new generation of iliac crest biopsy devices, including the Islam biopsy needle [86].

But needles developed for bone marrow biopsy are not necessarily well suited for IO infusion. The original reusable Jamshidi™ iliac crest biopsy needle (Fig. 1.18), for example, was quite long (e.g., 76–150 mm) with a tapered end designed to reduce crush artifact with marrow retrieval. These features also lengthened and narrowed the chamber through which fluids were infused, increasing resistance to flow. The modern Jamshidi™ needle typically used for IO infusion is disposable and much shorter than the reusable stainless steel model originally developed for iliac crest biopsy. The Illinois lancet tip modification, introduced in 1988 with the Monoject®

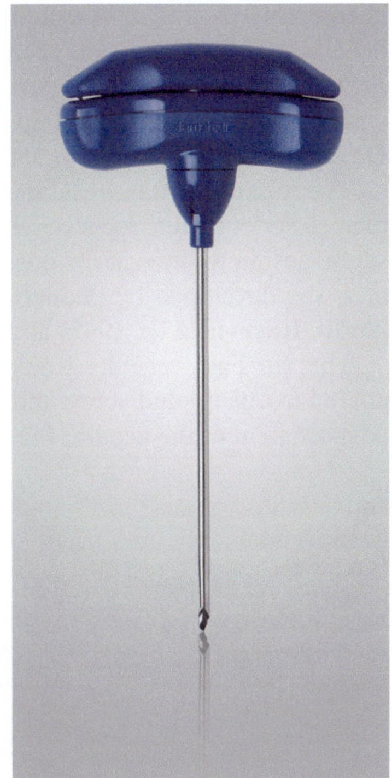

Fig. 1.17 Jamshidi™ needle for iliac crest biopsy. *(Image Courtesy of Becton, Dickson and Company. © 2023 Becton, Dickson and Company. All rights reserved.)* [85]

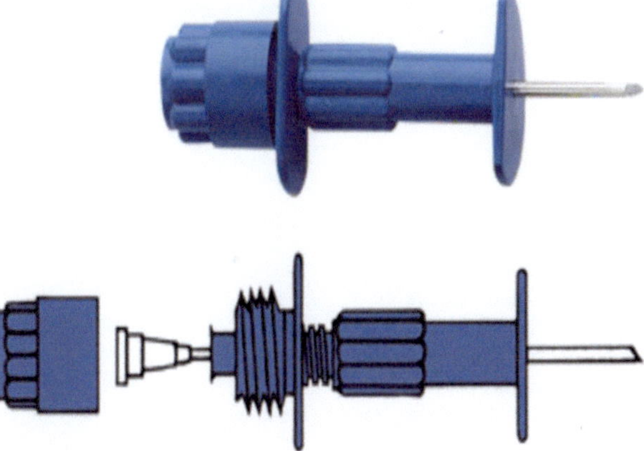

Fig. 1.18 Jamshidi™ modified Illinois disposable needle *(Image Courtesy of Becton, Dickson and Company. © 2023 Becton, Dickson and Company. All rights reserved.)* [87]

Illinois Needle (Sherwood Medical, St. Louis, Missouri), was later incorporated into the Jamshidi™ Illinois needle (Becton, Dickinson, and Company, Franklin Lakes, NJ).

With the resurgence of interest in manual IO devices, many new manual IO devices would become available for emergency care providers in the late 1980s and early 1990s. Cook Medical (Bloomington, Indiana) released the Cook intraosseous needle in 1986, available with various features including a 45° trocar, 35° lancet, or pencil point tip. The Cook needle with Dieckmann™ modification (Cook Medical) included two opposed side ports positioned near the needle cannula's distal tip to ensure proper flow when the tip is obstructed by bony cortex. The Cook needle with Dieckmann™ modification is shown in Fig. 1.19.

The Sussmane-Raszynski needle (Cook Medical) included a brass hub and base plate, a stylet with a trocar bevel (45° angle), and a cannula shaft with a fine needle-screw design to prevent dislodgement of the needle cannula (Fig. 1.20). This catheter was developed by pediatric intensivists **Jeffrey B. Sussmane** (b. 1955) and **Andre Raszynski** (b. 1948) at the Miami Children's Hospital (Miami, Florida).

The Sur-Fast™ needle (Cook Critical Care) was patented in 1996, featuring an angled trocar tip and screw threading along the length of the cannula to facilitate advancement of the needle (Fig. 1.21) [90].

Fig. 1.19 Cook manual IO needle with Dieckmann™ modification *(Image courtesy of Cook Medical. © 2023 Cook Medical. All rights reserved.)* [88]

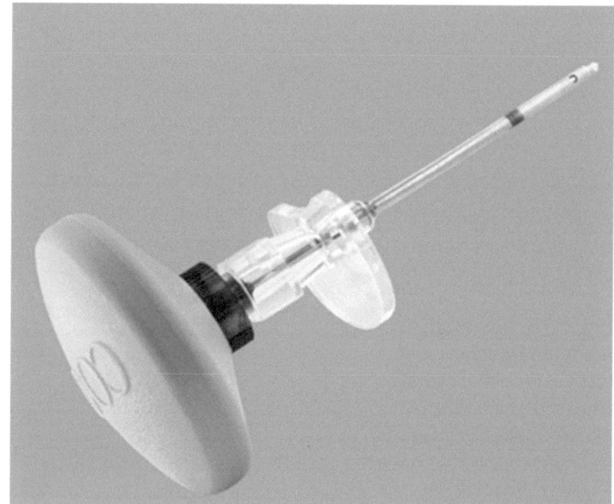

Fig. 1.20 Sussmane-Raszynski™ needle. *(Image courtesy of Cook Medical. © 2023 Cook Medical. All rights reserved.)* [89]

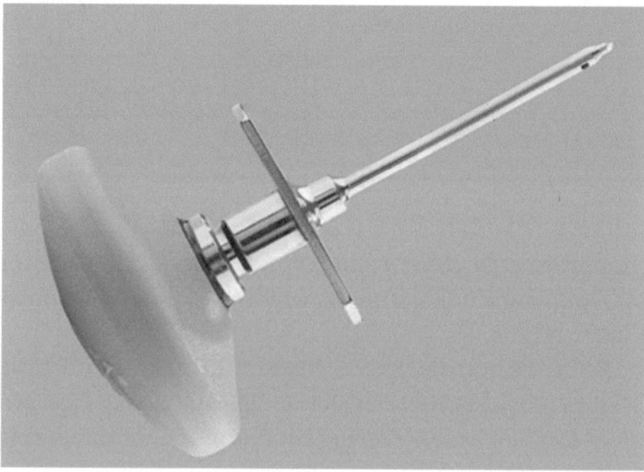

Fig. 1.21 Sur-Fast™ needle *(Image courtesy of Cook Medical. © 2023 Cook Medical. All rights reserved.)* [90]

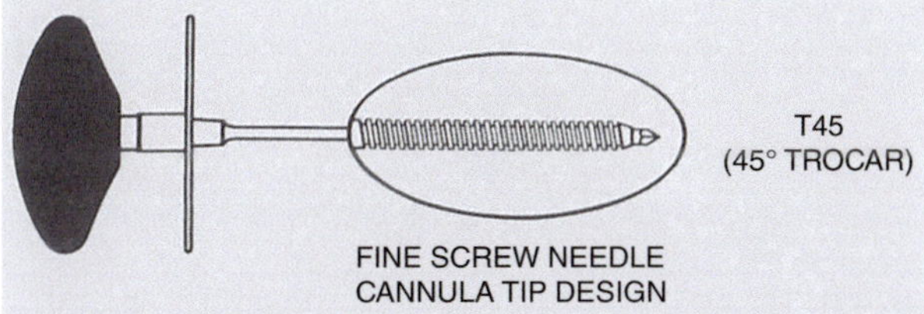

Fig. 1.22 The Near Needle Holder™ device. *(Image courtesy of Richard Near. © 2023 Near Manufacturing, Ltd. All rights reserved.)* [91]

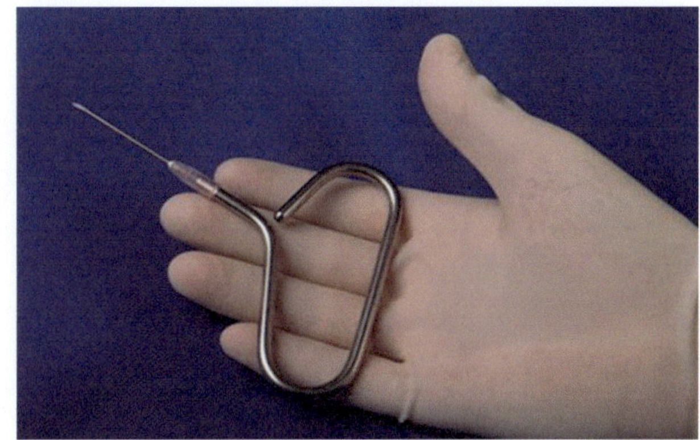

The entire Cook Medical portfolio of manual IO catheters, with the exception of the Dieckmann™ catheter, was discontinued by late 2022.

Novel devices to assist with manual IO catheter insertion have also been developed, including the Near Needle Holder™ (Near Manufacturing, Camrose, Alberta, Canada) (Fig. 1.22), a reusable handle allowing a standard hollow steel infusion needle to be inserted in the intraosseous space [92]. It was developed as a safe, inexpensive option to facilitate IO infusion in developing countries and other limited-resource areas. It should be noted that the Near Needle Holder™ is not FDA approved in the United States.

Pediatric IO infusion at the proximal tibia experienced a renaissance in the late 1980s, but it would be many years before the denser tibia of adult subjects was commonly targeted for IO cannulation. Meanwhile, manufacturers and investigator-clinicians began to revisit the sternal IO insertion site during the 1990s. The FAST-1® (First Access for Shock and Trauma) intraosseous infusion system, originally introduced by Pyng Medical (Vancouver, Canada) in 1998, was the first new sternal IO catheter to appear on the market in decades (Fig. 1.23). Pyng Medical was founded in 1986 by **Michael W. Jacobs** and colleagues, and this company led the early development of adult IO catheters during the 1990s. In its earliest days, Pyng had considered licensing the Sternal Access Vascular Entry (SAVE) manual IO infusion device from the US Army and University of California, which featured a self-tapping screw and stabilization features to prevent over-advancement. Ultimately, they found that a novel approach was needed, leading to the development of the FAST-1® system.

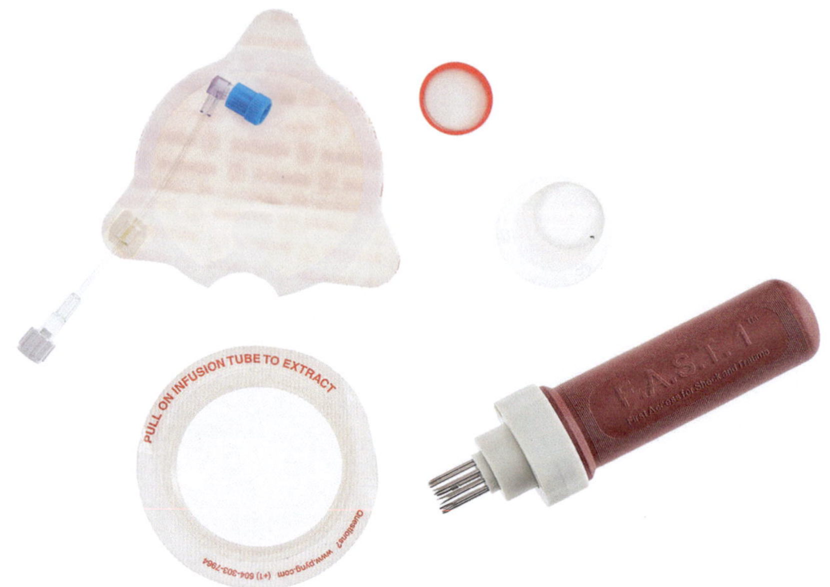

Fig. 1.23 The FAST-1® intraosseous system . *(Image courtesy of Teleflex Incorporated. © 2023 Teleflex Incorporated. All rights reserved.)* [93]

The FAST-1® device is placed manually, inserted gradually by continuous direct pressure on the sternum with an array of 10 stabilizer needles and central infusion catheter. A report on the first 50 uses of this device featured a 78% first-attempt success rate, with no complications noted on up to 2-month follow-up [94]. The FAST-Responder® (Fig. 1.24) introduced by Pyng Medical in 2014, the FAST Tactical®, and the FastX® were short-lived variants of the FAST-1® device that were ultimately phased out after Teleflex acquired Pyng in 2017.

Difficulties in cannulating the denser bones of adult subjects led to the development of myriad new devices in the late 1990s intended to facilitate IO device insertion in adult subjects. Early efforts to develop a drill-assisted IO catheter focused primarily on anterior iliac crest sampling for marrow biopsy [28, 96, 97] and were largely unsuccessful. However, several augmented mechanical devices would be developed during the late 1990s, including the Bone Injection Gun (BIG®) (WaisMed) and the EZ-IO® (Vidacare Corporation™).

The Bone Injection Gun (BIG®) was developed by Israeli orthopedic surgeon **Marc Waisman**, the founder of WaisMed (Caesarea, Israel) at Technion Entrepreneurial Incubator Co. Ltd. (TEIC) in 1994 (Fig. 1.25). Waisman's invention featured a tension-loaded spring used to inject a steel IO cannula into the bone with a trigger release. Early applications of this device focused on regional intraosseous anesthesia [99], but the potential for IO infusion of systemic therapies was apparent early in the device's development [100]. Although the company obtained U.S. Food and Drug Administration (FDA) approval for use of this device with IO infusion in 1999, the company ceased operating in 2000 due to financial difficulties

Fig. 1.24 The FAST-Responder®. *(Image courtesy of Teleflex Incorporated. © 2023 Teleflex Incorporated. All rights reserved.)* [95]

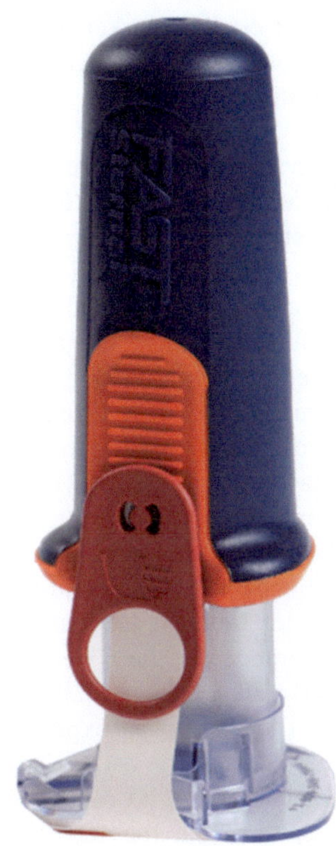

Fig. 1.25 Bone Injection Gun (BIG®), shown in pediatric (red) and adult (blue) sizes. *(Image courtesy of Safeguard Medical. © 2023 Safeguard Medical. All rights reserved.)* [98]

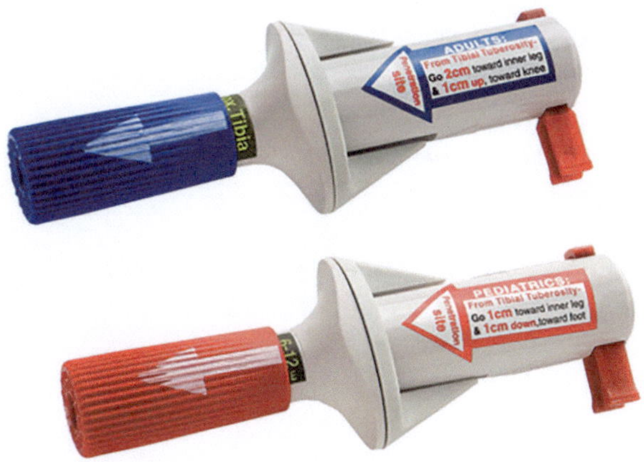

before ever bringing the BIG® to the market [101]. In June 2004, WaisMed was acquired by the PerSys group (founded in 1988, in Houston, Texas), and the device soon became commercially available. Since then, this device has been extensively utilized by the U.S. Army for military resuscitation and continues to be advertised in the civilian market as the "world's first automatic IO device" [101]. It is available in both adult (15-gauge) and pediatric (18 gauge, 23.6 mm length) sizes. The PerSys group was acquired by Safeguard Medical™ in 2021.

Around the same time that the BIG® was being developed in Israel, an American physician-inventor was working on a very different IO catheter. **Larry J. Miller** (b. 1938) (Fig. 1.26), an emergency physician at Baptist Healthcare System (San Antonio, Texas), had been working for some time on an intraosseous catheter infusion system. Miller received his MD from the University of Michigan (1965) and completed his emergency medicine residency at Cook County Medical Center before joining Baptist (1973–2004) and serving as Medical Director for a variety of EMS agencies in South Texas (1978–2015). His experiences with difficult vascular access in the prehospital and emergency department environments convinced him that better methods were needed for IO placement in adults. The Osteoport®, an implantable IO chemotherapy infusion port with a self-sealing silicone septum, had been invented by pharmacist **John G. Kuhn** and oncologist **Daniel D. Von Hoff** at the University of Texas Health Science Center (Houston, Texas) and was patented by the University in 1988. Miller founded LifeQuest Medical (San Antonio, Texas) in 1989 to seek FDA clearance for the Osteoport®, although the device never reached market due to early FDA concerns about implantable silicone devices.

The Osteoport® experience provides fascinating insight into the use of IO catheters during the early 1990s. According to Miller, LifeQuest applied to the FDA for use of the IO route for therapeutic infusion in 1992, which was met with a response that the IO route had not been previously approved for medication administration. The FDA then contacted James Cook from Cook Medical and

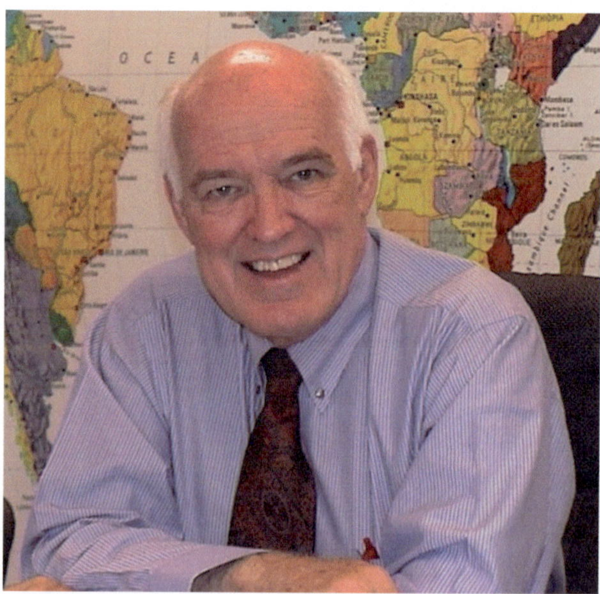

Fig. 1.26 Larry J. Miller, inventor of the EZ-IO® system. *(Image courtesy of Dr. Larry J. Miller. © 2023 Larry J. Miller. All rights reserved)*

advised him that they would need to remove the Cook IO catheter from the market as the FDA had not approved IO medication infusion. Cook issued a call for action to emergency physicians, yielding 750 letters from EM physicians suggesting that removal of IO devices from FDA approval would result in the deaths of "thousands of children." Upon receiving these responses, the FDA recanted their rejection of IO infusion but suggested that the LifeQuest application represented a different application. In order to prove that IO infusion was equivalent to IV infusion, LifeQuest funded a $5 million study to demonstrate that IO morphine was equivalent to IV morphine [102]. Even after this study was completed, Miller was required to contact the FDA regarding every other medication that was to be administered through an IO catheter. This missive apparently resulted in 59 additional calls to the FDA yielding 59 new medications approved for IO infusion. Although none of these other 59 drugs received the same level of FDA pharmacokinetic scrutiny as morphine, they were all subsequently approved. In this way, the Von Hoff study cleared the path for FDA approval of IO infusion for other drugs as well.

On behalf of LifeQuest, Miller also purchased the patent (#5,176,643) for the "First Med System" IO device from **George C. Kramer, PhD**, at the University of Texas Medical Branch, Galveston (Texas), in 1992. This device was similar to the BIG®, in that it was spring-loaded, but the medications (e.g., epinephrine) were preloaded into the device. In late 1992, LifeQuest Medical launched its initial public offering (stock ticker LQMD) at $10.50/share. Despite the enthusiasm generated by LifeQuest's IPO, neither the Osteoport® nor the First Med System were ultimately developed into a commercial product before the company was shuttered.

Miller's experience with developing the Osteoport® inspired him to continue experimenting with different methods of accessing the bone marrow. He tried various means of powering the insertion into cadaver bones, including nail guns and drills, and developed myriad different needle tips and other adjuncts. As Miller stated in a 2009 interview with *Design News*, "We got cadaver bones and started trying different things. We shot the bones with a nail gun. That seemed to be a good idea until one of the engineers shot himself through the finger" [103]. Originally, Miller hoped to use a medical drill to create the hole in the bone and place a standard catheter through the hole, but this method ultimately failed due to difficulties finding the hole again. He recalls being inspired in his device design by his father, an automotive engineer. "I woke up one night and had the answer. I remembered my dad had a tiny, hollow, oil-cooled drill. I figured we could use that kind of drill and hook an IV to it" [103].

Miller subsequently founded Vidacare™ LLC (San Antonio, Texas) in 2001, along with paramedic **David "Scotty" Bolleter**, Chief Financial Officer **Eric Eisbrenner**, and engineer **Bob Titkemeyer**, but his device was not yet fully developed when tragedy struck. On 30 January 2003, Miller's friend, paramedic, and 16th District International Association of Fire Fighters (IAFF) Vice President **Nick Davila** died in a traffic accident after difficulty receiving emergent venous access. This loss strengthened Miller's resolve to develop a powered IO device for use in the prehospital environment.

The device that Miller had in mind included a reusable 9-volt battery-operated drill with a removable single-use IO catheter. Vidacare was struggling financially by the summer of 2002, when Miller approached his attorneys about obtaining the patent. As Miller recalls,

> I built a prototype of my powered IO concept, that we called the VidaPen, which looked like a battery powered Dremel drill with a detachable IO needle. With this crude prototype we were able to show potential investors how it worked, using fake bones. The prototype was also the basis for filing patents. I thought we had solid patents and licenses from the University of Texas to add value to our company and give investors the comfort they needed to risk their investment capital.
>
> At last, we arranged for a venture capital investor to come visit us in San Antonio to learn more about our technology and our vision for the future. Of course he wanted to see validation of our patents, if we had freedom to operate, and rights to patent our innovative technology. I had already completed two world-wide patent searches and found nothing resembling the VidaPen. But before our investor's visit, I hired a Washington DC Patent firm to do one final patent search and certify by letter that our patent was valid.
>
> To my horror and dismay, this patent firm found a previous patent that was almost identical to the device I had invented and the patent I had filed. The reason we never found it before was because the patent was filed with the wrong name. We searched for 'intraosseous,' whereas the other patent was filed with a hyphen: 'intra-osseous.' My heart sank, because I knew with this new discovery, our company, Vidacare, had no value and it would be a waste of time for the potential investor to come visit us.
>
> Eric Eisbrenner, my business partner said, "Let's not give up yet. Maybe we can buy the patent or partner with the patent owner." So, we got our patent lawyers to analyze the patent, its status, and the owner. They found good news and bad news. The patent had been abandoned due to non-payment. Further, the patent was still good because the two-year grace period for reinstating the patent was still in effect. The bad news was that the grace period was about to expire in 2 weeks. After that, the technology would be public, and anyone could use it rendering my patents useless and the EZ-IO a distant dream.

Apparently, Miller's idea of drilling a catheter into the target bone had already been patented by pediatrician **Norman Myer Rosenberg** (1938–2009) of Wayne County General Hospital (Detroit, Michigan) in 1996. Rosenberg had recently retired after 25 years as Director of the Detroit Children's Hospital emergency department. When Miller reached out to Rosenberg,

> On the one hand I was reluctant to tell him why I needed the patent because … I felt he would be a tough business man, asking millions for his patent. I was broke. But, on the other hand, if I did not fully disclose my motives, he might not be interested. I felt I had nothing to lose. So, I briefly explained the situation. I asked him if we could meet in person, since he lived close to my mom and I believed a person-to-person conversation would be more productive. He said I could come by in a couple of weeks. I said, "No! I will be there first thing in the morning," as I booked my flight from San Antonio to Detroit. He said to meet him at Wendy's restaurant in Brighton [Michigan].
>
> Our meeting went well. He was a kind and lovely man. He explained that as a children's emergency physician he saw the tremendous need for a powered IO device and so he spent $15,000 to patent his concept. He then presented his patents to several medical device companies, including Cook, Medtronic, and Baxter. While they all expressed in interest, none were willing to buy his idea or develop his product. For that reason he abandoned his patent and did not want to spend more money on a futile idea. He was delighted that at last someone was serious about developing his ideas. We talked about what it would take for me to buy his patents. He was agreeable, but said before he could make any final decisions, I would have to speak with his wife, Bonnie, who was an emergency room nurse [104].

Miller was ultimately successful in negotiating a deal with Rosenberg, and the delayed renewal of patent was granted on 9 September 2002—one day before it would have expired. This first patent for Vidacare served as the foundation for over 144 other patents granted to the company in developing the EZ-IO® and OnControl® lines of IO catheters. Rosenberg received 50,000 shares of Vidacare stock for his patent and remained active in the company, facilitating cadaver studies and contributing to the development of the product lines. A photograph of Eisbrenner, Rosenberg, Rosenberg, and Miller is provided in Fig. 1.27.

The VidaPen® device (Fig. 1.28) originally developed by Vidacare was remarkably similar in appearance to Rosenberg's patent design, featuring a long, straight handle housing the motor, gears, and a rechargeable battery. But this design would soon be abandoned in favor of a more traditional "drill" handle design and a new name—the EZ-IO®.

The EZ-IO® infusion system (Fig. 1.29) would include a reusable 1200 rpm driver, which connected magnetically to a single-use 304 stainless steel catheter and internal stylet. The catheter's plastic hub would be color-coded to indicate the catheter's length (i.e., yellow for 45 mm, blue for 25 mm, pink for 15 mm) and made of medical grade polycarbonate. A sternal version of the EZ-IO® catheter (green hub, 7.5 mm length) was introduced in 2011 but discontinued in 2014. Black lines at 10 mm increments (apart from the line closest to the hub being at 5 mm) along the length of the catheter were intended to aid the provider in gauging the depth of insertion. The catheter is then secured to the skin surface after placement with the EZ-Stabilizer® adhesive dressing. The EZ-IO® system received FDA approval in 2004, as the first battery-powered device marketed for therapeutic IO infusion. A study of the first 250 insertions of the device reported a 97% placement success rate, with 94% of insertions requiring less than 10 s to complete [106]. By the time of Vidacare's acquisition by Teleflex Incorporated

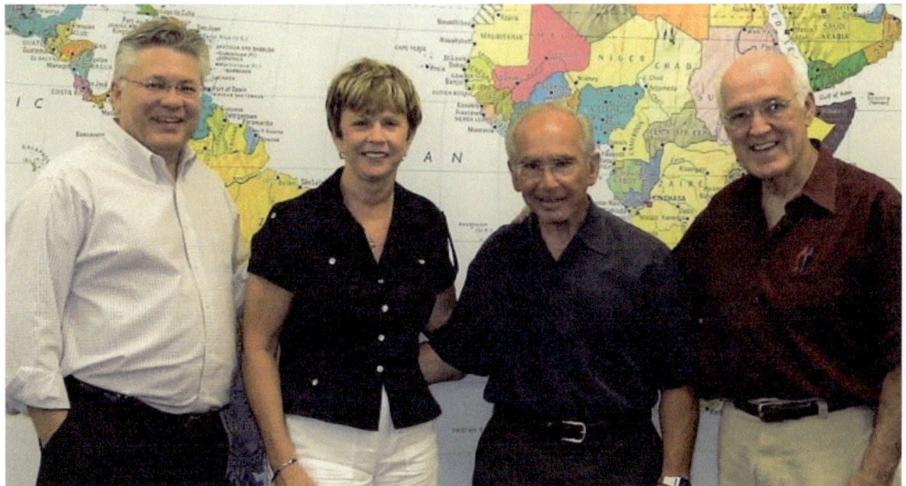

Fig. 1.27 (Left to right) Eric Eisbrenner, Bonnie Rosenberg, Norman Rosenberg, Larry Miller. *(Image courtesy of Dr. Larry J. Miller. © 2023 Larry J. Miller. All rights reserved)*

Fig. 1.28 The VidaPen® *(Image courtesy of Dr. Larry J. Miller. © 2023 Larry J. Miller. All rights reserved)*

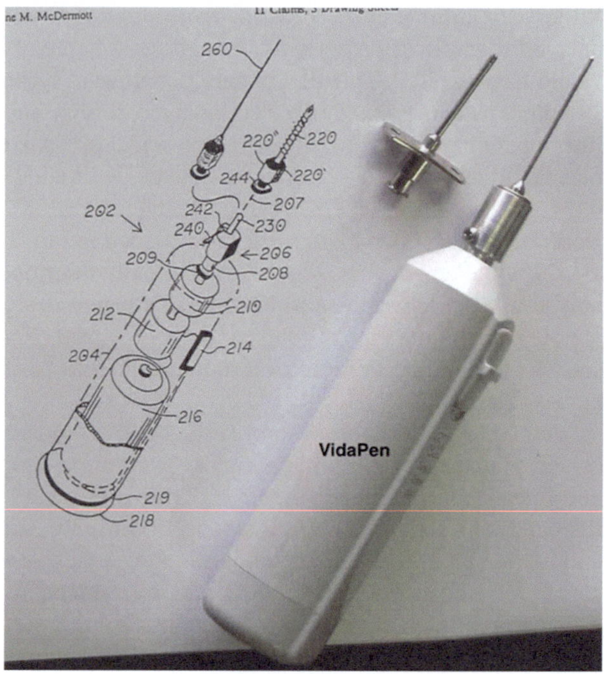

Fig. 1.29 The EZ-IO® intraosseous infusion system, including three catheter lengths, infusion tubing, and EZ-Stabilizer®. *(Image courtesy of Teleflex Incorporated. © 2023 Teleflex Incorporated. All rights reserved.)* [105]

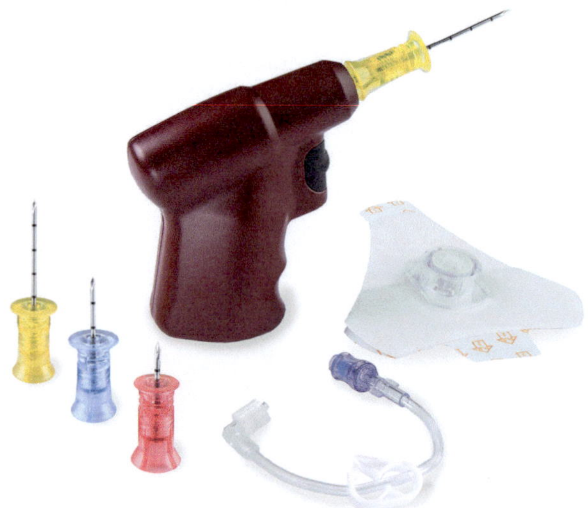

(Wayne, Pennsylvania) in 2014 for just under $300 million, more than 4 million EZ-IO® devices had been sold in over 60 countries, including 750,000 units in 2013 alone [104].

One of the ways in which the EZ-IO® line of IO catheters evolved over time was through improvements to the educational materials used to train providers on their insertion. A great deal of the credit for improving providers' ability to visualize the use and insertion of the EZ-IO® catheter is attributed to illustrators **David Baker** and **Sam Newman**, then working for the University of Texas Health Science Center (San Antonio, Texas). These two medical innovators created many of the advanced 2-D and 3-D images used for videos and other training materials for the EZ-IO® line of products. As Mr. Baker recalls,

> Thinking back on the years of involvement with Dr. Miller, Scotty, and the folks at Vidacare, I feel it was a very successful public-private partnership between the university and Vidacare over a length of time, 2003 to 2015 for me, in my largely 2-D illustration work. Sam Newman joined a bit later and added his years of very specialized animation and 3-D modeling skills to enhance the teaching aspect for Vidacare (later Teleflex) just as computer animation and web training videos were becoming more mainstream and accessible. We grew with the graphics/visualization technology just as Vidacare did with its bioengineering technology, so it was mutually beneficial to both parties (*Communication between D. Baker and the authors, 2023, unreferenced*).

A side-by-side comparison of the early 2-D (left) and later 3-D (right) images used to demonstrate EZ-IO® placement at the proximal tibia (Fig. 1.30) demonstrates the advanced visualization techniques that were used to improve Vidacare's IO device educational materials. These materials undoubtedly influenced the acceptance and use of the EZ-IO® device from its earliest days and contributed to the growth of IO use during the early 2000s.

Scotty Bolleter, one of the co-founders of Vidacare LLC and a co-inventor of the EZ-IO® system, was already a practicing flight paramedic and international expert on prehospital care when he joined Miller in developing and marketing the EZ-IO® device (Fig. 1.31). He was working for San Antonio AirLIFE when he met Miller, an emergency physician at Baptist Health System Hospitals during a trauma resuscitation in the late 1990s. As Bolleter puts it,

> There I was, minding my own business when [Dr. Miller] walks up with an idea. The idea seemed realistic and BETTER than the central lines (or nothing) that we had. Mind you, we were good at IV and central venous access … just needed something else faster.
>
> In 2003, I agreed to help with education and training [at Vidacare], creating the manuals (student and instructor), as well as the training videos. We started using PowerPoints with audio "on line," which at the time was novel. From there, I worked on improving the training materials—validating usage, developing protocols for usage adoption (think Eagles), then worked with Larry and team as we developed new sites (i.e., distal tibia, proximal humerus, sternum), new needles (i.e., 7.5-, 15- and 45-mm sets), and wrote the grant to create a new smaller driver (*Communication between S. Bolleter and the authors, 2023, unreferenced*).

During his 10 years with the company that would come to be known as Vidacare, Bolleter focused his efforts primarily on education and training, promoting IO access through better understanding of the anatomy and physiology of IO catheter placement and use throughout the United States, Russia, China, and the Middle East.

Many of the earliest innovations and manufacturer instructions developed for the EZ-IO® system were based upon Bolleter and Miller's work in the cadaver lab or

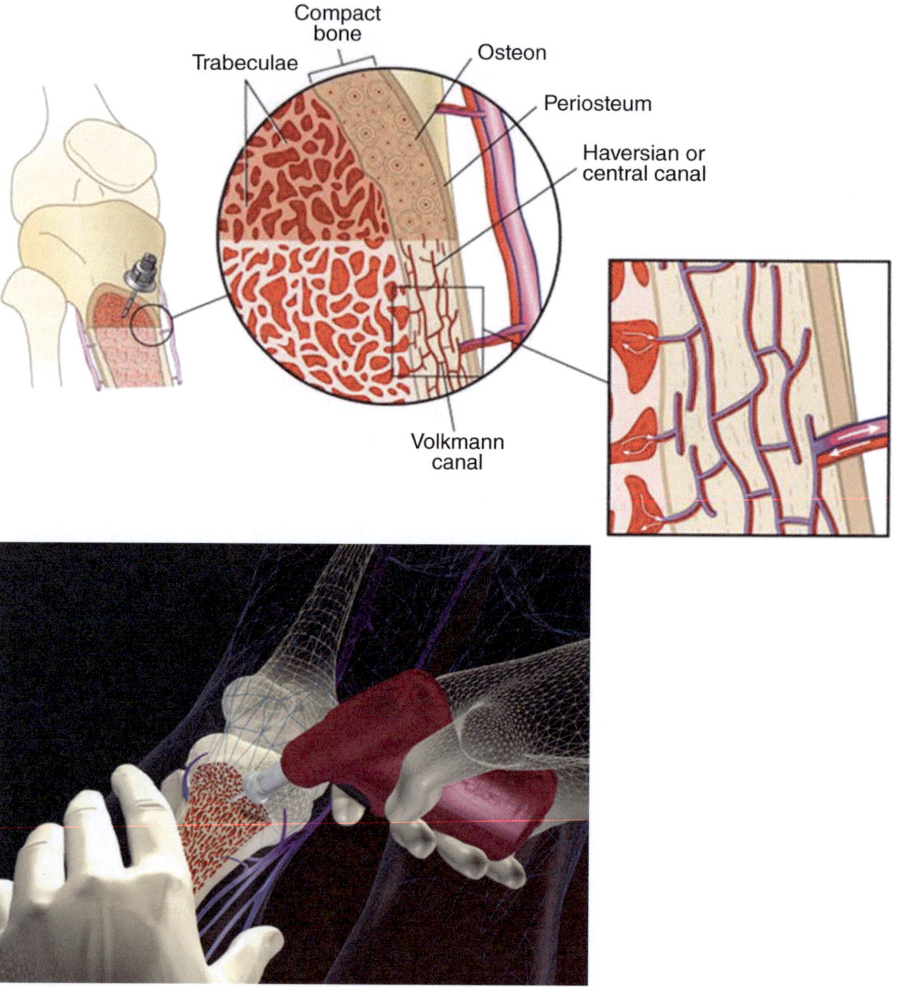

Fig. 1.30 Original Vidacare illustration of the IO space (left) and the reimagined EZ-IO® insertion technique, as illustrated by Baker and Newman (right) (*Images courtesy of David Baker & Sam Newman. © 2023 University of Texas Health Science Center, San Antonio. All rights reserved*)

with other instructional aids, including plastic bones and even raw eggs. One of the selling points for the EZ-IO® driver was the catheter's relatively atraumatic insertion technique, alleged to be less injurious to the bony cortex than that of their primary competitor, the spring-loaded BIG®. Vidacare illustrated their atraumatic insertion by encouraging learners to practice placing an EZ-IO® on an uncooked egg, demonstrating that the shell of the egg could remain unbroken with placement. At an American College of Emergency Physicians (ACEP) annual scientific assembly conference in the early 2000s, Bolleter was staffing the Vidacare booth when he was approached by a conference attendee.

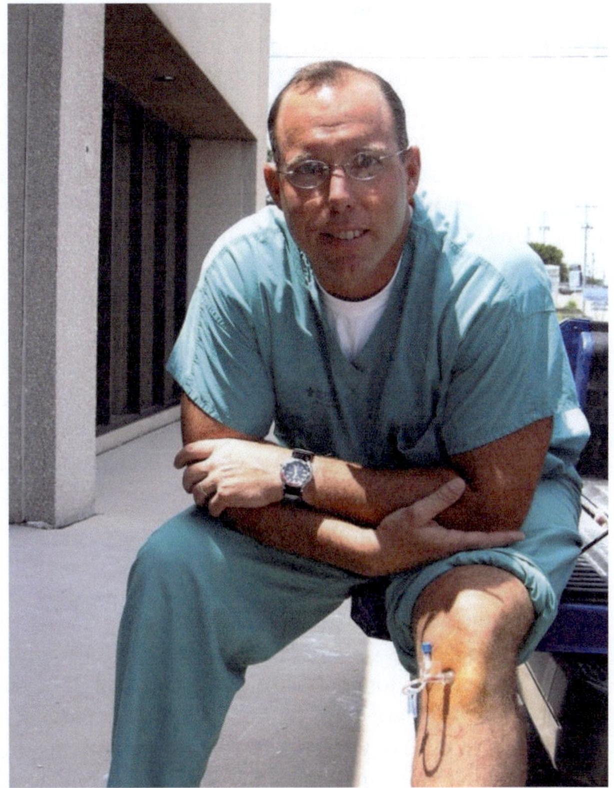

Fig. 1.31 Scotty Bolleter, demonstrating a proximal tibial IO catheter *(Image courtesy of Scotty Bolleter. © 2023 Scotty Bolleter. All rights reserved)*

Out of nowhere walks up this wee little nondescript gentleman. He asked if there is a "Scotty in the booth."

I said, "Hello, I'm Scotty—can I help you?"

To which he asked, "Are you the guy that shows people how to place an IO in a raw egg?" I said, "Yes sir, I am"… (and of course, continued to talk which is a fault of mine).

To which he stops me (with the wave of his hand), and says, "Well, I'm James Orlowski, and I taught IO with a chicken bone … (pause) … SO NOW, we know which came FIRST!!!! Don't we?" *(Communication between S. Bolleter and the authors, 2023, unreferenced).*

Miller and Bolleter would go on to recruit the "father of modern IO infusion" as a scientific advisor for Vidacare in May 2002, nearly 30 years after he helped bring the technique back into mainstream use in the United States.

In 2009, Bolleter returned to his work as a paramedic, but remained active in the development of new resuscitative devices. Later working with North American Rescue, LLC (Greer, South Carolina), Bolleter went on to invent the simplified pneumothorax emergency air release (SPEAR) system, Air Release System (ARS) pneumothorax decompression device, bougie-aided cricothyroidotomy (BAC) kit, and surgical intervention kit (SIK) [107]. At present, Bolleter is Chair of the Centre for Emergency Health Sciences, an emergency medicine research and training institution located in Spring Branch, Texas.

Although the sternum and proximal tibia had been popular IO infusion sites for decades, providers began to explore the proximal humerus site in the late 2000s, with FDA clearance achieved in 2006. Early clinical humeral IO insertions were performed primarily using the 25 mm EZ-IO® catheter [108, 109], as the 15 mm catheter was felt to be too short for use in adult subjects. In 2008, emergency physician **Marcus Eng Hock Ong** and colleagues at Singapore General Hospital (Bukit Merah, Singapore) reported their results from a prospective observational study comparing 11 humeral IO insertions to 24 tibial insertions and demonstrating no significant difference in flow rates or the rate of successful placement [109]. Another study published by emergency physician **James H. Paxton** and colleagues at Henry Ford Hospital (Detroit, Michigan) in 2009 compared humeral IO insertion to central venous and peripheral venous catheter insertion among trauma resuscitation patients in the emergency department [110, 111]. Although Ong and colleagues had reported no needle dislodgements or extravasations in their study, Paxton found that the 25 mm needles were not long enough to be seated appropriately in obese adult patients and would frequently dislodge. Consequently, the Henry Ford team utilized 68 mm OnControl® IO catheters (Vidacare, LLC) in five of the more obese study subjects. The use of these longer IO catheters reduced the dislodgement/extravasation rate from 40% to 20%, confirming that longer catheters were needed for many adult patients at the humeral insertion site [110, 111]. Partly in response to these findings, Vidacare released its 45 mm (yellow hub) EZ-IO® catheter in 2009, with the recommendation that this longer needle be used for adult humeral insertions.

In 2013, Vidacare launched its Tactically Advanced Lifesaving Intraosseous Needle (TALON™) device (Fig. 1.32), a manually inserted alternative to the EZ-IO® line. As a manually inserted device, the TALON™ was FDA cleared for sternal insertion (unlike the drill-assisted EZ-IO®) allowing providers in austere military environments more versatility in site selection. This catheter is 15 gauge in diameter, with a length of 38.5 mm. A similar product, the Manual EZ-IO® catheter, was

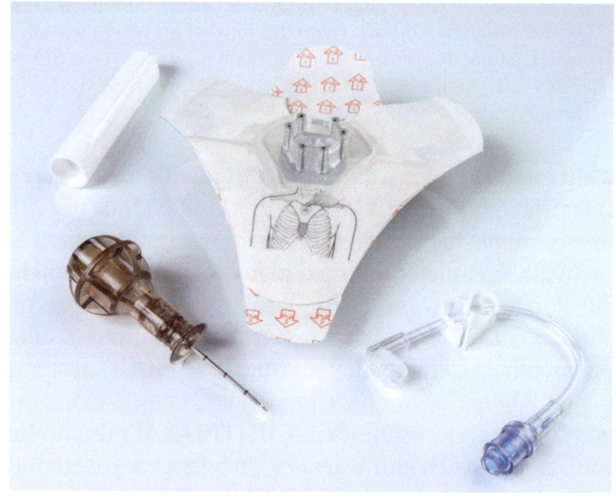

Fig. 1.32 The TALON™ device. *(Image courtesy of Teleflex Incorporated. © 2023 Teleflex Incorporated. All rights reserved.)* [112]

originally released in 2005 featuring 25 and 15 mm lengths, but the device was lengthened to 38.5 mm in 2019. Unlike the TALON™, which is more expensive and marketed to the military, the Manual EZ-IO® is not FDA cleared for sternal insertion.

WaisMed (now a subsidiary of PerSys Medical) released its upgraded version of the BIG® catheter in 2014, known as the NIO® (Next Generation Intraosseous) device. The NIO Adult® (NIO-A) catheter (Fig. 1.33) was the first iteration of the device, with a 15-gauge 42 mm stainless steel trocar needle and cannula, brass 360 nickel-plated hub, and Makrolon® Rx2530 polycarbonate casing. The NIO® line would soon grow to include the NIO Pediatric® (NIO-P) (38.1 mm length, 18 gauge) device in 2016, featuring an adjustable depth of insertion (14 mm for subjects 3–9 years old, 18 mm for subjects 9–12 years old). The NIO Infant® (NIO-I), developed for patients between gestational age 36 weeks (weight ≥2.3 kg) and 3 years old, received FDA clearance in November 2019. More recently, PerSys has released a GO IO™ intraosseous start kit to accompany the NIO® devices, which includes a NeedleVise, IV extension set, secure IV strap, alcohol prep pads, and patient bracelet.

The BD™ Intraosseous Powered Driver (Fig. 1.34) was introduced by Becton, Dickinson, and Company (Franklin Lakes, NJ) in 2020, including a battery-powered driver and five different lengths of IO catheter (15, 25, 35, 45, and 55 mm). According to the manufacturer, the driver can be recharged to last 12× longer than the non-rechargeable EZ-IO® driver, providing 70 catheter insertions at 10 s each on a fully charged battery. In June 2022, BD issued a voluntary recall notice for this IO system due to observed difficulties separating the stylet from the IO needle, failure in deployment of the needle safety mechanism, and difficulties separating the needle from the driver [115].

The SAM IO® device was introduced by SAM Medical (Tualatin, Oregon) in March 2020 (Fig. 1.35). This manually driven device is advanced into the bone through repeated compression of a trigger. As with the EZ-IO® device, catheters are available in three color-coded needle lengths: 15 mm (pink hub), 25 mm (blue), and 45 mm (yellow).

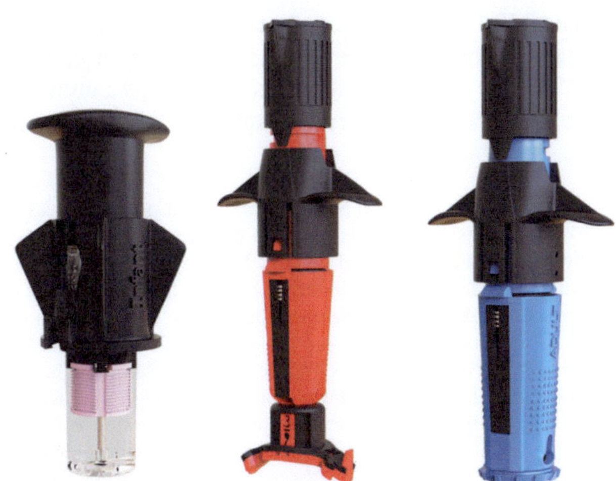

Fig. 1.33 (Left to right) The NIO Infant®, NIO Pediatric®, and NIO Adult® devices. *(Image courtesy of Safeguard Medical. © 2023 Safeguard Medical. All rights reserved.)* [113]

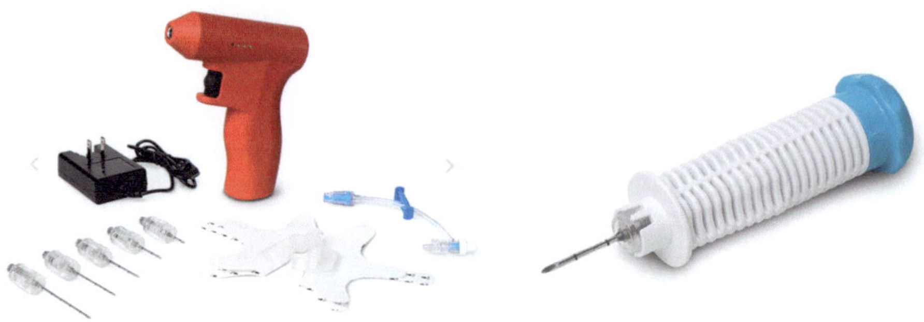

Fig. 1.34 The BD™ Intraosseous Powered Driver (left) and manual driver (right). *(Images courtesy of Becton, Dickson and Company. © 2023 Becton, Dickson and Company. All rights reserved.)* [114]

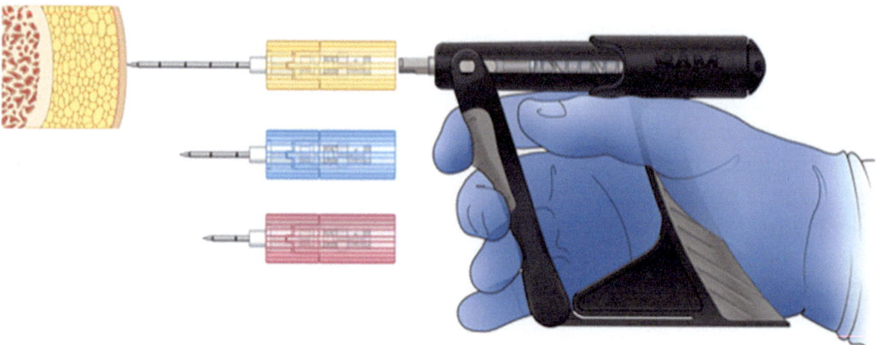

Fig. 1.35 SAM IO® Intraosseous system. *(Images courtesy of SAM Medical. © 2023 SAM Medical. All rights reserved.)* [116]

The SAM IO® system combines the versatility of multiple needle lengths seen in existing semiautomatic devices with increased user control during the insertion process. But the development of this device was a culmination of significant effort on the part of SAM Medical founder and CEO, **Sam Scheinberg**, and others. As Scheinberg puts it,

The development of the SAM IO, like most products, was not a straight line but one of zigs and zags. It began as part of a broader medical device platform originally invented by **Shawn Fojtik** (Distal Access LLC, Park City, Utah). Early in his career, Shawn worked in sales and marketing for Black and Decker. He learned that while electrical drills are fast, the end user could not easily "feel" when a drill bit crossed between hard and softer materials. For example, it can be difficult to feel when a power drill bit breaks through drywall into an open space between two boards … or when an IO powered needle assembly unexpectedly "hubs", pushing through the medullary cavity into the opposite cortex. We have all experienced that sudden loss of resistance and confidence when you pop or push a drill bit forward into the unknown. Likewise, we have also noticed we can much more securely manually punch through drywall with a Phillips head screwdriver using a back and forth oscillation action similar to what we use when inserting Cook or Jamshidi IO trocars. This is not only a safer and more tactile technique, but also produces a cleaner hole.

When Shawn entered the medical field, he was intrigued with the idea of marrying the speed of an electric drill with the feel and control of a manual device. The big idea was to increase the delicate touch for the end user while eliminating the durability, charge, maintenance, and expense considerations associated with power drivers. The first SAM IO prototypes would only oscillate. For example, the driver would spin a needle exactly three or five revolutions clockwise followed by three or five revolutions counterclockwise. While oscillation is effective at slowly and cleanly starting a pilot hole, it is not as effective or as fast as unidirectional clockwise drilling. The addition of a simple ratcheted slider solved this problem. It gave the SAM IO driver the flexibility to controllably oscillate during the slow creation of a pilot hole and then to automatically rapidly convert to unidirectional "clockwise only" fast drilling when the needle encounters resistance.

The Distal Access spinning devices were originally used to resect soft blood clots, uterine polyps, and fibroid tumors. An old friend of ours and legend in the EMS world, **Richard "Doc" Clinchy**, who originally consulted with Pyng Medical Corp (Vancouver, Canada) to introduce the FAST-1 sternal IO device, noticed the Distal Access product platform and mentioned to us that it would be demonstrated at an EMS World meeting in Las Vegas. My wife/business partner, Cherrie, and I visited the small 10′ by 10′ booth where we played with an early prototype using simulated bones. Both of us could see the tremendous potential. We gathered all of our team members around that little booth and the rest, as they say, is history (*Communication between S. Scheinberg and the authors, 9 November 2023, unreferenced*).

Dr. Scheinberg (Fig. 1.36), a board-certified orthopedic surgeon, had served as a trauma surgeon in Vietnam and recognized the need for improved care of trauma victims in the civilian world. His interest in advancing care for trauma victims led him to found The Seaberg Company (doing business as SAM Medical Products, Inc.) in 1984, with the introduction of the company's first commercial product, the SAM™ Splint, in 1985. Since that time, SAM Medical has introduced a variety of other trauma care innovations, including a pelvic sling (2003), soft shell splint (2005), chest seal (2010), junctional tourniquet (2013), ChitoSAM® hemostatic dressing (2013), extremity tourniquet (2017), bleeding control kit (2018), and ThoraSite anatomic landmark guide (2021).

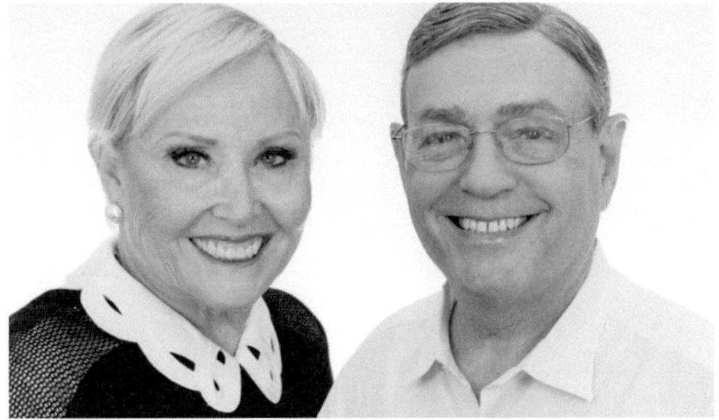

Fig. 1.36 Sam and Cherrie Scheinberg. *(Image courtesy of Sam Scheinberg. © 2023 Sam Scheinberg. All rights reserved)*

Conclusion

Much has changed over the last century of intraosseous infusion, led by an enthusiastic cadre of pioneering clinician-researchers (Fig. 1.37). Despite its humble beginnings in the animal lab, the intraosseous infusion route has proven its value to the practice of emergency medicine and inspired generations of forward-thinking researchers and clinicians to continue to advance the science of resuscitation through new devices, new insertion sites, and new approaches. The study of intraosseous infusion has truly been a worldwide effort, with collaborators spanning decades and across international boundaries to refine and improve these techniques. Although challenges remain, it is hard to imagine a future of emergent vascular access that will not include continued growth and development of this valuable approach for indirect vascular access.

Key Concepts
- Early intraosseous cannulation efforts focused primarily on bone marrow biopsy for diagnostic purposes.
- Therapeutic intraosseous infusion was initially performed most commonly at the sternum in adults and the proximal tibia in children. The tibial site was selected in children because the sternum was felt to be unsafe due to the risk of iatrogenic injury.
- Although intraosseous infusion reports seldom appeared in the English-language medical literature from 1950 to 1984, the approach was still commonly reported in the non-English medical literature during this period.
- Various devices have historically been used to achieve intraosseous infusion, including peripheral intravenous cannulae, spinal needles, and specialized manual or mechanical intraosseous cannulae.
- The civilian IO market is currently dominated by mechanical intraosseous devices, although manual devices remain popular for military and pediatric applications.

Date	Event
1903-1905	First reports of diagnostic bone marrow biopsies in living patients
1916	Drinker describes the circulation of the canine tibia
1922	Doan describes "functionally dormant" network of capillaries existing within the marrow space that may be recruited
	Sternal trephination techniques are introduced for bone marrow biopsy diagnosis
1934	Josefson reports campolon injection at the human sternum to treat pernicious anemia
1940	Henning reports on sternal IO infusion techniques for resuscitation
	Tocantins describes the IO resuscitation of shock patients, including early use of the proximal tibia and distal femur in children
1942	Papper reports IO absorption rates similar to peripheral intravenous infusion
	Macht reports the "depot effect," with delayed absorption of IO medications suspended in oil
World War II	Turkel needle used extensively by US and European combat medics
1944	Bailey and Gimson introduce versions of a "winged cannula" IO device
1971	Jamshidi™ needle introduced
1984	Orlowski publishes "My Kingdom for an Intravenous Line" editorial
	Berg publishes first report of continuous IO vasopressor infusion
1986	First mention of IO devices in Advanced Cardiac Life Support (ACLS) guidelines for pediatric cardiac arrest
	Cook IO needles introduced
1992	First mention of IO devices in Advanced Cardiac Life Support (ACLS) guidelines for adult cardiac arrest
1994	First automatic IO device introduced (BIG®, Waismed)
1998	FAST-1® (Pyng Medical) manual sternal IO device introduced
2004	First drill-powered IO device (EZ-IO®, Vidacare) introduced
2014	NIO® device (Waismed) introduced
2020	BD® IO device (Becton, Dickinson) introduced
	SAM IO® device (SAM Medical) introduced

Fig. 1.37 Timeline of historical events in the history of intraosseous cannulation

References

1. Müller F. Deutsch Med Zeitung 1901;22:349.
2. Pianese G. Sull'anemia splenica infantile (anemia infantum leishmania). Gazz internaz med e chir. 1905;265.
3. Wolff A. Ueber eine methode zur untersuchung des lebender knochenmarks. Deutsche med Wchnschr. 1903;10:165.
4. Drinker CK, Drinker KR. A method for maintaining an artificial circulation through the tibia of the dog, with a demonstration of the vasomotor control of the marrow vessels. Am J Phys. 1916;40(4):514–21. https://doi.org/10.1152/ajplegacy.1916.40.4.514.
5. Drinker CK, Drinker KR, Lund CC. The circulation in the mammalian bone-marrow. Am J Physiol. 1922;62(1):1–92.
6. Lab partners, life partners. Harvard T.H. Chan School of Public Health—News; 2023.
7. Doan CA. The circulation of the bone marrow. Contrib Embryol. 1922;14:27–45.
8. The Ohio State University, University Libraries. Historical reflections: the medical heritage center blog; 2014. https://library.osu.edu/site/mhcb/. Accessed 30 May 2023.
9. Seyfarth C. Eine einfache methode zur diagnostichen entnahme von knochenmark beim lebenden. Arch fur Schiffs-und Tropen-Hygiene, Pathologie und therapie exotischer Krankheiten. 1922;26:337–41.
10. Anirkin MI. Die intravitale untersuchungsmethodik des knochenmarks. Folia Haematol. 1929;38:233–40.
11. Josefson A. A new method of treatment: intraosseous injection. Acta Med Scand. 1934;81:550–64.
12. Young RH, Osgood EE. Sternal marrow aspirated during life: cytology in health and in disease. Arch Intern Med (Chicago). 1935;55(2):186–203. https://doi.org/10.1001/archinte.1935.00160200016002.
13. Benda R. Reseignements fournsi par les injections intramédullaires de sang humaine chez le cobaye. Sang. 1937;11:659.
14. Benda R, Debray C, Bourrée J. Injection du système veineux du cobaye par voie médullaire osseuse: Resultats qu'il est possible d'en attendre. Bull et mém Soc Méd d hôp de Paris. 1937;53:662.
15. Benda R, Orinstein E. Depitre: Injections intra-médullaires osseuses de substances opaques chez l'homme. Sang. 1940;14:172.
16. Leandro M. Tocantins. Image from the History of Medicine (IHM). Jefferson Medical College of Philadelphia; 1955. https://jdc.jefferson.edu/historical_photos/241/. Accessed 30 May 2023.
17. Tocantins LM, O'Neill JF, Jones HW. Infusion of blood and other fluids via the bone marrow. JAMA. 1941;117(15):1229–34.
18. Tocantins LM, O'Neill JF, Price AH. Infusions of blood and other fluids via the bone marrow in traumatic shock and other forms of peripheral circulatory failure. Ann Surg. 1941;114(6):1085–92. https://doi.org/10.1097/00000658-194112000-00015.
19. Tocantins LM, Price AH, O'Neill JF. Infusions via the bone marrow in children. Penn Med J. 1943;46:1267–73.
20. Tocantins LM, O'Neill JF. Complications of intra-osseous therapy. Ann Surg. 1945;122(2):266–77.
21. Tocantins LM, O'Neill. Infusion of blood and other fluids into the circulation via the bone marrow. Proc Soc Exp Biol Med. 1940;45:782–3.
22. Papper EM. The bone marrow route for injecting fluids and drugs into the general circulation. Anesthesiology. 1942;3(3):307–13.
23. Guzman JG. Trabajos sobre Meduloterapia. Rev Med Del Hosp Gen. 1941;3:370.
24. Baravalle N, Alvarez A. Transfusion de Sangre por via de la Medula Osea. An Cirurgia. 1942;8:251.

25. Henning N, Korth J. Die diagnostische sternalpunktion. Einen neue untersuchungsmethode des knochenmarks in vivo. Klin Wochenschr. 1934;34:1219–20.
26. Henning N. Die sternalinjektion als ersatz fuer die intrasternale injektion. Bergmann, Muenchen: Verhandlungen der Deutschen Gesellschaft fuer Innere Medizin; 1940. p. 319–20.
27. Henning N. Die intrasternale injektion und transfusion als ersatz fuer die intravenösen methoden. Dtsch Med Wochenschr. 1940;27:737–9.
28. Parapia LA. Trepanning or trephines: a history of bone marrow biopsy. Br J Haematol. 2007;139(1):14–9. https://doi.org/10.1111/j.1365-2141.2007.06749.x.
29. Henning N. Ueber die intrasternale bzw. intraossale injektion und infusion. Dtsch Med Wochenschr. 1943;41/42:720–2.
30. Henning N. Anzeigen, technik und erfolge der intrasternalen injektion. Ther Ggw. 1944;4/5:130–1.
31. Lamprecht W. Zweckmaessiges sternal-besteck fuer infusion, transfusion und narkose. Dtsch Med Wochenschr. 1949;51:1380–1.
32. Goerig M, Agarwal-Koslowski K. The bone marrow as a site for the reception of infusions, transfusions and anaesthetic agents. Int Congr Ser. 2002;1242:105–12.
33. Emanuel M. Papper, circa 1985. University of Miami Louis Calder Memorial Library collection. Accessed 12 Dec 2022.
34. Papper EM, Rovenstine EA. Utility of marrow cavity of sternum for paternal fluid therapy. War Med. 1942;2:277–83.
35. B-29 Crewman Save a Life in the Air by New Method. The Detroit News; 1945.
36. Bailey H. Bone marrow as a site for the reception of infusions, transfusions, and anesthetic agents. Br Med J. 1944;1:181–2.
37. Ellison JB. Bone-marrow transfusion. Br Med J. 1944;1:266.
38. Craig R. A history of syringes and needles. The University of Queensland Australia; 2018.
39. Behr G. Bone-marrow infusions. Br Med J. 1944;1(4338):305.
40. O'Neill JF, Tocantins LM, Price AH. Further experiences with the technique of administering blood and other fluids via the bone marrow. N C Med J. 1942;3:495–500.
41. Ravitch MM. Suppurative anterior mediastinitis in an infant following intrasternal blood transfusion: operation and recovery. Arch Surg. 1947;47(3):250–7.
42. Dardinski VJ. Sternal transfusions in infants. Med Ann Dist Columbia. 1945;14(5):236–7.
43. Napier LE, Gupta PC. Sternum puncture. The findings in normal Indians. Ind Med Gaz. 1938;73(1):1–7.
44. Gimson JD. Bone-marrow transfusion in infants and children. Introducing a specially designed needle. Br Med J. 1944;1(4352):748–9.
45. Macht DI. Studies on intraosseous injections of epinephrine. Am J Phys. 1942;38:269.
46. Morrison M, Samwick AA. Intramedullary (sternal) transfusion of human bone marrow. JAMA. 1940;115(20):1708–11.
47. Wile UJ, Schamberg IL. Pulmonary fat embolism following infusions via the bone marrow. J Invest Dermatol. 1942;5:173–7.
48. Wright CS, Sams WM. Udo Julius Wile, MD 1882-1965. Arch Dermatol. 1966;93(1):1–2. https://doi.org/10.1001/archderm.1966.01600190007001.
49. Turkel H. Emergency infusion through the bone. Mil Med. 1984;149(6):349–50.
50. Frederick A. Coller, MD, FACS, 1887-1964. https://www.facs.org/about-acs/archives/past-highlights/collerhighlight/. Accessed 5 Mar 2024.
51. Churchill ED. Modern surgery in combat areas. Med Bull N Afr Theat Op. 1944;1:7.
52. Turkel H, Bethell FH. Biopsy of bone marrow performed by new and simple instrument. J Lab Clin Med. 1943;28:1246–51.
53. Heinild S, Tyge S, Tudvad F. Bone marrow infusion in childhood. J Pediatr. 1947;30:400–12.
54. Kalinovskaia EN. Vnutrikostnoe perelivanie krovi i lekarstvennykh zhidkostei [Intraosseous transfusion of blood and medicinal solutions]. Sov Med. 1953;17(9):25–6. Russian.
55. Berg EJ. Intra-ossale anaesthesietechniek [Technic of intra-osseous anesthesia]. Rev Belge Stomatol. 1954;51(4):533–4. Dutch.

56. Spivak LI. Vnutrikostnye vlivaniia lekarstvennykh veshchestv i krovi v psikhiatriches-koi praktike [Intraosseous administration of drugs and blood in psychiatric practice]. Zh Nevropatol Psikhiatr Im S S Korsakova. 1958;58(2):215–7. Russian.

57. Atiasov NI. Intra-osseous infusions in extensive burns. Ortop Travmatol Protez. 1962;23:58–62. Russian.

58. Boiadzhiev S, Filipov S, Momchev M. Prilaganeto na regionalnata intravenozna analgeziia za vutrekostnoto aplitsirane na antibiotik pri osteomielit na dolen kraĭnik [Use of regional intravenous analgesia for the intraosseous administration of antibiotic in osteomyelitis of the lower extremity]. Khirurgiia (Sofiia). 1977;30(6):530–2. Bulgarian.

59. Millam D. The history of intravenous therapy. J Intraven Nurs. 1996;19(1):5–14.

60. Seldinger SI. Catheter replacement of the needle in percutaneous arteriography; a new technique. Acta Radiol. 1953;39(5):368–76. https://doi.org/10.3109/00016925309136722.

61. Parrish GA, Turkewitz D, Skiendzielewski JJ. Intraosseous infusions in the emergency department. Am J Emerg Med. 1986;4:59–63.

62. Valdes MM. Intraosseous fluid administration in emergencies. Lancet. 1977;1(8024):1235–6.

63. Shoor PM, Berryhill RE, Benumof JL. Intraosseous infusion: pressure-flow relationship and pharmacokinetics. J Trauma. 1979;19(10):772–4.

64. Waisman M, Bursztein-De Myttenaere S, Goldberger Y, Heifetz M. Intra-osseous regional anesthesia as an alternative to intravenous regional anesthesia. Harefuah. 1982;102(6):227–9. Hebrew.

65. Turkel H. Intraosseous infusions. Am J Dis Child. 1983;137(7):706.

66. Standards for cardiopulmonary resuscitation (CPR) and emergency cardiac care (ECC). 3. Advanced life support. JAMA 1974;227(7):852–860.

67. Standards and Guidelines for cardiopulmonary resuscitation (CPR) and emergency cardiac care (ECC). JAMA 1980;244(5):453–509.

68. Standards and Guidelines for cardiopulmonary resuscitation (CPR) and emergency cardiac care (ECC). JAMA. 1986;255(21):2905–2984.

69. American Heart Association. National conference on standards and guidelines for cardiopulmonary resuscitation and emergency cardiac care. Standards and guidelines for cardiopulmonary resuscitation (CPR) and emergency cardiac care (ECC). Part VI: pediatric advanced life support. JAMA. 1986;255:2961–4.

70. American Heart Association. Guidelines for cardiopulmonary resuscitation emergency cardiac care. Adult advanced cardiac life support. JAMA. 1992;268(16):2199–241.

71. Berg RA. Emergency infusion of catecholamines into bone marrow. Am J Dis Child. 1984;138(9):810–1. https://doi.org/10.1001/archpedi.1984.02140470010003.

72. Orlowski JP. My kingdom for an intravenous line. Am J Dis Child. 1984;138(9):803. https://doi.org/10.1001/archpedi.1984.02140470003001.

73. Orlowski JP, Julius CJ, Petras RE, Porembka DT, Gallagher JM. The safety of intraosseous infusions: risks of fat and bone marrow emboli to the lungs. Ann Emerg Med. 1989;18(10):1062–7. https://doi.org/10.1016/s0196-0644(89)80932-1.

74. Orlowski JP, Porembka DT, Gallagher JM, Van Lente F. The bone marrow as a source of laboratory studies. Ann Emerg Med. 1989;18(12):1348–51. https://doi.org/10.1016/s0196-0644(89)80274-4.

75. Orlowski JP, Porembka DT, Gallagher JM, Lockrem JD, VanLente F. Comparison study of intraosseous, central intravenous, and peripheral intravenous infusions of emergency drugs. Am J Dis Child. 1990;144(1):112–7. https://doi.org/10.1001/archpedi.1990.02150250124049.

76. Spivey WH, Crespo SG, Fuhs LR, Schoffstall JM. Plasma catecholamine levels after intraosseous epinephrine administration in a cardiac arrest model. Ann Emerg Med. 1992;21(2):127–31. https://doi.org/10.1016/s0196-0644(05)80145-3.

77. Spivey WH, Unger HD, Lathers CM, McNamara RM. Intraosseous diazepam suppression of pentylenetetrazol-induced epileptogenic activity in pigs. Ann Emerg Med. 1987;16(2):156–9. https://doi.org/10.1016/s0196-0644(87)80005-7.

78. Spivey WH, Lathers CM, Malone DR, Unger HD, Bhat S, McNamara RN, Schoffstall J, Tumer N. Comparison of intraosseous, central, and peripheral routes of sodium bicarbonate

administration during CPR in pigs. Ann Emerg Med. 1985;14(12):1135–40. https://doi.org/10.1016/s0196-0644(85)81015-5.

79. Schoffstall JM, Spivey WH, Davidheiser S, Lathers CM. Intraosseous crystalloid and blood infusion in a swine model. J Trauma. 1989;29(3):384–7. https://doi.org/10.1097/00005373-198903000-00019.

80. Silverman I. New biopsy needle. Am J Surg. 1938;40(3):671–2.

81. Favorite GO. Instrument for obtaining bone marrow. J Lab Clin Med. 1939;25:199–201.

82. Reddy DG. New needle for obtaining undiluted bone marrow. Am J Clin Path. 1952;22:1137–41.

83. Klima R, Rosegger H. Zur methodik der diagnostschen sternalpunktion. Klinische Woechenschrift. 1935;14:541–2.

84. Jamshidi K, Windschitl HE, Swaim WR. A new biopsy needle for bone marrow. Eur J Haematol. 1971;8(1):69–71.

85. Reusable Jamshidi™ needle for iliac crest biopsy. Becton, Dickson and Company. Accessed Jan 2023.

86. Islam A. New sternal puncture needle. J Clin Pathol. 1991;44(8):690–1. https://doi.org/10.1136/jcp.44.8.690.

87. Jamshidi™ modified Illinois disposable needle. Becton, Dickson and Company. Accessed Jan 2023.

88. Cook manual IO needle with Dieckmann modification. Cook Medical. Image provided by manufacturer.

89. Sussmane-Raszynski needle. Cook Medical. Image provided by manufacturer.

90. Sur-Fast™ needle. Cook Medical. Image provided by manufacturer.

91. The Near Needle Holder™. Richard Near, Near Manufacturing Ltd. Image provided by the manufacturer.

92. Kalechstein S, Permual A, Cameron BM, Pemberton J, Hollaar G, Duffy D, Cameron BH. Evaluation of a new pediatric intraosseous needle insertion device for low-resource settings. J Pediatr Surg. 2012;47(5):974–9. https://doi.org/10.1016/j.jpedsurg.2012.01.055.

93. The FAST-1® intraosseous system. Teleflex Incorporated. Image provided by the manufacturer.

94. Macnab A, Christenson J, Findlay J, Horwood B, Johnson D, Jones L, et al. A new system for sternal intraosseous infusion in adults. Prehosp Emerg Care. 2000;4(2):173–7.

95. The FAST-Responder®. Teleflex Incorporated. Image provided by the manufacturer.

96. Burkhardt R. Bone and bone tissue, colour atlas of clinical histopathology. New York: Springer; 1971.

97. Parapia LA, Cox J, Brown G. Powered biopsy needle. British Patent Application No. 8817008.9; 1988.

98. The Bone Injection Gun (BIG®), adult and pediatric sizes. Safeguard Medical. Accessed Mar 2023.

99. Waisman M, Roffman M, Bursztein S, Heifetz M. Intraosseous regional anesthesia as an alternative to intravenous regional anesthesia. J Trauma. 1995;39(6):1153–6.

100. Waisman M, Waisman D. Bone marrow infusions in adults. J Trauma. 1997;42(2):288–93.

101. Brinn D. Israeli device goes straight to the bone. Israeli21c [Internet]. [31 Jul 2005, updated 13 Sep 2012; cited 19 December 2022]. https://www.israel21c.org/israeli-device-goes-straight-to-the-bone/.

102. Von Hoff DD, Kuhn JG, Burris HA, Miller LJ. Does intraosseous equal intravenous? A pharmacokinetic study. Am J Emerg Med. 2008;26:31–8.

103. *Design News* [Internet]. Informa Markets (Santa Monica, CA). Anatomy of a life saver. https://www.designnews.com/anatomy-life-saver-0.

104. Miller L. Letter from LJ Miller to JH Paxton, dated 2022 Dec 7.

105. The EZ-IO® intraosseous infusion system, including three catheter lengths, infusion tubing and EZ-Stabilizer®. Teleflex Incorporated. Accessed Feb 2023.

106. Miller L. Adult IO arrives: the solution to difficult vascular access. JEMS. 2005:1–35.

107. North American Rescue, LLC. [Internet]. Our Products. https://www.narescue.com/. Accessed 14 Feb 2023.

108. Horton MA, Beamer C. Powered intraosseous insertion provides safe and effective vascular access for pediatric emergency patients. Pediatr Emerg Care. 2008;24(6):347–50. https://doi.org/10.1097/PEC.0b013e318177a6fe.
109. Ong ME, Chan YH, Oh JJ, et al. An observational, prospective study comparing tibial and humeral intraosseous access using the EZ-IO. Am J Emerg Med. 2009;27(1):8–15.
110. Paxton JH, Knuth TE, Klausner HA. Proximal humerus intraosseous infusion: a preferred emergency venous access. J Trauma. 2009;67(3):606–11. https://doi.org/10.1097/TA.0b013e3181b16f42.
111. Knuth TE, Paxton JH, Myers D. Intraosseous injection of iodinated computed tomography contrast agent in an adult blunt trauma patient. Ann Emerg Med. 2011;57(4):382–6. https://doi.org/10.1016/j.annemergmed.2010.09.025. Epub 2010 Dec 15
112. The TALON™ device. Teleflex Incorporated. Image provided by the manufacturer.
113. The NIO Infant®, NIO pediatric® and NIO adult® devices. Safeguard medical. Image provided by the manufacturer.
114. The BD™ Intraosseous Powered Driver (left) and manual driver (right). Becton, Dickson and Company. Image provided by the manufacturer.
115. Kannuchamy S. [Internet] BD announced voluntary recall for intraosseous products. XTalks [28 June 2022; cited 22 December 2022]. https://xtalks.com/bd-announced-voluntary-recall-for-intraosseous-products-3134/.
116. SAM IO® Intraosseous system. SAM Medical. Image provided by the manufacturer.

Anatomy and Physiology of Intraosseous Infusion

2

Andrew Mizerowski and James H. Paxton

Introduction

Unlike the more common method of **direct** infusion of medications and fluids through a peripheral intravenous (PIV) or central venous catheter (CVC) into the venous drainage system of the human cardiovascular system, intraosseous (IO) infusion utilizes an **indirect** infusion of substances by depositing substances into the intramedullary space for eventual uptake by the venous drainage system of the bone. Historically, the **long bones** of the human body including the tibia, humerus, and femur have been preferred as catheterization sites for IO infusion. However, the sternum (a flat bone), clavicle, radius, and calcaneus (a short bone), among others, have also been studied. Although each site has different physiological properties that uniquely impact the infusion of medications and fluids, the principle of IO infusion remains similar in all cases. This chapter explores the basic principles behind IO infusion, including common mechanisms relating to bony anatomy and physiology that enable this technique to be effectively used for the treatment of critically ill patients.

Bone Anatomy

Long bones are comprised of three main parts: the **diaphysis** or middle of the bone, the **metaphysis** (i.e., proximal and distal to the diaphysis), and the **epiphysis** (i.e., proximal and distal to the metaphysis). Most of the **medullary cavity** resides within the boundaries of the diaphysis. The medullary cavity is comprised of a combination of yellow marrow and red marrow. **Yellow marrow** is composed largely of

A. Mizerowski (✉) · J. H. Paxton
Department of Emergency Medicine, Wayne State University School of Medicine, Detroit, MI, USA
e-mail: hh9947@wayne.edu; james.paxton@wayne.edu

   43
J. H. Paxton (ed.), *Intraosseous Vascular Access*,
https://doi.org/10.1007/978-3-031-61201-5_2

Fig. 2.1 Bone anatomy, as it relates to intraosseous infusion

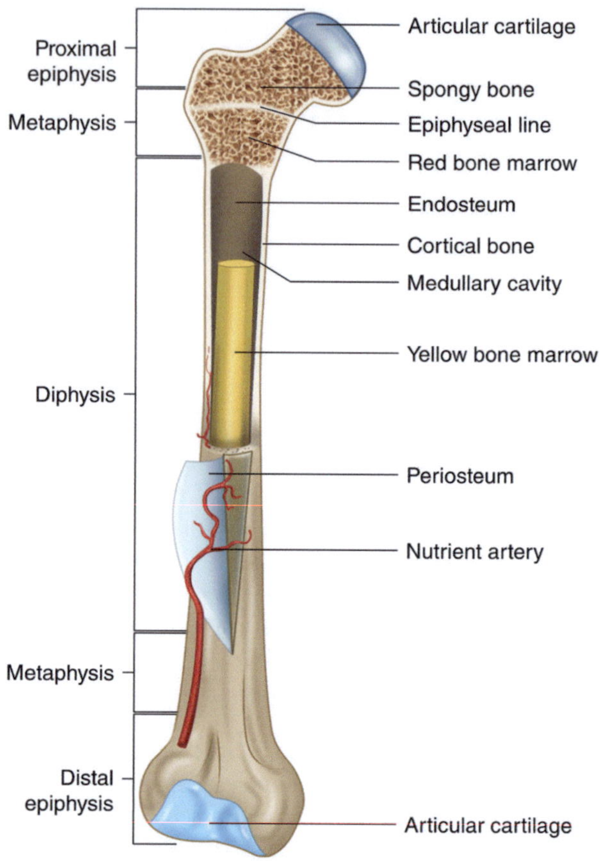

adipocytes within a connective tissue meshwork that additionally supports blood vessels. **Red marrow**, in contrast, consists primarily of hematopoietic cells (i.e., blood stem cells) organized within a loose connective tissue stroma that supports an extensive blood supply [1]. The diaphysis surrounding the medullary cavity is composed of cortical (i.e., compact) bone, while the metaphysis and epiphysis consist primarily of trabecular (i.e., spongy) bone positioned deep to the cortex. The outermost surface of bone consists of the **periosteum**, a highly vascularized, densely innervated connective tissue layer containing both osteoclasts and osteoblasts. The periosteum covers almost the entirety of long bones except at surfaces where bones articulate with one another. Just below the periosteum is the **cortex**, which consists of three layers: the outer circumferential lamellae, the interstitial lamellae, and the inner circumferential lamellae. The interstitial lamellae tend to arrange into **Haversian canals**, bony channels surrounding perforating blood vessels, and nerve fibers. This anatomy is illustrated in Fig. 2.1.

The **endosteum** is a highly vascularized connective tissue layer also containing osteoclasts and osteoblasts and is in contact with both lamellar bone and the

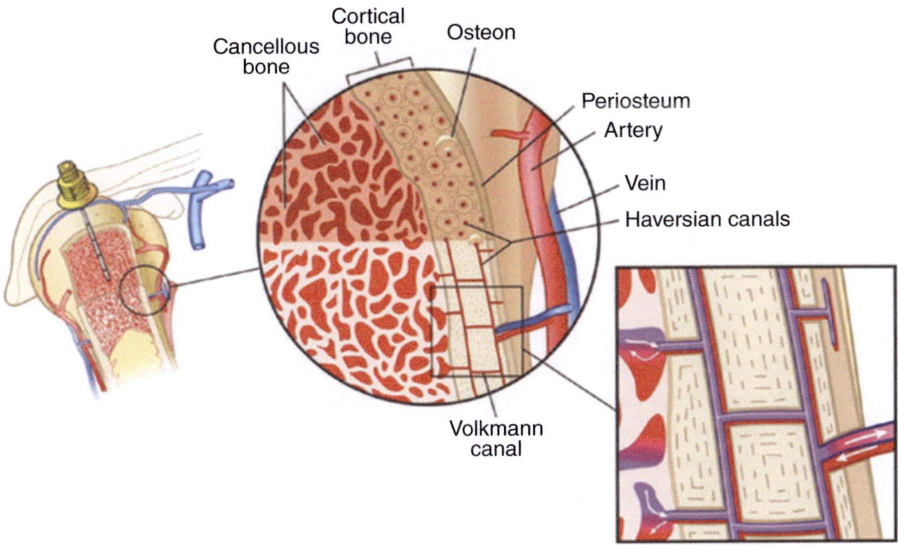

Fig. 2.2 Intraosseous vascular anatomy. (Image courtesy of David Baker & Sam Newman. © 2023 *University of Texas Health Science Center, San Antonio. All rights reserved*)

medullary cavity [1]. Oxygenated blood is supplied to the medullary cavity via **nutrient arteries**, with their number depending upon the size of the bone. These arteries enter the bone through **nutrient foramina** to supply the ascending and descending portions of the marrow cavity before branching into radial arteries. The radial arteries supply the bone marrow and the inner one-third of compact bone before further branching into spiral arteries, which anastomose with the metaphyseal arteries. **Sinusoids** in bone represent the transition point between the human arterial and venous systems. After oxygen in the blood has been extracted by the bone and its contents, deoxygenated blood is removed from the bone via numerous collecting veins. Metaphyseal vessels are separated early in life from epiphyseal vasculature by the epiphyseal growth plate. Upon closure of the growth plate, anastomosis of these vessels occurs. Periosteal supply is accomplished in part by the nutrient artery and by the periosteal arteries, which travel within the **Haversian canals**. Haversian canals communicate with each other via **Volkmann canals** [2]. The relationship between these vascular channels is demonstrated in Fig. 2.2.

Blood delivery to human bones is very efficient, with the skeletal system receiving between 5.5% and 11% of cardiac output [2]. Early in life, these blood vessels fuel the rapid growth of long bones from their transition as chondrocytes (i.e., cells that secrete cartilage and become embedded in it) to mature bony tissue. Even after bones cease to grow in size, this rich blood supply is needed to promote continued remodeling of the bone throughout the human life cycle.

Although the anatomy of flat or short bones differs slightly from that of long bones, their structure closely resembles the epiphysis of long bones. Both flat and short bones are composed of a thin layer of cortical bone surrounding trabecular bone. As humans age, the medullary cavities tend to become less hematopoietically active, with red marrow gradually replaced by yellow (i.e., adipose) marrow. This transition occurs more slowly in flat (e.g., sternum) and short (e.g., calcaneus) bones than in long bones (e.g., humerus, femur, tibia) so that **a higher proportion of red marrow is found to reside within the trabecular bone of adults when compared to the long bones** [1].

Neurohormonal Regulation

Modulation of the blood supply to bone is accomplished by both sympathetic neural and neurohumoral mechanisms. Sympathetic control is modulated through the release of endogenous catecholamines, mainly **norepinephrine** and, to a smaller extent, epinephrine. Catecholamines interact with prejunctional and postjunctional adrenergic receptors on the smooth muscle vasculature to mediate vasoconstriction and vasodilation. The two main categories of adrenergic receptors are alpha (α) and beta (β) adrenergic receptors, and both come in a variety of subtypes. Postjunctional α-1 and α-2 receptors are known to be the two primary mediators of vasoconstriction. The density of these receptors and receptor subtypes varies widely between different vascular beds. The postjunctional β-2 receptor subtype has been shown to be implicated in mediating vasodilation, although the role of prejunctional β-receptors in bony vasomotor control remains largely unknown. Activation of the prejunctional α-2 adrenergic receptors induces inhibition of norepinephrine release through the process of feedback inhibition. Neurohumoral mechanisms are carried out by stimulation of the adrenal glands to secrete mainly epinephrine (and some norepinephrine), along with the stimulation of the renin-angiotensin aldosterone system (RAAS). The RAAS system ultimately increases blood volume, increases peripheral resistance through vasoconstriction, and can increase sympathetic neural transmission [3].

The interaction between marrow vasculature and neural stimulation has been extensively studied. An early investigation by Stein et al. published in 1958 documented the vasoactive effects of endogenously synthesized catecholamines, including norepinephrine and epinephrine [4]. This study was one of the first to demonstrate that the decrease in bone marrow pressure seen with peripheral intravenous injections of epinephrine and norepinephrine may be due to the vasoconstriction of nutrient arteries. Subsequent investigations have reported similar findings [5, 6]. The clinical implications of these findings are reflected in certain emergency situations such as cardiac arrest, which is associated with increased sympathetic activity. The perfusion of bone marrow in such circumstances is limited [7], ultimately affecting the administration of medications that are infused intraosseously. However, studies of vasopressor administration in the treatment of cardiac arrest have shown incongruent results when comparing the pharmacokinetics of IO versus IV routes of infusion. Some authors have shown no significant difference in maximal concentration (Cmax) and time to maximal concentration (Tmax) between IO and IV administration of epinephrine [6], while others have reported that PIV administration of epinephrine is associated with a significantly greater Cmax and Tmax when compared to IO administration [8]. It is unclear whether these discrepancies are due to differences in adrenergic receptor density at the nutrient arteries or rather due to the effect of infused epinephrine on adrenergic receptors at the marrow arterioles.

Factors Influencing Vascular Supply to Bone

Investigations of several other endogenous molecules, such as bradykinin, adenosine, vasopressin, and metabolic byproducts, have provided compelling evidence regarding their influence on bone marrow vascular resistance. Notably, the peptide bradykinin has been shown to decrease vascular resistance, resulting in increased blood flow within the bone marrow space [9]. This effect aligns with bradykinin's well-known vasodilatory actions observed during the inflammatory process. Likewise, the ubiquitous nucleoside adenosine has also been found to increase bone marrow blood flow [6] by causing relaxation of the arterial smooth muscle [10].

Vasopressin demonstrates a unique effect on bone perfusion, generating both vasodilatory and vasoconstrictive effects. In general, the determination of vasculature effect is predicted by the receptor that a substance is acting upon. As vascular beds often contain more than one receptor type, the net effect of a vasoactive substance will depend upon which receptor displays the greater density at that site. Vasoconstrictive responses are carried out by V1 vascular receptors [11], KATP [12] channels, NO signaling pathway, and potentiation of vasoconstrictor agents [13]. Vasodilation, by contrast, is primarily mediated by endothelial oxytocin receptors [14]. The density of these various receptors at different marrow beds remains unknown. One study by Volker et al. measured plasma concentrations of vasopressin following IO and IV infusion, finding that the plasma concentrations achieved were not found to be significantly different [15]. Similarly, Burgert et al. did not observe a significant difference in Tmax or Cmax between IO and IV infusion of vasopressin [16].

Common metabolic byproducts such as carbon dioxide (CO_2) and hydrogen ions (H^+) can accumulate in the blood and even in bone through metabolic activity. In conditions such as hypercapnia and acidosis, it has been demonstrated in anesthetized canines that blood flow to the sternum, ribs, and femoral marrow is increased [17].

The blood supply to bone is intimately tied to the effectiveness of IO infusion. Exogenously administered molecules have the ability to induce an increase in blood flow to the bone. For example, certain parathyroid hormones (e.g., PTH 1-34, PTH 1-84, and PTHrP) have been shown to have vasodilatory effects on the peripheral nutrient artery of rat femoral bones via nitric oxide (NO) and endothelial cell-mediated mechanisms [18]. Evidence of the potent vasodilatory capacity of PTH and PTHrP opens the door for investigation into its utilization in IO infusion regimens.

Just as the blood supply to bone can change in the acute setting, it can also change over the long term. Chronic changes of blood supply to the bone likely

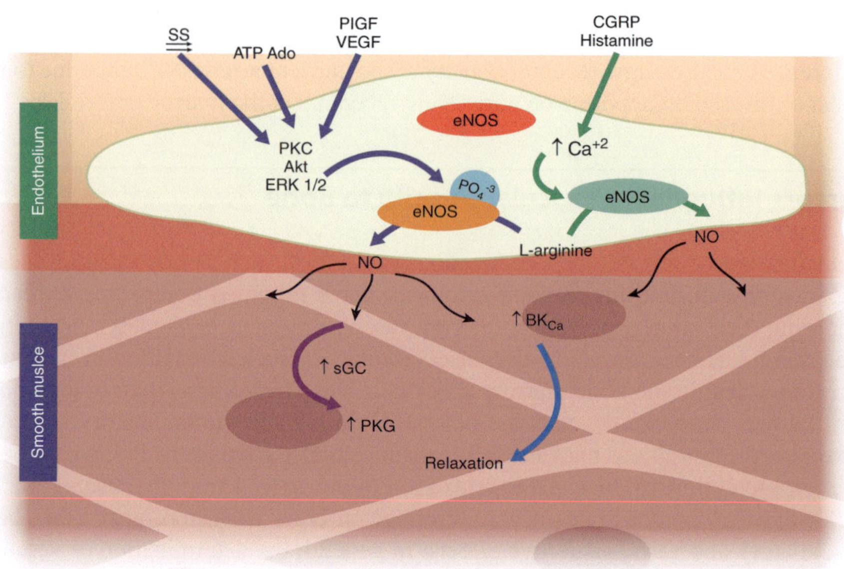

Fig. 2.3 Nitric oxide-dependent vasodilation
Notes: SS Shear stress, *ATP* Adenosine triphosphate, *Ado* Adenosine, *PlGF* Placental growth factor, *VEGF* Vascular endothelial growth factor, *CGRP* Calcitonin gene-related peptide, Ca^{+2} Ionized calcium, *eNOS* Endothelial nitric oxide synthase, *PKC* P rotein kinase C, *Akt* Akt serine/threonine protein kinase, *ERK 1/2* Extracellular signal-related kinases 1/2, *NO* Nitric oxide, *sGC* Soluble guanylyl cyclase, *PKG* Protein kinase G, *BKCa* Large-conductance Ca^{+2}-activated K^+ channel, PO_4^{-3} Phosphate

impact the effectiveness of IO infusion. Some of the factors to consider include mechanical loading or exercise, presence of specific hormones (e.g., estrogen), and aging. Chronic exercise, both weight-bearing and non-weight-bearing, has been shown to increase blood flow due to increased NO-dependent vasodilation in rats [19]. This mechanism is depicted in Fig. 2.3.

During exercise, increased blood flow generates a shear stress (SS) on endothelial cells. A downstream cascade following the shear stress further activates the kinases protein kinase c (PKC), Akt, and extracellular signal-related kinases 1/2 (ERK 1/2), leading to phosphorylation of endothelial nitric oxide synthase (eNOS) and generation of nitric oxide. Nitric oxide induces smooth muscle relaxation either through large-conductance Ca^{+2}-activated K^+ (BKCa) channels or through a series of reactions that upregulate cyclic GMP (cGMP)-dependent protein kinase G (PKG). In addition, a host of other molecules depicted in Fig. 2.3 are generated during exercise and increase NO production. Other theories suggest that the increased blood flow from consistent exercise is a result of perfusion to a greater percentage of the bone [20]. As the demand on bone increases, the supply of oxygen and nutrients must also increase.

Estrogen is known to have a major impact on bone health in females. Large changes in estrogen levels occur during puberty and menopause. Interestingly, endothelial cells have estrogen receptors on their surface. A study by Griffith and colleagues investigated the effects of reduced estrogen on bone vascularity. They demonstrated that acetylcholine-mediated, endothelium-dependent vasodilation was impaired, and phenylephrine-induced contraction was enhanced in ovariectomized rats [21]. Vascular endothelial growth factor, VEGF, a signaling protein important for vascular growth, has also been observed to decrease in ovariectomized rats [22].

Throughout an individual's lifetime, blood supply to bone does not remain stagnant, but continuously changes. During development, children's bones require a lot of energy, which is accomplished by an increase in blood flow to the bone [23]. Further aging effects on medullary perfusion were investigated by Prisby et al. Advanced age has been shown to be associated with a reduced capacity of endothelial dependent vasodilation in femoral bones mainly attributed to the NO signaling pathway [24]. With a reduced vasodilator capacity associated with aging, so comes an increased reliance upon the periosteal vascular network [25]. Increased reliance on the periosteal vascular network can lead to a reduced medullary flow rate and diminished effectiveness of IO infusion.

These discoveries shed light on the complex regulatory mechanisms governing bone marrow perfusion from the acute setting to chronic changes and offer potential insights into therapeutic interventions targeting vascular function.

Intraosseous Pressure and Flow

The baseline intraosseous pressure (IOP) of long bones is highly variable between sites and is likely dependent upon several intrinsic physiological parameters. Forward flow of substances into the intramedullary space is only accomplished when infusion pressures exceed the IOP of the target bone. However, different bones have different IOPs and therefore different tolerances for IO infusion. Baseline IOP values were investigated in a study by De Lorenzo et al. with the following results: tibia (mean 17.4, SD 8.2 mmHg), femur (18.4, SD 3.8 mmHg), humerus (15.7 ± 1.8 mmHg), and sternum (5.7 ± 0.5 mmHg) [26]. These measurements were calculated at baseline and varied based on increases and decreases in blood pressure. This study showed that IO infusion into the diaphysis was drained by a single nutrient foramen, while those infusions introduced at the metaphysis or epiphysis were drained by multiple channels, suggesting that infusion sites near the ends of long bones tend to be more aggressively extracted, possibly due to the presence of an enriched drainage system. Interestingly, the only site that showed even a weak correlation with MAP ($r = 0.65$) in this study was the femur, which also showed the highest IOP among those animals tested [27]. Of course, these results were shown in a swine model, which may limit predictions of IO flow rates among human subjects as it is possible that human and porcine IOPs differ. What is clear from this study, and likely also true in human subjects, is that **different bones**

within the same subject have different IOPs. Moreover, those bones with lower IOPs likely enjoy better uptake of infused substances from the medullary cavity, especially when the infusion is introduced near the proximal or distal portions of the long bone. Gravity infusion may not be sufficient to overcome a bone's intrinsic IOP and generate forward flow of infusates. In clinical practice, pressurized infusion may be necessary to achieve an acceptable flow rate, especially at sites with a high intrinsic IOP. An extreme example demonstrating the fluctuation in IOP can be seen during hemorrhagic shock, as the body works to divert blood flow toward vital organs, with arterial vasoconstriction causing a decrease in bone marrow pressures of 70–80% [4–6]. Factors that likely influence the flow rate achievable at a specific infusion site include the size and shape of the medullary cavity, the total sinusoidal cross-sectional area, and the site's proximity to large veins.

The discontinuous capillaries of the medullary cavity are known as **sinusoids**. They allow medications and fluids to enter and make their way into central circulation because they are composed of endothelial cells lacking an organized basement membrane and junctional proteins [28]. **Starling forces** control the exchange of fluids between the capillary intravascular space and the interstitial fluid found between extravascular cells. These forces include the osmotic pressure exerted by proteins and other large molecules in the plasma (i.e., **oncotic pressure**) and **hydrostatic pressure**, which is exerted by a fluid at rest due to the force of gravity. **Starling's equation** describes the net flow resulting from the combined effects of these forces (Fig. 2.4). In this equation, the flow per unit time is labeled the fluid flux (J_v) and is defined as the difference between hydrostatic ($P_c - P_t$) and oncotic ($\pi_c - \pi_t$) gradients. The symbol P_c represents intravascular hydrostatic pressure, P_t represents interstitial hydrostatic pressure, π_c represents intravascular oncotic pressure, and π_t represents interstitial oncotic pressure. The **filtration coefficient** (K_t)

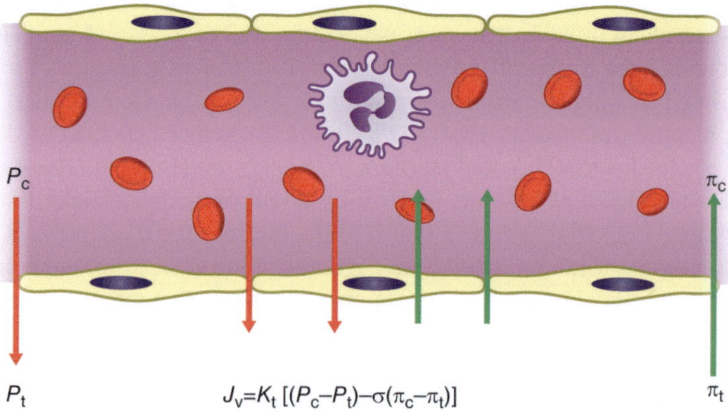

Fig. 2.4 Starling's equation, which describes the exchange of fluid between the intravascular and interstitial spaces in human capillaries *Notes:* J_v Transendothelial solvent filtration volume per second, K_t Filtration coefficient, P_c Capillary hydrostatic pressure, P_t Interstitial fluid hydrostatic pressure, σ Reflection coefficient, π_c Capillary osmotic pressure, π_t Interstitial osmotic pressure

quantifies the conductance or relative ease of fluids to cross the membrane, while the **reflection coefficient** (σ) defines the permeability of the membrane, which is often related to pore size. In order to drive fluid into the sinusoids, a higher hydrostatic pressure (or lower oncotic pressure) must exist within the interstitium than that found within the sinusoids.

A physiologic limit to the fluid flow rates achievable with IO infusion does exist, but it is not known how this maximal flow rate compares to that achievable with peripheral IV infusion. Warren et al. investigated the IV infusion rate of normal saline compared to the IO infusion rate in a pediatric model at many sites including the humerus, femur, tibia, and medial malleolus under normovolemic and hypovolemic conditions. They also tested the effect of gravity infusion versus pressurized infusion (at 300 mmHg). In this porcine model, the average flow rate for all conditions was as follows: peripheral IV 23.6 ± 7.7 mL/min, humeral IO 22.3 ± 8.8 mL/min, femoral IO 16.5 ± 7.8 mL/min, medial malleolus IO 12.1 ± 7.2 mL/min, and proximal tibial IO 8.8 ± 6.3 mL/min. This study suggests that **humeral IO infusion most closely approximates IV infusion**, with proximal tibial infusions performing the worst. Pressurized infusion resulted in an increase of 2–4 times the rates of infusion for both peripheral IV and IO in both the hypovolemic and normovolemic swine models. In addition, this study demonstrated a 32% decreased flow rate on average under hypovolemic conditions when compared to normovolemic subjects for both peripheral IV and IO infusions [27].

The impact of pressurized infusion on IO flow rates was also studied by Lairet et al. in a porcine model. Investigating high pressures (i.e., those above 300 mmHg), the mean infusion flow rate for the tibia was 103 mL/min (±48.1 mL/min), distal femur 138 mL/min (±65.3 mL/min), and proximal humerus 213 mL/min (±53.2 mL/min) [29]. In this study, the proximal humerus flow rate was significantly greater than both the distal femur and proximal tibia. More recent studies demonstrate inconsistent findings between the flow rates at the proximal tibia and distal humerus. Certain studies found significant differences in flow rate between the two sites in both clinical [30] and cadaveric [31] models. On the other hand, further cadaveric [32] and clinical [33] studies did not find significant differences between these two sites.

Schoffstall et al. studied the infusion flow rates of saline and blood comparing larger and smaller pigs. The outcome was an increase in flow rates under pressurized infusion in the larger pigs, but only with the use of a 13-gauge needle and not with an 18-gauge needle [34]. Thus, it appears that the caliber of the IO catheter may also influence flow rates, although the degree to which a narrow IO catheter size restricts flow is unknown.

Factors Influencing Bioavailability

Proximity to the central venous circulation likely affects the degree to which IO infusates exit the marrow via the venous system. Each injection site has a different route to central circulation that ultimately affects the pharmacokinetics and potentially the intended clinical efficacy of the infusion. Intraosseous infusions at the sternum drain into the **internal thoracic vein**, thence to the **subclavian vein**, thence the **brachiocephalic vein**, and finally the **superior vena cava** before reaching the heart. In terms of distance, more proximal sites of IO infusion (e.g., proximal humerus, sternum) are closer to central circulation compared to more distal insertion sites (e.g., iliac crest, distal femur, proximal tibia, calcaneus). The implications of this principle can be seen in a pharmacokinetic investigation of drug delivery during cardiopulmonary resuscitation in a porcine model by Hoskins et al. In this study, the sternal and tibial IO routes were compared to central venous infusion. Evans blue and indocyanine green dyes were administered along with a 0.014 mg/kg bolus of epinephrine. Comparing the two IO groups (i.e., sternal and proximal tibial), the time to maximal concentration of tracer was significantly lower (53 ± 11 s) for the sternal versus the tibial (107 ± 27 s) route. The authors also found that the time to maximal concentration of tracer was not significantly different between sternal IO and central venous delivery routes (97 ± 17 s and 70 ± 12 s, respectively). It is important to keep in mind that this study was measuring concentrations of dye tracer and not the exogenously administered epinephrine, which may demonstrate different pharmacokinetic effects based on interactions with bone marrow and vasculature [35].

Interestingly, there is evidence suggesting that red blood cells contain a moderate level of P-450-like activity producing conjugation reactions (e.g., methylation, acetylation, glutathione conjugation) [36]. Thus, increased duration of a drug within the bloodstream allows for greater metabolism of this drug before reaching its target site.

Depot Effect

Investigations into chloramphenicol and vancomycin administration via the IO and peripheral IV routes demonstrated a significant decrease in the maximal concentration of both antibiotics when delivered through the IO route [37]. Important implications for these findings, particularly vancomycin, are due to the largely indicated use of the antibiotic in situations of community-acquired pneumonia, meningitis, and skin and soft tissue infection and when infection is of unknown origin [38]. The mechanism contributing to the decreased maximal concentration from IO administration is not well understood. Vancomycin's lipid solubility, protein binding, and calcium binding properties may play a role in the observed results. The results that were observed for chloramphenicol point toward likely deposition in the bone marrow, also known as the **depot effect**. Chloramphenicol is highly lipid soluble, rendering it susceptible to reduced uptake from the bone marrow, especially yellow marrow, with markedly reduced uptake from the sinusoids. A more recent study investigating plasma concentrations following IO and PIV antibiotic administration in a septic shock model showed no significant difference in plasma concentrations of cefotaxime and gentamicin [39]. Both gentamicin and cefotaxime are freely soluble in water, suggesting minimal deposition in the bone marrow [40, 41].

The depot effect may be most prominently seen in long bones with a high concentration of yellow marrow. After age 5, red marrow is gradually replaced with yellow marrow in humans. While yellow marrow contains approximately 95% fat cells and 5% nonfat cells, red marrow contains 60% hematopoietic cells and 40% fat cells [42]. The adult pattern of marrow distribution is observed after 25 years of age, with yellow marrow predominating within the appendicular skeleton other than the proximal humerus and femoral metaphysis [43]. Even among adults, red marrow is much more prominent in the axial skeleton, sternum, ribs, and anterior superior iliac crests. However, red marrow distribution decreases with advancing age in the humerus and femur metaphysis and, albeit with a weaker trend, in the axial skeleton, sternum, and ribs [42].

A recent study of rocuronium by Loughren et al. measured the time to complete neuromuscular blockade in swine and found no significant difference in the time required to achieve blockade between subjects treated with the IO and IV routes. The authors did note a significantly longer recovery time after drug infusion among the IO group when compared to the IV group [44]. Atropine, a lipophilic drug, was the subject of an investigation by Prete et al. In this study, the authors compared maximal concentrations and time to achieving maximal concentration following drug administration via the tibial IO, peripheral IV, and endotracheal routes. The time to maximal plasma concentration was significantly shorter, and maximal plasma concentrations were significantly greater with the IV route when compared to the IO and endotracheal routes. They also found that the atropine concentration remained higher in the plasma from 5 to 30 min after IO administration [45]. These data suggest that atropine is slowly released from the bone marrow after IO infusion via the depot effect.

Orlowski et al. investigated the pharmacokinetics of hydrophilic solutions, specifically 50% dextrose in water and calcium chloride. This group compared the infusion of these solutions through the distal femoral IO, peripheral IV, and central venous routes. They found no significant difference between the three routes regarding blood glucose levels following administration of 0.25 g/kg of 50% dextrose in water. Additionally, no significant difference was noted for a change in ionized calcium concentration over time after administration of calcium chloride between the three groups [46]. Interestingly, when investigating lidocaine hydrochloride, a moderately hydrophilic drug [47], a significantly reduced maximal concentration was observed following distal femoral IO infusion compared to both peripheral IV and central venous infusion. There are multiple potential reasons for this finding. As lidocaine is only moderately hydrophilic, a certain amount of the drug could have been deposited in the bone marrow. However, nuance to this discussion is important. Lidocaine is a weakly basic molecule with a pKa of 7.7, which means that at physiological pH of 7.4, only about 25% of the lidocaine molecules will be unionized [48]. Flat bones demonstrate a pH-like blood, but long bones have a lower pH ranging from 6.7 to 6.9 [49]. The lower pH of long bones means that there will be a higher fraction of unionized lidocaine. Comparing ionized and unionized molecules, typically the unionized forms will demonstrate greater lipid solubility. These findings suggest that **the pH of the marrow space being utilized and the pKa of the medication are important considerations in regard to the drug solubility with IO infusion**.

Conclusion

Perfusion of the bone marrow space relies on blood flow through the nutrient arteries, while drainage is facilitated by collecting veins. Infusates are able to access the central circulation through the marrow sinusoids, which act as a transition point between the arterial and venous circulatory systems. At the sinusoids, fluid uptake is regulated by Starling's equation, which underscores various controlling factors. It is important to note that the vascular supply to bone is not static. Rather, it can change acutely in response to neurohormonal control and endogenous molecules such as vasopressin, adenosine, bradykinin, and metabolic byproducts. Chronic changes in bone vascular supply are influenced by factors such as aging, estrogen exposure, and exercise. Another critical predictor of IO infusion capacity is the bone's intraosseous pressure, which must be overcome to facilitate forward fluid flow into the marrow space. Clinicians must recall that the composition of bone marrow evolves over time, transitioning from mostly hematopoietic cells (i.e., red marrow) to predominantly fat cells (i.e., yellow marrow) as patients age. Consequently, the sequestration of IO infusates within the marrow and soft tissues depends to a large degree on their lipid solubility profile, with increasingly lipophilic molecules showing greater deposition and reduced uptake into the central circulation. Despite significant progress in understanding intraosseous physiology, the physiologic factors controlling IO infusion rates and uptake into the central circulation remain worthy of further investigation.

Key Concepts
- Neurohormonal regulation of the bone vasculature is accomplished by many mechanisms, including the release of endogenous catecholamines.
- Endogenous molecules such as bradykinin, adenosine, and vasopressin have been shown to induce bony vasodilation.
- Vasopressin can induce both vasoconstriction and vasodilation, depending upon the receptor density at the site of action.
- Forward flow of fluid into the marrow space is greatest during pressurized infusion under normovolemic conditions.
- The bioavailability of infused medications is influenced by the site of infusion, with factors including distance to central circulation, extent of deposition in the marrow, and marrow pH.
- Hemorrhagic shock and other hypovolemic states can decrease blood flow to and from the intraosseous space, which may reduce the availability of IO-infused medications and fluids.

References

1. Standring S, Gray H. Gray's anatomy: the anatomical basis of clinical practice. 42nd ed. Philadelphia, PA: Elsevier; 2021.
2. Marenzana M, Arnett TR. The key role of the blood supply to bone. Bone Res. 2013;1(3):203–15.

3. Thomas GD. Neural control of the circulation. Adv Physiol Educ. 2011;35(1):28–32.
4. Stein A, Morgan H, Porras R. The effect of pressor and depressor drugs on intramedullary bone-marrow pressure. J Bone Joint Surg. 1958;40(5):1103–10.
5. Voelckel WG, Lurie KG, McKnite S, Zielinski T, Lindstrom P, Peterson C, et al. Comparison of epinephrine with vasopressin on bone marrow blood flow in an animal model of hypovolemic shock and subsequent cardiac arrest. Crit Care Med. 2001;29(8):1587–92.
6. Johnson D, Garcia-Blanco J, Burgert J, Fulton L, Kadilak P, Perry K, et al. Effects of humeral intraosseous versus intravenous epinephrine on pharmacokinetics and return of spontaneous circulation in a porcine cardiac arrest model: a randomized control trial. Ann Med Surg. 2015;4(3):306–10.
7. Mann DL, Bristow MR. Mechanisms and models in heart failure. Circulation. 2005;111(21):2837–49.
8. Burgert J, Gegel B, Loughren M, et al. Comparison of tibial intraosseous, sternal intraosseous, and intravenous routes of administration on pharmacokinetics of epinephrine during cardiac arrest: a pilot study. AANA J. 2012;80(4 Suppl):S6–10.
9. Schneider T, Drescher W, Becker C, Schlack W, Sager M, Assheuer J, et al. The impact of vasoactive substances on intraosseous pressure and blood flow alterations in the femoral head: a study based on magnetic resonance imaging. Arch Orthop Trauma Surg. 1998;118(1–2):45–9.
10. Burnstock G, Ralevic V. Purinergic signaling and blood vessels in health and disease. Pharmacol Rev. 2013;66(1):102–92. https://doi.org/10.1124/pr.113.008029.
11. Yauger YJ, Johnson MD, Mark J, Le T, Woodruff T, Silvey S, et al. Tibial intraosseous administration of epinephrine is effective in restoring return of spontaneous circulation in a pediatric normovolemic but not hypovolemic cardiac arrest model. Pediatr Emerg Care. 2020;38(4):1166–72.
12. Wakatsuki T, Nakaya Y, Inoue I. Vasopressin modulates k(+)-channel activities of cultured smooth muscle cells from porcine coronary artery. Am J Physiol Heart Circ Physiol. 1992;263(2):491–6.
13. Holmes CL, Landry DW, Granton JT. Science review: vasopressin and the cardiovascular system part 2—clinical physiology. Crit Care. 2004;8(1):15.
14. Thibonnier M, Conarty DM, Preston JA, Plesnicher CL, Dweik RA, Erzurum SC. Human vascular endothelial cells express oxytocin receptors. Endocrinology. 1999;140(3):1301–9.
15. Wenzel V, Lindner KH, Augenstein S, Voelckel W, Strohmenger HU, Prengel AW, et al. Intraosseous vasopressin improves coronary perfusion pressure rapidly during cardiopulmonary resuscitation in pigs. Crit Care Med. 1999;27(8):1565–9.
16. Burgert JM, Johnson AD, Garcia-Blanco J, Fulton LV, Loughren MJ. The resuscitative and pharmacokinetic effects of humeral intraosseous vasopressin in a swine model of ventricular fibrillation. Prehosp Disaster Med. 2017;32(3):305–10.
17. Gross PM, Heistad DD, Marcus ML. Neurohumoral regulation of blood flow to bones and marrow. Am J Physiol Heart Circ Physiol. 1979;237(4):440–8.
18. Benson T, Menezes T, Campbell J, Bice A, Hood B, Prisby R. Mechanisms of vasodilation to PTH 1–84, PTH 1–34, and PTHRP 1–34 in rat bone resistance arteries. Osteoporos Int. 2016;27(5):1817–26.
19. Dominguez JM, Prisby RD, Muller-Delp JM, Allen MR, Delp MD. Increased nitric oxide-mediated vasodilation of bone resistance arteries is associated with increased trabecular bone volume after endurance training in rats. Bone. 2010;46(3):813–9.
20. Stabley JN, Moningka NC, Behnke BJ, Delp MD. Exercise training augments regional bone and marrow blood flow during exercise. Med Sci Sports Exerc. 2014;46(11):2107–12.
21. Griffith JF, Wang Y-XJ, Zhou H, Kwong WH, Wong WT, Sun Y-L, et al. Reduced bone perfusion in osteoporosis: likely causes in an ovariectomy rat model. Radiology. 2010;254(3):739–46.
22. Zhao Q, Shen X, Zhang W, Zhu G, Qi J, Deng L. Mice with increased angiogenesis and osteogenesis due to conditional activation of HIF pathway in osteoblasts are protected from ovariectomy induced bone loss. Bone. 2012;50(3):763–70.
23. Brookes M. Blood flow rates in compact and cancellous bone, and bone marrow. J Anat. 1967;101(Pt 3):533–41.

24. Prisby RD, Ramsey MW, Behnke BJ, Dominguez JM, Donato AJ, Allen MR, et al. Aging reduces skeletal blood flow, endothelium-dependent vasodilation, and no bioavailability in rats. J Bone Miner Res. 2007;22(8):1280–8.
25. Brookes M. Sequelae of experimental partial ischaemia in long bones of the rabbit. J Anat. 1960;94:552–61.
26. De Lorenzo RA, Ward JA, Jordan BS, Hanson CE. Relationships of intraosseous and systemic pressure waveforms in a swine model. Acad Emerg Med. 2014;21(8):899–904.
27. Warren DW, Kissoon N, Sommerauer JF, Rieder MJ. Comparison of fluid infusion rates among peripheral intravenous and humerus, femur, malleolus, and tibial intraosseous sites in normovolemic and hypovolemic piglets. Ann Emerg Med. 1993;22(2):183–6.
28. Sarin H. Physiologic upper limits of pore size of different blood capillary types and another perspective on the dual pore theory of microvascular permeability. J Angiogenes Res. 2010;2:14. https://doi.org/10.1186/2040-2384-2-14.
29. Lairet J, Bebarta V, Lairet K, Kacprowicz R, Lawler C, Pitotti R, et al. A comparison of proximal tibia, distal femur, and proximal humerus infusion rates using the EZ-IO intraosseous device on the adult swine (*Sus scrofa*) model. Prehosp Emerg Care. 2013;17(2):280–4.
30. Miller L, Philbeck T, Montez D, Puga T. 467: a two-phase study of fluid administration measurement during intraosseous infusion. Ann Emerg Med. 2010;56(3):S151.
31. Pasley J, Miller CHT, DuBose JJ, Shackelford SA, Fang R, Boswell K, et al. Intraosseous infusion rates under high pressure. J Trauma Acute Care Surg. 2015;78(2):295–9.
32. Hammer N, Möbius R, Gries A, Hossfeld B, Bechmann I, Bernhard M. Comparison of the fluid resuscitation rate with and without external pressure using two intraosseous infusion systems for adult emergencies, the CITRIN (Comparison of InTRaosseous infusion systems in emergency medicINe)-study. PLoS One. 2015;10(12):e0143726. https://doi.org/10.1371/journal.pone.0143726.
33. Ong ME, Chan YH, Oh JJ, Ngo AS-Y. An observational, prospective study comparing tibial and humeral intraosseous access using the EZ-IO. Am J Emerg Med. 2009;27(1):8–15.
34. Schoffstall J, Spivey W, Davidheiser S, Lathers C. Intraosseous crystalloid and blood infusion in a swine model. J Trauma. 1989;29(3):384–7.
35. Hoskins SL, do Nascimento P, Lima RM, Espana-Tenorio JM, Kramer GC. Pharmacokinetics of intraosseous and central venous drug delivery during cardiopulmonary resuscitation. Resuscitation. 2012;83(1):107–12.
36. Cossum PA. Role of the red blood cell in drug metabolism. Biopharm Drug Dispos. 1988;9(4):321–36.
37. Fitzgerald J. Evaluation of intraosseous vs intravenous antibiotic levels in a porcine model. J Emerg Med. 1992;10(1):107.
38. Talan DA, Moran GJ, Abrahamian FM. Severe sepsis and septic shock in the emergency department. Infect Dis Clin N Am. 2008;22(1):1–31.
39. Strandberg G, Larsson A, Lipcsey M, Michalek J, Eriksson M. Intraosseous and intravenous administration of antibiotics yields comparable plasma concentrations during experimental septic shock. Acta Anaesthesiol Scand. 2015;59(3):346–53.
40. O'Neil MJ, editor. The Merck index: an encyclopedia of chemicals, drugs, and biologicals. RSC Publishing; 2013. p. 810.
41. Aid 1996—aqueous solubility from MLSMR Stock Solutions—PubChem [Internet]. National Center for Biotechnology Information. PubChem Compound Database. U.S. National Library of Medicine; 2010 [cited 2022 Oct 8]. https://pubchem.ncbi.nlm.nih.gov/bioassay/1996#section=Data-Table
42. Blebea JS, Houseni M, Torigian DA, Fan C, Mavi A, Zhuge Y, et al. Structural and functional imaging of normal bone marrow and evaluation of its age-related changes. Semin Nucl Med. 2007;37(3):185–94.
43. Vande Berg BC, Malghem J, Lecouvet FE, Maldague B. Magnetic resonance imaging of normal bone marrow. Eur Radiol. 1998;8(8):1327–34.
44. Loughren M, Banks S, Naluan C, Portenlanger P, Wendorf A, Johnson D. Onset and duration of intravenous and intraosseous rocuronium in swine. West J Emerg Med. 2014;15(2):241–5.

45. Prete MR, Hannan CJ, Burkle FM. Plasma atropine concentrations via intravenous, endotracheal, and intraosseous administration. Am J Emerg Med. 1987;5(2):101–4.
46. Orlowski JP. Comparison study of intraosseous, central intravenous, and peripheral intravenous infusions of emergency drugs. Arch Pediatr Adolesc Med. 1990;144(1):112.
47. Yalkowsky SH, He Y, Jain P. Handbook of aqueous solubility data. CRC Press; 2016.
48. Beecham GB, Nessel TA, Goyal A. Lidocaine—StatPearls—NCBI bookshelf [internet]. National Library of Medicine. National Center for Biotechnology Information; 2021 [cited 2022 Oct 9]. https://www.ncbi.nlm.nih.gov/books/NBK539881/
49. Nikolaeva LP. Features of acid–base balance of bone marrow. Acta Medica Int. 2018;5(2):55.

Indications and Contraindications 3

Jacob C. Lenning and James H. Paxton

Introduction

The fundamental indications and contraindications for intraosseous (IO) vascular access have not changed significantly since this technique was first utilized in human patients during the late 1930s and 1940s [1]. Intraosseous vascular access was heavily employed and researched during the World War II era [2–4]. However, there was a lull in utilization until renewed interest during the 1980s led to multiple landmark case reports describing the successful use of IO infusion to resuscitate critically ill pediatric patients [5, 6]. Since that time, many research studies and case reports have been published detailing specific uses and complications of IO catheter placement.

Drawing from this growing body of medical literature, many summaries and reviews have been written over the past 80 years suggesting specific indications and contraindications for IO access. In 1985, the Pediatric Advanced Life Support (PALS) pediatric resuscitation guidelines from the American Heart Association (AHA) became the first set of major clinical guidelines to include indications for IO vascular access [7, 8]. Today, many modern resuscitation guidelines provide recommendations regarding the use of IO devices for both adult and pediatric patients.

In general, **most resuscitation guidelines recommend the use of intraosseous vascular access when peripheral intravenous (PIV) vascular access is**

J. C. Lenning (✉)
Department of Emergency Medicine, Western Michigan University Homer Stryker
M.D. School of Medicine, Kalamazoo, MI, USA
e-mail: jacob.lenning@wmed.edu

J. H. Paxton
Department of Emergency Medicine, Wayne State University School of Medicine,
Detroit, MI, USA
e-mail: james.paxton@wayne.edu

deemed by the provider to be exceedingly difficult or impossible. The basis for this recommendation likely originated from the earliest studies on the clinical use of IO vascular access for therapeutic purposes, now validated by more than 80 years of research and anecdotal evidence. As early as 1941, Tocantins conducted multiple animal trials and human studies in which he utilized IO vascular access for the administration of fluids, blood products, and various medications. In his report, Tocantins concluded that "the intramedullary route is indicated whenever veins are not available" [1]. Current resuscitation guidelines employ similar language. The most recent executive summary of the AHA guidelines for cardiopulmonary resuscitation and emergency cardiovascular care states that "intraosseous access may be considered if attempts at intravenous access are unsuccessful or not feasible" (Class IIb, LOE B-NR) [9]. The European Resuscitation Council (ERC) guidelines for resuscitation also suggest that providers should "consider intraosseous access if attempts at intravenous access are unsuccessful or intravenous access is not feasible" [10]. Importantly, current resuscitation guidelines do not limit the use of IO vascular access to cardiopulmonary arrest, but rather suggest this approach as an alternative to PIV vascular access in any cases of circulatory failure [11, 12] or other potentially life-threatening medical conditions [13].

Most resuscitative medications that can be delivered through the peripheral IV route are considered to be safe and effective when given intraosseously [14]. Some authors have even suggested that "all intravenous medications can be administered intraosseously" [15, 16], although such claims are anecdotal and not supported by evidence from human clinical trials. A comprehensive list of the many medications that have been administered via IO infusion in human subjects has been previously published [7, 17] and is also provided in a separate chapter of this book.

The potential for soft tissue necrosis following the extravasation of noxious substances (e.g., vasoconstricting medications and hypertonic saline) and other serious complications suggest a more restrictive approach to the use of IO infusion [1, 18, 19]. However, the frequency of these complications is a matter of some debate [20, 21]. Intraosseous infusion is also associated with a "depot effect" for certain medications, resulting in altered pharmacokinetics, diminished efficacy, and the potential need for higher doses when administering those substances via the intramedullary space [22–25].

Many diagnostic studies traditionally facilitated by direct venous access can also be safely and reliably performed with IO access. For example, results from many serum laboratory tests utilizing marrow-derived blood have been shown to closely approximate serum values [15]. Additionally, case reports of computed tomography (CT) studies performed using IO administration of contrast have demonstrated this method to be an acceptable alternative to IV contrast injection [26].

Not surprisingly, modern manufacturers of IO devices generally endorse broad utilization of these devices. The manufacturers of the EZ-IO® device suggest the use of that device for "medical conditions when immediate vascular access is required, but standard IV access is challenging or impossible," and describe the device as a "safe, fast, and effective method of delivering lifesaving fluids or medication when vascular access is difficult to obtain in emergent, urgent, or medically necessary situations" [27]. The Bone Injection Gun (BIG®) and Next-Generation IO (NIO®) manufacturers simply promote their devices as "quick, safe … immediate vascular access" [28]. Of course, clinical practice guidelines and manufacturer recommendations cannot be applied to all clinical circumstances, so some degree of familiarity with the approach and insight into the existing medical literature are required to translate these recommendations to clinical practice.

Considering the versatility of this approach, the simplest way to define the scope of indications for intraosseous infusion would be to **consider IO vascular access for any clinical scenario in which vascular access is emergently needed but cannot otherwise be safely and efficiently obtained**, whether for the administration of fluids and medications or for the performance of diagnostic studies. However, such a broad indication is ambiguous, providing little guidance to clinicians when making medical decisions for their patients. Providers must consider the advantages, disadvantages, complications, and contraindications of this approach when determining whether IO vascular access is truly indicated for their patient based upon factors unique to the patient's condition including the need for emergent access. While the ease and speed of IO catheter placement do represent important advantages of this technique, the relative disadvantages of IO infusion (e.g., patient discomfort, limited flow rates, potential complications) must also be weighed against these benefits. While specific contraindications to IO infusion have been suggested over the years, a lack of consensus exists in the existing medical literature as to whether these suggested restrictions are *absolute* contraindications or merely *relative* contraindications.

The goal of this chapter is to identify factors that clinicians must consider in their determination of whether IO vascular access is appropriate for their patient based upon the existing medical evidence. Given the broad utility of IO devices, it is not necessarily the diagnosis, but rather patient factors such as acuity of illness, age, and comorbid health status that will ultimately inform the clinician's decision on whether IO vascular access is appropriate for their patient (Fig. 3.1).

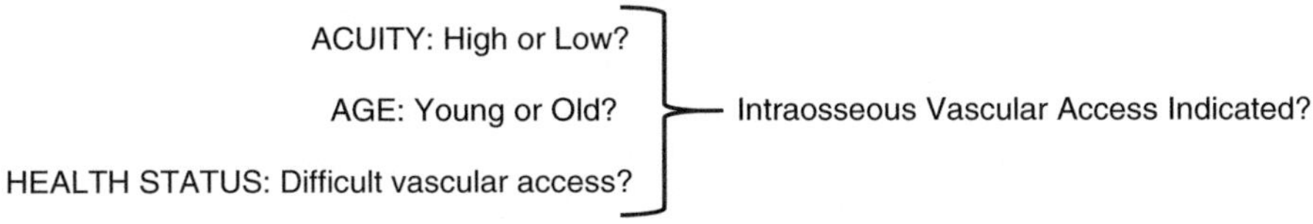

Fig. 3.1 Patient factors supporting the appropriateness of intraosseous vascular access

Acuity of the Presenting Condition

Most modern emergency care providers consider intraosseous vascular access to be a valuable alternative to direct venous access for patients facing an acute, life-threatening emergency. The higher success rate and faster deployment speed of IO devices when compared to peripheral intravenous (PIV) and central venous catheter (CVC) devices represent a significant clinical advantage when immediate pharmacological therapy or rapid diagnostic testing are required.

However, determinations on the acuity of a patient's presenting condition are not limited to the potential for loss of life. Other considerations, such as the potential for **persistent loss of function** (e.g., limb-threatening injury, stroke, ischemic organ failure), may be important determinants of the appropriateness of immediate IO infusion versus delayed IV infusion of medications and fluids. Ultimately, the acuity of a patient's condition depends upon many factors. These may include the **relative advantage of early intervention upon the patient's medical condition**, such as the need for thrombolytic therapy in treating pulmonary embolism or ischemic stroke or the need for early volume resuscitation and antibiotic therapy in septic patients. As with many clinical decisions, **the decision of which vascular access approach to use should be informed by the perceived benefits of immediate intervention, weighed against the potential need for other forms of vascular access later in the patient's clinical management**. Patients who require central venous access, for example, may require "bridging" access with an IO catheter until their definitive access device (e.g., CVC) can be placed. Patients with low intravascular volume may benefit from a similar bridging approach in order to facilitate subsequent PIV or CVC placement by expanding the target vessels to better accommodate direct venous cannulation.

Success Rates and Speed of Vascular Access Methods

In general, PIV vascular access can be achieved successfully and rapidly in most patients. First-pass success rates for PIV vascular access are typically around 70–76% with overall (i.e., including the potential for multiple failed attempts) success rates of up to 99% [29–31]. Ultrasound assistance has also been shown to significantly improve first-pass success rates. One meta-analysis reporting vascular access attempts for over 1600 patients reported overall first-pass success rates for conventional PIV and US-guided PIV (US-PIV) vascular access to be 70% and 80%, respectively [29]. However, **PIV vascular access can be increasingly difficult in critically ill patients, especially when performed using conventional methods**. Recent studies have suggested an overall success rate for PIV vascular access of only 80% in hypotensive medical patients and as low as 42% in trauma patients in need of resuscitative thoracotomy [32, 33]. The time required to achieve useable venous access is an important consideration when assessing first-pass and overall success rates, as providers may not consider alternative vascular access methods until they have already invested a great deal of time in attempting PIV access. The law of diminishing returns suggests that the likelihood of achieving useable PIV access decreases with each failed attempt, yet many providers remain fixated upon the search for a suitable target vein as time passes, to the detriment of their critically-ill patient. While PIV access is adequate and appropriate for the treatment of many acute medical conditions, situational awareness is needed to recognize when a delay in obtaining PIV access may begin to compromise patient safety and reduce the likelihood of a successful resuscitation. Once the delay in establishing PIV access has become unacceptable, providers owe it to both themselves and their patients to consider whether alternative means of achieving vascular access may be warranted.

Central venous catheter placement is often required for the resuscitation of unstable patients, but can be challenging in hypotensive or dehydrated patients. The first-pass success rate for CVC placement using ultrasound guidance is approximately 87%, although overall success rates up to 98% have been reported [34, 35]. However, CVC placement success rates are much lower without the use of ultrasound guidance. One study reported a first-pass success rate of only 23% employing conventional external anatomic landmark guidance [35]. Another study investigating vascular access success rates in patients undergoing resuscitative thoracotomy reported a success rate of only 46% for CVC placement [33]. In addition to the potential for failed device placement, providers must also consider the known complications of central venous access and greater time required for line placement in their decision algorithm. Although IO and PIV cannulation can generally be achieved clinically in less than 1 min, CVC placement can take much longer [33]. While some patients experiencing a critical illness may require central venous access for the infusion of vasopressors or invasive monitoring techniques, these patients may also benefit from initiation of therapy with PIV or IO line placement while their CVC placement is being attempted. This can allow providers to initiate early medication or fluid infusion, thereby augmenting systemic blood pressure, increasing intraluminal volume, and potentially facilitating subsequent venous access attempts.

One reason why IO vascular access is often preferred in acute life-threatening emergencies is that **IO cannulation success rates do not appear to be affected by low-flow or vasoplegic shock states that typically make venous cannulation more difficult** [36]. Many authors have compared the intraosseous space to a "noncollapsible vein" because the rigid bony compartment does not collapse with loss of intraluminal pressure, unlike thin-walled target veins [37]. While arteries have a rigid layer of smooth muscle that marginally resists collapse, veins are highly dependent upon intravascular volume to maintain their patency. Consequently, venous access can be exceedingly difficult or even impossible for patients with cardiac arrest, profound hypovolemia, or other conditions characterized by hypotension and/or hypovolemia. It is important to remember that blood pressure is not always a direct reflection of intravascular volume status. Shock states, for example, can be associated with vasoplegia that preferentially affects the arterial system, leading to hypotension with or without hypovolemia. Similarly, patients with comorbid hypertension can have a "normal" blood pressure even while experiencing profound dehydration or blood loss. Thus, providers should consider appropriate diagnostic methods such as dynamic ultrasound assessment of cardiac output and vena caval collapsibility when evaluating a patient's fluid volume status. Early identification of patients with low intravascular volume can help clinicians to accurately assess the likelihood of successful direct venous cannulation, which could inform earlier consideration of indirect venous access techniques.

The reported first-pass success rates for modern IO cannulation techniques in adult subjects range from 72% to 97% [38, 39] (Table 3.1). However, first-pass success rates are typically lower for sternal IO device placement than for other sites, ranging from 72% to 81% [39, 40]. By comparison, first-pass success rates for tibial and humeral IO device placement range from 82% to 97% [38, 41]. In trials comparing first-pass success rates for tibial and humeral IO device placement, tibial IO catheter insertion appears to be the most reliable [41, 42], although these studies likely incorporate a familiarity bias as the proximal humerus site has traditionally been less commonly used in clinical practice. As with any vascular access device, familiarity leads to competency in placement. For this reason, providers who intend to utilize IO cannulation in their practice should familiarize themselves with each of the standard IO insertion sites available at their institution. This will allow greater flexibility in site selection, which becomes especially important when clinical circumstances preclude the use of a familiar insertion site.

Under standardized conditions, such as those provided by vascular access simulators and with select hemodynamically stable patients, the difference in placement times between PIV catheters and IO devices appears to be minimal. In one study using training manikins, the average time from opening packaged materials to the initiation of medication infusion was 20 s less with IO than with PIV access (50 s (SD 9) vs. 70 s (SD 30)) [44]. This difference in mean times (i.e., 20 s) alone is reported to be statistically significant in this study, but could be considered to be clinically insignificant. However, this time advantage imparted by IO catheter insertion may appear to be understated when one considers the standard deviation (SD) values reported by the authors, which are more than three times greater for PIV access when compared to IO access. Given that a range of two standard deviations from the mean includes 95% of all time values, 95% of all IO catheters were placed within 32–68 s in this study, while 95% of all PIV catheters were placed within 10–130 s, suggesting that **the range of reported times required for PIV placement is much broader than that associated with IO device placement**. While IO catheter placement was almost always achievable in less than 1 min in this study, PIV placement required more than 2 min in some cases. Thus, the 20-s difference in mean placement times may substantially underestimate the potential delay associated with PIV insertion for outlier patients, which is shown to occasionally exceed 70 s. For patients experiencing cardiac arrest or life-threatening hypotension, an

Table 3.1 Range of first-pass success rate for various methods of vascular access in adult patients

Method of vascular access	Range of first-pass success rates
PIV	30–80% [29, 43]
CVC	23–87% [34, 35]
IO	72–97% [38, 39]

additional delay of 70 s before administering first medication or fluids could potentially worsen clinical outcomes. These data illustrate an important consideration for providers attempting to interpret the results of published studies comparing times to vascular access for different devices. When applying the results of these studies to clinical practice, **the mean time may be less important than the standard deviation or range of times required for access to be established**. While mean times do allow us to compare techniques, the real value of IO device placement (in comparison to PIV catheter placement) is its reliability, which is often reflected in a tighter range of time values for IO catheter placement in the existing literature. It is important to note that manikin models provide the same "patient" conditions to multiple providers, with the wide variation in placement times likely due to differences in provider competence, including familiarity with the model and skill at vascular access device placement.

Real-world conditions are rarely ideal, and studies evaluating the placement of PIV and IO devices under clinical (i.e., non-simulated) conditions are more likely to reflect the high variability that exists among patients independent of provider skill. In one study of adult patients undergoing resuscitative thoracotomy, successful IO vascular access was found to be approximately 15 s faster than PIV access (23 s vs. 38 s) on average, but the overall success rate of catheter placement was much higher with IO than with PIV (95% vs. 42%). These results suggest that **IO catheter placement is both faster and more reliably obtained than PIV catheter placement in patients with hypotension due to cardiovascular collapse** [33]. In another observational study including both medical and trauma patients in an emergency department setting, the mean time from skin sterilization to line placement with the ability to infuse fluids was 1.5 min, compared to 3.6 min with PIV access [45].

Other studies have demonstrated that the time from provider arrival on scene to successful vascular access and medication administration is faster for IO versus PIV vascular access. One out-of-hospital cardiac arrest study with paramedics reported median time from arrival to vascular access to be 4.6 min (IQR 3.6, 6.2) for tibial IO vascular access and 5.8 min (IQR 4.1, 8.0) for PIV vascular access [46]. As with other studies, the range of times required for PIV was much greater than that for tibial IO placement, suggesting that PIV access times varied more widely than IO placement times due to the study's inclusion of patients with extraordinarily difficult peripheral venous access. Another recent in-hospital study examining vascular access by rapid response nurses reported mean time from arrival to first medication to be 1.7 min for IO vascular access and 3.1 min for PIV vascular access, although standard deviations were not reported [47]. One potential confounder when considering studies that report time to first medication is the general IO manufacturer recommendation to flush all newly-placed lines with 10 mL of 0.9% normal saline and to provide a slow infusion (over 2 minutes) of 2 mL (40 mg) of 2% lidocaine. Neither of these preliminary steps are required with PIV catheters, which could bias estimates of time to first dose for a specific medication if the study does not report whether these additional preliminary steps were taken. It is worth noting that this guidance to flush the line with syringe injection of saline is intended to "clear a path" within the marrow space for subsequent fluid infusion, and is not likely needed when other medications are being infused under syringe pressure with a saline flush to follow. Similarly, lidocaine infusion is intended for pain control in awake patients and is generally not performed with cardiac arrest patients, who constitute the vast majority of reported IO use cases.

Central venous access requires more steps than the other forms of vascular access and has been shown to require significantly more time than required for either IO or PIV vascular access. Reported times for obtaining CVC vascular access typically range from 8 to 16 min, compared to 1.5 to 2 min for IO access in the same studies [45, 48]. One study of patients undergoing resuscitative thoracotomy reported an average time of only 3.6 min to obtain CVC vascular access; however, this seems to be the exception, and notably, the average time to obtain IO vascular access was only 39 s in this study population [33]. It is clear from review of the medical literature that the time required to place any form of vascular access is highly provider-dependent, and can vary widely between studies. Thus, it is imperative that clinicians reflect upon their own individual catheter placement times, and not rely heavily upon placement times reported by other groups when developing a personalized algorithm for vascular access device selection.

The speed and ease of IO placement offer advantages in the stabilization of critically ill patients due to the close proximity of target sites to large deep-tissue veins [49]. For example, the intramedullary space of the proximal tibia empties directly into the popliteal vein and femoral vein, thence through the common femoral vein into the inferior vena cava [50]. Early animal studies have already demonstrated that dye injected into the tibia can reach the heart in less than 10 s under normal physiologic conditions [51]. One recent human subject study in healthy volunteers reported that the average time required for dye injected into the proximal humerus to reach the superior vena cava is about 3 s [52]. However, some pharmacokinetic studies have demonstrated lower peak serum concentrations and delayed time to peak serum concentrations for certain medications when administered via tibial IO versus PIV or CVC routes, due to prolonged egress from the bone marrow, a phenomenon termed the "**depot effect**" [53]. Infusion via IO insertion sites closer to the central circulation, such as the proximal humerus and sternum, appears to be associated with a lesser depot effect [54, 55].

Notwithstanding the potential for altered pharmacokinetics with the use of specific medications, the ability of IO infusion to rapidly deliver therapeutics to the central circulation provides a lifesaving alternative when PIV and CVC vascular access cannot be easily obtained. Therefore, IO vascular access appears to be appropriate for any acute, life-threatening situation in which rapid and reliable vascular access is required. Examples of such conditions include (1) cardiopulmonary emergencies, (2) shock and circulatory emergencies, (3) traumatic emergencies, and (4) select neurological or toxicologic emergencies (Table 3.2). These categories are described in greater detail in the following sections.

Table 3.2 Examples of emergent conditions for which intraosseous vascular access is appropriate

Category	Examples
Cardiopulmonary emergencies	Cardiac arrest
	Myocardial infarction
	Arrhythmia
	Acute respiratory failure
Shock and circulatory emergencies	Hypovolemic shock
	Distributive shock
	Septic shock
	Obstructive shock
	Pulmonary embolism
Traumatic emergencies	Hemorrhagic shock
	Neurogenic shock
	Airway obstruction
	Traumatic brain injury
Neurologic and toxicologic emergencies	Status epilepticus
	Overdose
	Toxic ingestion
	Environmental exposure
	Hypoglycemia

Cardiopulmonary Emergencies: Cardiac Arrest

Much of the recent literature regarding indications for IO vascular access pertains to cardiopulmonary emergencies, specifically out-of-hospital cardiac arrest (OHCA). Intraosseous vascular access is particularly useful in the management of cardiac arrest due to its ease and speed of placement combined with the fact that all medications commonly required for OHCA resuscitation can be given safely and effectively via IO infusion [14]. **Epinephrine** is perhaps the most common medication used to treat cardiac arrest, but other medications, including atropine, amiodarone, lidocaine, calcium chloride, calcium gluconate, sodium bicarbonate, dextrose, and naloxone, have also been safely and effectively administered via IO infusion [7, 56, 57]. Multiple case reports have even demonstrated the feasibility of initiating targeted temperature protocols with iced saline delivered intraosseously once return of spontaneous circulation (ROSC) has been achieved [58, 59].

The utility of IO vascular access during OHCA when other methods of vascular access cannot be readily obtained is well established. However, **the timing of IO device placement in OHCA remains controversial**, and current recommendations by authoritative resuscitation guidelines actually provide very little guidance on when the decision to place an IO catheter (versus direct venous access) should be made. Although IO device placement can generally be achieved faster than PIV or CVC line placement, yielding shorter times to first medication administration, this benefit has not yet been shown to consistently yield improved clinical outcomes such as ROSC or favorable neurological outcomes.

The 2010 American Heart Association (AHA) guidelines for Advanced Cardiac Life Support (ACLS) state that "it is reasonable for providers to establish IO access if IV access is not readily available (Class IIa, LOE C)" and the executive summary of the same guidelines emphasized "early" IO device placement, although **what constitutes early placement is not clearly defined** [60, 61]. However, subsequent studies questioning the equivalency of IO to PIV vascular access in the management of OHCA have led the AHA to change its recommendations with the 2020 ACLS guidelines, now suggesting that "it is reasonable for providers to first attempt establishing IV access for drug administration in cardiac arrest (Class 2a, LOE B-NR). IO access may be considered if attempts at IV access are unsuccessful or not feasible" (Class 2b, LOE B-NR) [9].

These recommendations regarding the timing of IO device placement in OHCA are based largely upon conclusions drawn from published observational studies and secondary analyses of data obtained for other purposes from randomized controlled trial (RCT) data. Meta-analyses of these data suggest that an "IO-first" approach may be inferior to a "PIV-first" approach when viewed through the lens of various clinically relevant endpoints including ROSC, rates of survival, and favorable neurologic outcomes [62–70]. While a few small studies do suggest noninferiority for the IO-first approach [71–73], the scarcity of large, well-designed RCTs focusing primarily upon the choice of vascular access device (rather than other clinical interventions) has prevented the development of a consensus of opinion on the equivalency of IO and PIV access. Most of the studies purporting to compare PIV to IO infusion of ACLS medications for OHCA are secondary analyses of data collected by registries for other purposes, which leads to many potentially fatal flaws in their design. For example, current OHCA management guidelines recommend that a proximal peripheral vein or central vein be used to deliver resuscitative medications, with antecubital veins being the most commonly used for this purpose by emergency care providers. It has been well-established for decades that subdiaphragmatic (e.g., leg and foot) peripheral veins are not optimal candidate veins for use in OHCA management, and these veins are rarely (if ever) used. In states of profound hypotension, such as cardiac arrest receiving external chest compressions, distal arterial perfusion and venous return are severely compromised. Yet the vast majority of published reports on IO use for OHCA focus almost exclusively on the proximal tibial IO site, which is a subdiaphragmatic location and quite distant from the heart. Although this site has traditionally been the most commonly used for OHCA management, it is also suboptimal from a physiologic perspective and should not be expected to perform as well as a site closer to the central circulation. Even when other IO sites (e.g., sternum, proximal humerus) are included in these analyses, subgroup analyses are generally not performed and all IO sites are considered to be equivalent. This fallacy of equivalency between IO sites is not supported by any clinical evidence and undermines our efforts to accurately assess the potential value of non-tibial IO sites in the treatment of OHCA.

Studies suggesting the inferiority of IO vascular access in OHCA management also require careful appraisal due to heterogeneity in their study designs. While the reported times to vascular access or medication administration for both IO and PIV vascular access in these studies are typically very similar for both methods, a few studies have reported longer average times for IO vascular access than for PIV access, which seems improbable on a grand scale considering the well-documented challenges associated with PIV cannulation among cardiac arrest patients. Therefore, any clinical advantage of rapid IO placement is nullified in many of these studies as confounding variables causing delayed access may have also influenced patient outcomes. Regardless, these studies suggest that **if the times to initial vascular access and first medication administration are similar, infusion through an appropriately placed proximal PIV is likely superior to distal tibial IO infusion of medications for OHCA.**

Based upon the available evidence, **it is reasonable to prioritize PIV line placement for OHCA if an appropriate (i.e., proximal) peripheral vein can be cannulated immediately.** However, if adequate PIV access is delayed or deemed to be impossible, providers should consider rapid placement of an IO catheter for medication and fluid infusion until alternative venous access can be established. **The definition of what constitutes a "delayed" or "impossible" access must be determined by the provider,** as existing professional guidelines do not agree on definitions for these concepts. Two failed PIV access attempts may appear to be a prudent metric for many providers, while others may prefer a time-limit constraint (e.g., 2 min). Such a linear, consecutive approach to vascular access decision-making is especially important when resuscitation teams have limited manpower [74]. However, if multiple providers are available to assist with obtaining vascular access, a simultaneous approach may be more appropriate, with different providers attempting PIV and IO access at the same time. Although clinical studies are lacking, some preclinical data exist to support the importance of early IO epinephrine administration over delayed PIV administration. One recent swine study showed that IO epinephrine administration at 1 min postarrest was associated with improved rates of ROSC and 24-h survival when compared to a delayed PIV infusion at 8 min postarrest [75].

At present, the only clearly-defined recommendation on the timing of IO access comes from the European Resuscitation Council (ERC) pediatric guidelines, which suggest that direct intravenous access is preferred for pediatric circulatory failure and recommend that **alternative forms of vascular access (e.g., IO) be pursued after two failed PIV attempts or 5 min of failed direct venous access attempts** [11]. But even this attempt to define acceptable delay with PIV insertion accommodates a wide range of practice patterns, as two failed PIV attempts may occur very quickly, and some providers may be uncomfortable managing OHCA in a pediatric patient without vascular access for 5 minutes. Consequently, the provider's level of expertise and familiarity with each available method of establishing vascular access should be considered when deciding upon the proper time to redirect efforts towards IO catheterization.

General Cardiopulmonary Emergencies

Cardiac arrest is only a small subset of all cardiopulmonary emergencies. Any cardiopulmonary emergency in which immediate vascular access is necessary and alternative methods have already failed or are not considered feasible could represent an indication for IO vascular access. Examples include life-threatening arrhythmias and respiratory emergencies requiring immediate endotracheal intubation.

Amiodarone and lidocaine are commonly administered via the intraosseous route during cardiac arrest but can be administered for additional indications such as life-threatening wide-complex tachyarrhythmias. Other antiarrhythmics and rate control agents such as adenosine and diltiazem have also been safely given intraosseously for narrow-complex tachyarrhythmias [53, 76, 77].

Intraosseous vascular access can also be indicated in acute respiratory failure when intubation and mechanical ventilation are required. Many common sedative and paralytic agents such as fentanyl, etomidate, ketamine, propofol, rocuronium, vecuronium, and succinylcholine have been administered intraosseously [78–80]. In the treatment of other respiratory emergencies such as acute asthma exacerbation, magnesium sulfate and other supportive treatment can be given via an IO catheter [81].

Shock and Circulatory Emergencies

Acute hypotension due to shock and circulatory emergencies is another indication for IO vascular access, especially if PIV or CVC vascular access attempts have failed or are delayed. Unlike thin-walled veins, the intraosseous space does not collapse during hypovolemic or shock states [37], making IO vascular access an important bridging method that can be used for therapies to increase intravascular volume and blood pressure until direct venous access can be obtained [36].

In states of hypovolemic and septic shock, crystalloid solutions such as 0.9% normal saline and lactated Ringer's solution, albumin-containing solutions, and blood products can all be given intraosseously [80, 82–86]. For septic, cardiogenic, and neurogenic shock patients requiring vasopressors, commonly utilized vasopressors such as epinephrine, norepinephrine, dobutamine, dopamine, and vasopressin have all been administered via the IO route, although the risks of IO vasopressor infusion likely mirror those of PIV infusion including extravasation and subsequent soft tissue injury [5, 14, 86, 87]. Many antibiotics such as penicillin, ampicillin, and vancomycin can also be given intraosseously [79, 86, 88]. The treatment of obstructive shock due to acute pulmonary embolism with fibrinolytic agents and heparin boluses have been reported [89]. Fibrinolytics have also been administered intraosseously in the treatment of acute myocardial infarction [89, 90].

Traumatic Emergencies

Time-sensitive trauma-related emergencies such as airway or respiratory compromise, hemorrhagic shock, neurogenic shock, severe burns, and traumatic brain injury are all potential indications for IO vascular access. The prompt treatment of these traumatic emergencies often requires immediate vascular access for fluid or blood product resuscitation, vasopressor initiation, and mediation administration. Therefore, the American College of Surgeons (ACS) Advanced Trauma Life Support (ATLS) guidelines state that "if peripheral access cannot be obtained, consider placement of an intraosseous needle for temporary access," suggesting the use of IO vascular access as a bridging device until definitive PIV or CVC vascular access can be obtained [91].

The utility of IO vascular access for large-volume resuscitation, specifically with blood products, has been debated in the literature. The most frequently cited concern is that the limited flow rates often reported with IO vascular access devices (often half of what is reported with PIV infusion) may not be sufficient for rapid and large-volume administration [92–95]. A more detailed discussion of the flow rates achievable with IO infusion is provided in a separate chapter in this book.

It has also been theorized that the high infusion pressure required to deliver viscous blood products via the intraosseous space may cause hemolysis of blood products [96]. However, **numerous studies have demonstrated successful intraosseous administration of blood products**, including the infusion of packed red blood cells (pRBCs) and whole blood, without evidence of hemolysis [94, 95, 97]. Both civilian and military trauma reports have confirmed the efficacy of blood product resuscitation via IO cannulae when immediate venous access cannot be obtained [98, 99]. In fact, the military literature has demonstrated that a variety of blood products, including pRBCs, fresh frozen plasma, cryoprecipitate, and platelets, appear to be safe and effective when administered intraosseously [99]. Whole-blood autotransfusion via IO catheter in the setting of traumatic hemothorax has been performed in the battlefield [100]. Additional research is needed to determine whether the use of devices to increase infusion pressure (e.g., syringe infusion, rapid-infusion pumps) may lead to increased red blood cell lysis, although there seems to be adequate evidence to suggest that gravity-driven infusion of blood products through an IO catheter is not associated with significant hemolysis.

Indications for IO vascular access in the trauma patient are not limited to volume fluid resuscitation. Specific medications commonly utilized in the treatment of trauma patients can also be administered intraosseously. For example, IO tranexamic acid infusion has been shown to be effective in swine models of hemorrhagic shock and has been administered in battlefield scenarios without reported complications [99, 101, 102]. Vasopressors such as norepinephrine and epinephrine, which may be indicated to supplement volume resuscitation or to treat neurogenic shock, have been given via IO infusion. Furthermore, many commonly used sedatives and paralytics have been successfully infused via the IO route to assist in airway management. In cases of severe traumatic brain injury, both hypertonic saline and mannitol have been given via IO cannula in the effort to temporize intracranial hypertension [21, 80, 103]. The potential risk of soft tissue necrosis following extravasation of hypertonic medications might support a more restrictive use of these medications via the IO route, although the frequency of this complication appears to be low [18, 20]. Ultimately, the potential risks and benefits of IO infusion for the undifferentiated trauma patient must be considered on a per-patient basis.

Neurologic and Toxicologic Emergencies

Guidelines for the treatment of **status epilepticus** emphasize the early administration of benzodiazepines, generally recommended as first-line agents [104, 105]. Which specific benzodiazepine is recommended depends upon whether intravenous access has been obtained. Lorazepam is preferred if intravenous access has been achieved, although midazolam is favored for intramuscular administration and diazepam is recommended when rectal administration is required. Despite studies demonstrating the safe and effective IO administration of benzodiazepines (e.g., midazolam and diazepam in humans, and lorazepam in swine) to treat status epilepticus, recommendations on IO administration of anti-epileptics are absent from current guidelines [86, 87, 106]. Second-line antiepileptic agents, including phenytoin and levetiracetam, have been safely given via the IO route in humans [80, 107]. The IO administration of valproic acid has been demonstrated to reach noninferior serum levels when compared to IV administration in a swine model [108]. Propofol, a third-line antiepileptic, has been administered intraosseously for sedation, but there are no known reports in which propofol was administered as an IO continuous infusion for the treatment of status epilepticus in humans [79]. Intraosseous phenobarbital, another third-line agent, has been demonstrated to be effective in swine models at the same doses recommended by existing treatment guidelines [23].

The absence of any specific recommendations regarding IO administration of antiepileptics likely stems from the lack of data comparing IO therapy to intramuscular and rectal benzodiazepine administration; consequently, these routes may be favored for these agents. For status epilepticus requiring second-line agents, when other forms of vascular access cannot be quickly obtained, IO administration is a viable option as based on evidence from the available case reports and should be considered indicated in such scenarios. However, there is insufficient evidence to support the administration of third-line anti-epileptic agents via the IO route.

Treatment of the **hypoglycemic** patient can be challenging for emergency providers, as vascular access is often difficult to obtain in these patients presenting comatose or with agitated confusion and diaphoresis due to the associated catecholamine response. Therefore, IO vascular access may be indicated for the treatment of hypoglycemia if other forms of vascular access cannot be quickly and safely achieved. Various concentrations of dextrose solutions (ranging from 5% to 50%) have been reported to be safely and effectively administered via the IO route [87, 109]. However, in the event of extravasation from the IO insertion site, **the risk of soft tissue necrosis is increased with more hypertonic formulations** [18]. Furthermore, the viscosity of more highly concentrated dextrose solutions can make IO infusion difficult due to the increased pressure required to push the solution through the bone marrow space into the central circulation. When glucagon is needed to treat hypoglycemia, the recommended routes of administration are either intramuscular or subcutaneous [110]. However, IO glucagon infusion has been reported, specifically in the setting of calcium channel blocker and beta-blocker overdose [111].

The specific indications for IO infusion of antidotes to treat acute overdose, toxic ingestion, and environmental exposures are numerous, and many common antidotes have been safely and effectively administered via this route. In general, IO vascular access is indicated in any poisoned patient requiring immediate antidote administration when other forms of vascular access are difficult or impossible to obtain. Specific antidotes that have been administered intraosseously include **atropine** for organophosphate poisoning, **hydroxocobalamin** for cyanide poisoning, **lipid emulsion** for calcium channel blocker overdose, **methylene blue** for methemoglobinemia, **naloxone** for opioid overdose, **prothrombin complex concentrate** for coagulopathy, **sodium bicarbonate** for sodium channel blocker overdose, and **scorpion antivenom** [112, 113]. The IO administration of pralidoxime for organophosphate poisoning has not been reported in humans; however, it has been demonstrated to be effective in a swine model [114]. Beyond specific antidotes, IO vascular access is also indicated in any extreme environmental condition in which other forms of vascular access would be difficult or impossible, such as search and rescue operations, military applications, and conditions requiring urgent evacuation [115, 116].

Diagnostic Studies

Values for many standard blood tests using intraosseous blood appear to be comparable to results obtained with peripheral or central venous blood. However, estimation of serum potassium and calcium levels has been repeatedly shown to be inaccurate using IO samples [117–119]. There is also conflicting evidence on the accuracy of IO blood levels for alanine transaminase (ALT), aspartate aminotransferase (AST), and lactate dehydrogenase (LDH) [120–124]. Therefore, these studies should be assumed to be unreliable when obtained via IO blood sampling. Complete blood count (CBC) components including red blood cell (RBC) count, hemoglobin, and hematocrit are known to be accurate with IO samples, but white blood cell (WBC) counts and platelet counts have been shown to be unreliable [118, 119, 122, 123]. Coagulation studies are also generally inaccurate when obtained via IO sampling [125]. The blood gas components of pH and pCO_2 are accurate, but pO_2 is inaccurate when measured in IO samples. Point-of-care I-STAT testing of lactic acid is also accurate [125, 126]. A summary of common laboratory tests previously evaluated in IO blood studies is provided in Table 3.3.

In general, laboratory tests performed with IO blood samples become inaccurate after medications have been administered through the IO catheter or after prolonged cardiopulmonary arrest/resuscitation efforts. Published studies suggest that acid-base values are likely to be inaccurate after 15 min of cardiac arrest resuscitation and most other values are inaccurate after 30 min of cardiopulmonary arrest and resuscitation [127, 128]. Therefore, **draws of IO blood for the determination of laboratory values should generally be performed immediately after IO catheter insertion, not later in the resuscitation effort**. It is also important for providers to consider that particulate matter within the bone marrow specimen (e.g., fat globules, bony spicules) may potentially damage equipment used to analyze blood samples in the central laboratory. Providers should indicate to their laboratory staff when blood samples have been acquired via IO aspiration to avoid inappropriate specimen processing and damage to analyzers. This effect may be less problematic for point-of-care (POC) analyzers, although evidence is limited in the existing medical literature and further study is needed.

Table 3.3 Reportedly accurate or inaccurate laboratory studies (as compared to same-subject venous blood levels) using blood obtained from bone marrow aspiration via intraosseous catheter

Accurate	Inaccurate
Sodium [117, 122]	Potassium [117–119]
Chloride [117, 119, 122]	Calcium [118, 119]
Magnesium [127]	pO2 [118, 122]
Phosphorus [122]	White blood cell count [119, 123]
Uric acid [122]	Platelet count [119]
Blood urea nitrogen (BUN) [117, 119]	PT/aPTT/INR [125]
Total bilirubin [122]	Lactate dehydrogenase (LDH)[a] [122, 124]
Albumin [119, 122]	Alanine transaminase (ALT)[a] [120–124]
Total protein [119, 122]	Aspartate aminotransferase (AST)[a] [120, 122]
Glucose [118, 119]	
pH [118, 129, 130]	
Bicarbonate (HCO_3^-) [118, 122, 129, 130]	
pCO_2 [118, 122, 126, 129, 130]	
Lactate [125, 126]	
Red blood cell count [119, 123]	
Hemoglobin [119, 122]	
Hematocrit [118, 119]	
Type and screen [131]	
Blood cultures [132]	

Notes: pH Potential of hydrogen, *PT* Prothrombin time, *aPTT* Activated partial thromboplastin clotting time, *INR* International normalized ratio, *pCO_2* Partial pressure of carbon dioxide, *pO_2* Partial pressure of oxygen
[a]Indicates conflicting reports

Emergent contrast-enhanced computed tomography (CT) studies can also be performed using IO contrast media injection. Numerous imaging protocols including CT angiogram of the head and neck, CT perfusion for suspected stroke, comprehensive trauma protocols, CT for pulmonary embolism, and standard contrast imaging of the chest/abdomen/pelvis utilizing contrast infused via IO catheters have been reported in the literature [133–139]. Multiple guidelines suggesting methods to safely administer contrast dyes via the IO route have been published [26, 140]. It should be noted that **gadolinium contrast agents, as commonly used in MRI studies, have not been shown to be compatible with IO infusion** [26].

Indications for Awake Patients

Intraosseous infusion is most commonly used in comatose patients, as critically ill patients experiencing life-threatening emergencies often present in a state of reduced consciousness. Many providers are justifiably concerned that IO insertion and subsequent infusion may be painful for sensate patients, even with the use of lidocaine or other analgesics. However, there are instances in which IO vascular access is indicated and appropriate for awake and stable patients.

Most of the case reports in which IO vascular access has been utilized in awake and stable patients come from the anesthesia literature, focusing upon patients who experienced failed vascular access attempts in the perioperative setting [79, 141]. Entire procedures have been performed with IO vascular access alone, including at least one case report describing the use of IO vascular access for the entire duration of an elective hysterectomy [142]. Regional anesthesia using IO lidocaine infusion has also been described [143]. Notably, in many of the cases reported in the anesthesia literature, either anesthetic gases, local anesthesia, or both were administered prior to placement of the IO catheter. Despite the paucity of available data on IO catheter use in awake patients, this modality may be indicated in a select group of patients who have been advised of the risks and benefits of its use, including the potential for pain with pressurized infusion. Patients with difficult venous access who have failed multiple PIV attempts may be willing to attempt IO infusion, and in such cases the recommended use of IO 2% lidocaine to anesthetize the marrow space should be employed. Additional systemic analgesics or sedatives may be indicated, depending upon the patient's perception of pain and anxiety with the procedure. An entire chapter of this book is dedicated to the topic of pain with IO infusion.

Age and Health Status

Extremes of age are known to be associated with difficult direct venous access, especially among very young or very old patients experiencing life-threating emergencies. Therefore, age may be a factor influencing the decision to employ IO vascular access. Very young (i.e., <2 years old) and very old patients characteristically have difficult vascular access. Increased difficulty in obtaining vascular access among pediatric patients is often directly related to their small size and early stage of development [144]. In older patients, difficulties with direct venous access often arise from the presence of chronic medical conditions that lead to vein fragility and scarring, such as diabetes mellitus, chronic steroid use, and chronic kidney disease [145].

Pediatric Patients

Obtaining direct venous access in the setting of a life-threatening medical emergency can be especially difficult among pediatric subjects [146]. Certain factors, including extremely young age and prematurity, have been directly correlated with difficult PIV vascular access among pediatric cohorts [144, 147]. In pediatric populations, **the level of difficulty that providers should expect to experience in establishing peripheral venous access correlates inversely with patient age** [144]. In one 3-year study of children treated at a dedicated pediatric hospital, the average time required to obtain direct venous access following cardiac arrest was 7.8 min, with 24% requiring >10 min to obtain access and 6% of subjects never able to receive venous access [147]. Considering that many emergency departments are more accustomed to treating adult patients, some authors have suggested that **IO vascular access should be considered to be first-line therapy in cases of pediatric cardiac arrest or other severe shock states when care providers are not adequately experienced in obtaining direct venous access for pediatric patients** [148].

Not surprisingly, pediatric resuscitation guidelines often emphasize early IO catheter placement. The American Heart Association (AHA) first included the following recommendation in their 2010 guidelines, and the suggestion remains unchanged in more recent updates: "IO access is a rapid, safe, effective, and acceptable route for vascular access in children, and it is useful as the initial vascular access in cases of cardiac arrest (Class I, LOE C) [149, 150]." The 2020 International Consensus for Pediatric Life Support states that IO vascular access is an acceptable alternative to direct venous access that should be considered early in critically ill children [151]. The European Resuscitation Council (ERC) guidelines, however, suggest that venous access should be preferred in the treatment of pediatric circulatory failure and propose first attempting PIV vascular access before considering the IO route. They recommend that **alternative forms of vascular access (e.g., IO cannulation) should be pursued after two failed PIV attempts or 5 min of failed direct venous access attempts** [11].

Other techniques of vascular access frequently described in the pediatric literature include peripheral venous cutdown and umbilical vein catheterization. **Peripheral venous cutdown** was commonly reported and endorsed in the 1980s and early 1990s, but is seldom mentioned in the modern medical literature due to advances in ultrasound guidance and other technologies that have obviated the need to perform this highly invasive procedure in all but the most extreme cases [152–156]. Previous studies have demonstrated that even highly trained pediatric surgeons require up to 11 min to perform peripheral venous cutdown, while IO vascular access can generally be achieved within a minute [154]. Umbilical vein catheterization (UVC) remains a common technique utilized by experienced neonatal providers in neonatal intensive care units. However, studies have shown that less specialized providers are likely to have higher success rates with IO vascular access than with UVC [155]. Therefore, **IO vascular access is considered an acceptable alternative to UVC in neonatal resuscitation guidelines and is indicated for neonates when providers are more skilled with IO placement than UVC placement** [12, 156].

Numerous reports of IO infusion in the treatment of neonates have been associated with a low rate of complications, although some studies suggest that success rates with IO vascular access may be directly related to patient size and age. One study reported lower IO cannulation success rates in infants <8 kg when compared to children greater than 8 kg [157]. Another study reported lower success rates in children <1 year of age when compared to children >1 year of age [158]. Other studies have found no association between pediatric patient age and IO catheter placement success rate [87, 159]. Generally, most studies have demonstrated IO placement success rates in children comparable to those seen with adults, including first-pass success rates approximating 80% and overall success rates as high as 100% [160, 161]. However, two separate studies evaluating IO placement in children using postmortem CT imaging report much lower placement success rates of 56%–65% among pediatric patients [158, 162]. This may seem to be quite low, but it remains higher than the rate of successful PIV placement in children, which has been reported to be as low as 53% [163]. Despite these challenges, IO infusion of medications and fluids has been shown to yield positive results for pediatric patients experiencing dehydration, systemic infection, traumatic injuries, cardiovascular emergencies, and diabetic ketoacidosis, among other conditions [1, 6, 80, 164, 165].

Older Patients and Patients with Chronic Medical Conditions

Vascular access is frequently challenging in older patients and patients with chronic medical conditions. Difficult vascular access is associated with conditions such as diabetes mellitus, extreme body habitus, extremity edema, concomitant cancer therapy, chronic kidney disease, sickle cell disease, connective tissue disorders, and a history of intravenous drug abuse [145, 166]. One study even correlated difficult vascular access with higher levels of systemic disease as indicated by the American Society of Anesthesiologists (ASA) physical classification system [145]. The Consortium on Intraosseous Vascular Access in Healthcare Practice suggests that IO vascular access is indicated in any patient with chronic disease requiring acute stabilization with otherwise limited vascular access for any reason such as arteriovenous fistulas, grafts, shunts, mastectomy, or obesity [167].

Contraindications

Very few contraindications are suggested by IO device manufacturers or found within the medical literature. Most proposed contraindications are relative, and very few should be considered absolute contraindications. In acutely ill patients with life-threatening emergencies, **most relative contraindications for IO catheter placement should be regarded as precautions prompting careful site selection and placement but should not prevent the appropriate utilization of IO devices**. The primary indication for establishment of IO vascular access is to provide lifesaving vascular access; therefore, relative contraindications can and should be considered in that context. Once a patient is stabilized and definitive vascular access has been obtained, the IO infusion device can be removed to reduce the risk of complications.

Absolute Contraindications

Absolute contraindications to IO vascular access include any abnormalities of the soft tissue, vasculature, or bone at or near the proposed site of placement that would impair proper function of the IO device or cause more harm than benefit to the patient. Absolute contraindications to IO catheter placement currently reported by IO device manufacturers include (1) inability to palpate bony landmarks; (2) infection at the site of insertion; (3) severe extremity injury, especially with disruption of the proximal vasculature; (4) fracture of the target bone; (5) previous orthopedic procedure involving the target bone; and (6) previously attempted IO device

Table 3.4 Proposed absolute and relative contraindications for intraosseous (IO) vascular access

Absolute contraindications	Relative contraindications
Inability to identify bony landmarks	Disorders or bony metabolism: For example, osteoporosis, osteopetrosis, osteogenesis imperfecta
Infection overlying or of the target bone	Overlying burn injury
Severe extremity injury, suspected to involve disruption of venous circulation	Hematologic disorders: For example, acute leukemia and myeloproliferative disorders
Fracture injury of the target bone	Immunosuppression
Previous surgery of the target bone	Septicemia
Previous attempt at IO placement of the target bone within the past 24 h	

placement at the target bone within the last 24 h (Table 3.4). In general, these absolute contraindications are actually **site-specific contraindications** and may simply require providers to select a different IO catheter insertion site (i.e., target bone) for infusion. Although providers may be concerned about the risk of bleeding for anticoagulated patients, or increased risk of bone fracture in osteopenic patients, **no such whole-patient absolute contraindications are currently endorsed or suggested by existing clinical practice guidelines**.

The inability to identify relevant external anatomic landmarks should be considered a contraindication for any landmark-based vascular access procedure not utilizing ultrasound or other alternative imaging modalities. In the case of IO devices, the inability to palpate bony landmarks may preclude attempts at device placement. However, the threshold for withholding attempts is likely provider- and patient-dependent. Excessive muscular tissue, adipose tissue, or edema over a proposed insertion site can obscure bony landmarks, but none of these alone are absolute contraindications for IO device placement. These factors should only be considered absolute contraindications if the provider is unable to palpate the bony landmarks needed to ensure proper insertion of the device [142]. Multiple studies have been conducted to help determine the optimal IO catheter length based on soft tissue depth [45, 168].

Infection at the proposed site of IO device insertion is typically considered an absolute contraindication because localized areas of infection can usually be avoided by simply choosing a different insertion site. Intraosseous devices should not be placed through areas of cellulitis, abscess, or bones with suspected osteomyelitis, as the IO catheter would act as a foreign body and provide an additional nidus for infection [169]. Theoretically, bacteria could be transferred from the soft tissues into the bone and systemic vasculature via the IO catheter [25]. In the case of osteomyelitis, bone composition may also be altered, resulting in increased risk of leakage and extravasation. Of course, similar site precautions apply to any other form of vascular access (e.g., PIV, CVC) as well. In the rare circumstance that no other site is available in life-threatening circumstances, soft tissue infection overlying the target bone is considered by some to be a relative contraindication to IO device placement [56, 170].

Anatomical disruptions of the target bone or of the proximal vasculature, whether from injury or procedure, are another absolute contraindication to IO device placement [56, 170]. Any acute fracture, chronic unhealed fracture, previous orthopedic surgery, or recent attempts at IO device placement might be associated with defects in the bony cortex and contribute to unintended extravasation of IO infusates. One study demonstrated that serum phenobarbital levels were lower in dogs with multiple IO device placement attempts in the same tibia when compared to dogs with only one attempt, presumably due to extravasation [171]. One recent case report documented the development of compartment syndrome after multiple liters of lactated Ringer's solution were infused through a tibial IO catheter following multiple failed attempts at IO placement on the same bone [172]. In the trauma setting, IO devices should not be placed in extremities for which there is concern for potential compartment syndrome due to the underlying injury as placement could worsen this limb-threatening condition [88, 169, 173].

Orthopedic surgeries involving implanted metals (e.g., joint replacements or internal fixation) may distort the local bone and soft tissue anatomy, and these materials could also damage the IO catheter during the placement attempt. Additionally, any injury or disruption of the proximal vasculature, whether within the extremity or more proximally within the trunk or pelvis, is a contraindication to the use of IO vascular access in that specific extremity. For example, IO devices should not be placed in a lower extremity with confirmed or suspected femoral vein injury or in the lower extremities of a patient with pelvic fracture and concern for associated vascular injury.

Relative Contraindications

Relative contraindications to IO vascular access are patient factors that increase the risk of IO device-related complications, but for whom the benefits of IO infusion may in some cases outweigh the risk of harm. Many of the relative contraindications to IO vascular access pertain to systemic disease states such as disorders of bony metabolism or hematologic and immunologic disorders. Frequently cited examples include osteoporosis, osteopetrosis, and *osteogenesis imperfecta* [25, 167]. Other proposed contraindications include acute leukemia, myeloproliferative disorders, septicemia, immunocompromised states, and bleeding disorders [132, 174]. Additional relative contraindications commonly mentioned in the literature include burn injury overlying the target bone and the awake patient (Table 3.4).

These theoretical concerns regarding IO device placement in patients with disorders of bony metabolism include an increased risk of fracture, displacement, and/or extravasation [25]. Osteoporosis is characterized by loss of bone density, osteopetrosis by an increase in density, and *osteogenesis imperfecta* by pathologic collagen production. The abnormal bone matrix characterized by all of these disorders increases the risk of fracture and may not provide a strong anchor for IO devices, which could lead to extravasation by leakage around the catheter or even catheter displacement. One identified case report described failed placement of an IO device in an adult patient with *osteogenesis imperfecta* due to loosening of the IO catheter immediately after insertion [175]. Notably, IO device manufacturers do not list osteoporosis as a contraindication to IO device placement due to the lack of observed complications in a study of 250 patients in which 113 of the patients were over the age of 60 years [38].

Some concern has also been raised about whether alterations in bone marrow composition due to hematologic disorders such as acute leukemia or **myeloproliferative disorders** might affect the function of IO vascular access devices. No evidence has been published to support these concerns. Additionally, immunocompromised states and **septicemia** have been suggested as relative contraindications. One case report described a patient who was started on immunosuppression therapy shortly after IO device placement including IO device removal following cardiac arrest and later developed severe osteomyelitis requiring below-knee amputation of the lower extremity [174]. Although the theoretical concern for patients with septicemia is that the IO device may become a nidus for infection and cause osteomyelitis, no reports of this complication have been reported.

Anticoagulation and **bleeding risks** are often considered when selecting sites for vascular access. Typically, compressible sites are chosen for vascular access in patients with an increased propensity for bleeding. Fortunately, all sites in which IO vascular access devices are placed are amenable to compression. Multiple case reports have been published describing patients on anticoagulation undergoing IO device placement and removal without complication [45]. Heparin boluses and fibrinolytic therapy have also been administered intraosseously without complications [89, 90].

Another relative contraindication for IO vascular access device placement is **thermal skin burn** overlying the proposed site of insertion. As with localized infection, areas of localized burn can easily be avoided if other sites are available for IO cannulation. However, in patients with diffuse burns, there may not be any unaffected skin, leaving no other option. One case report describes the successful placement of a sternal IO through a noticeable full-thickness chest burn. In this case, the device functioned appropriately and allowed for the administration of lifesaving therapies until a central venous catheter could be placed to provide definitive therapy [176].

Finally, one of the most common misconceptions about IO vascular access is that device placement is contraindicated in **awake and conscious patients** due to the perceived discomfort and the association of the devices with life-threatening emergencies. However, there are numerous reported cases of the devices being utilized in awake and stable adult and pediatric patients [79, 141, 142].

Conclusion

Intraosseous (IO) vascular access is indicated whenever emergent vascular access is necessary and other methods of vascular access have failed or are deemed impossible to obtain. The primary advantage of IO vascular access is the speed and ease of placement available with this route of infusion. Most medications suitable for peripheral intravenous infusion appear to be safe and effective when administered via the IO route, although medications requiring central venous infusion should not be given via IO cannula. Numerous laboratory studies and even contrast computed tomography studies can be performed using IO vascular access, although some laboratory studies are not reliable when assessed using IO blood. Specific indications for IO catheter insertion include acute life-threatening emergencies, extremes of age, and poor health status, all of which might contribute to scenarios requiring immediate vascular access or may be associated with otherwise difficult vascular access. Absolute contraindications for IO vascular access are few, and most are resolved by simply selecting a different site for IO catheter placement. While the benefits of IO vascular access often outweigh the risks associated with any relative contraindications, decisions to place an IO catheter should be informed by a balanced assessment of the risks and benefits unique to the individual patient's clinical condition.

Key Concepts
- Current resuscitation guidelines recommend the use of intraosseous devices for the treatment of life-threatening medical conditions when direct venous access is deemed by the provider to be exceedingly difficult or impossible.
- While specific contraindications to the use of IO infusion have been suggested, a lack of consensus exists on whether such conditions are absolute or merely relative contraindications to IO catheter placement.
- In studies comparing PIV to IO access, the mean time to access may be less important than the standard deviation or range of times required for access to be established.
- Absolute contraindications to IO catheter placement include fracture of the target bone, disruption of venous drainage within the target extremity at or proximal to the insertion site, inability to identify external landmarks for catheter insertion, previous surgery at the target bone, and previous IO catheter attempt in the target bone within 24 h.
- Providers should interpret the results of serum blood tests obtained using IO blood with caution and consider the relative limitations of this approach to blood sampling.

References

1. Tocantins L, O'Neill J, Jones H. Infusions of blood and other fluids via the bone marrow: application in pediatrics. JAMA. 1941;117(15):1229–34.
2. Heinild S, Sondergaard T, Tudvad F. Bone marrow infusion in childhood; experiences from a thousand infusions. J Pediatr. 1947;30(4):400–12. https://doi.org/10.1016/s0022-3476(47)80080-0.
3. Turkel H. Intraosseous infusion. Am J Dis Child. 1983;137(7):706. https://doi.org/10.1001/archpedi.1983.02140330088029.
4. McLaughlin TJ, Farmer JC. Resuscitation access and assessment: recurring themes of the intraosseous route. Crit Care Med. 2000;28(8):3109–10. https://doi.org/10.1097/00003246-200008000-00087.

5. Berg RA. Emergency infusion of catecholamines into bone marrow. Am J Dis Child. 1984;138(9):810–1. https://doi.org/10.1001/archpedi.1984.02140470010003.

6. Orlowski JP. My kingdom for an intravenous line. Am J Dis Child. 1984;138(9):803. https://doi.org/10.1001/archpedi.1984.02140470003001.

7. Paxton JH. Intraosseous vascular access: a review. Trauma. 2012;14(3):195–232. https://doi.org/10.1177/1460408611430175.

8. American Heart Association. National conference on standards and guidelines for cardio-pulmonary resuscitation and emergency cardiac care. Standards and guidelines for cardiopulmo-nary resuscitation (CPR) and emergency cardiac care (ECC). Part VI: pediatric advanced life sup- port. J Am Med Assoc. 1986;255:2961–4.

9. Merchant RM, Topjian AA, Panchal AR, Cheng A, Aziz K, Berg KM, et al. Part 1: executive summary: 2020 American Heart Association guidelines for cardiopulmonary resuscitation and emergency cardiovascular care. Circulation. 2020;142(16_Suppl_2):S337–S57.

10. Perkins GD, Graesner J-T, Semeraro F, Olasveengen T, Soar J, Lott C, et al. European resuscitation council guidelines 2021: executive summary. Resuscitation. 2021;161:1–60.

11. Van de Voorde P, Turner NM, Djakow J, de Lucas N, Martinez-Mejias A, Biarent D, et al. European resuscitation council guidelines 2021: paediatric life support. Resuscitation. 2021;161:327–87.

12. Aziz K, Lee HC, Escobedo MB, Hoover AV, Kamath-Rayne BD, Kapadia VS, et al. Part 5: neonatal resuscitation: 2020 American heart association guidelines for cardiopulmonary resuscitation and emergency cardiovascular care. Circulation. 2020;142(16_Suppl_2):S524–S50.

13. Gorski LA. Standard 63: intraosseous access devices. J Infus Nurs. 2008;31(3):146–7. https://doi.org/10.1097/01.NAN.0000317700.81642.27.

14. Buck ML, Wiggins BS, Sesler JM. Intraosseous drug administration in children and adults during cardiopulmonary resuscitation. Ann Pharmacother. 2007;41(10):1679–86. https://doi.org/10.1345/aph.1K168. Epub 2007 Aug 14.

15. Kleinman ME, Chameides L, Schexnayder SM, Samson RA, Hazinski MF, Atkins DL, et al. Pediatric advanced life support: 2010 American Heart Association guidelines for cardiopulmonary resuscitation and emergency cardiovascular care. Pediatrics. 2010;126(5):e1361–e99.

16. DeBoer S, Andrews D. Infant venous access:'counting fingers' and 'playing baseball'. Austr Emerg Nurs J. 2007;10(2):46–51.

17. DeBoer S, Russell T, Seaver M, Vardi A. Infant intraosseous infusion. Neonatal Netw. 2008;27(1):25–32. https://doi.org/10.1891/0730-0832.27.1.25.

18. Alam HB, Punzalan CM, Koustova E, Bowyer MW, Rhee P. Hypertonic saline: intraosseous infusion causes myonecrosis in a dehydrated swine model of uncontrolled hemorrhagic shock. J Trauma. 2002;52(1):18–25. https://doi.org/10.1097/00005373-200201000-00006.

19. Doud EA, Tysell JE. Massive intramedullary infusions. JAMA. 1942;120(15):1212–3.

20. Bebarta VS, Vargas TE, Castaneda M, Boudreau S. Evaluation of extremity tissue and bone injury after intraosseous hypertonic saline infusion in proximal tibia and proximal humerus in adult swine. Prehosp Emerg Care. 2014;18(4):505–10. https://doi.org/10.3109/10903127.2014.912704. Epub 2014 May 15.

21. Farrokh S, Cho SM, Lefebvre AT, Zink EK, Schiavi A, Puttgen HA. Use of intraosseous hypertonic saline in critically ill patients. J Vasc Access. 2019;20(4):427–32. https://doi.org/10.1177/1129729818805958. Epub 2018 Oct 17.

22. Pollack CV Jr, Pender ES, Woodall BN, Tubbs RC, Iyer RV, Miller HW. Long-term local effects of intraosseous infusion on tibial bone marrow in the weanling pig model. Am J Emerg Med. 1992;10(1):27–31. https://doi.org/10.1016/0735-6757(92)90120-m.

23. Jaimovich DG, Shabino CL, Ringer TV, Peters GR. Comparison of intraosseous and intravenous routes of anticonvulsant administration in a porcine model. Ann Emerg Med. 1989;18(8):842–6. https://doi.org/10.1016/s0196-0644(89)80208-2.

24. Jaimovich DG, Kumar A, Francom S. Evaluation of intraosseous vs intravenous antibiotic levels in a porcine model. Am J Dis Child. 1991;145(8):946–9. https://doi.org/10.1001/archpedi.1991.02160080124035. Erratum in: Am J Dis Child 1991;145(11):1241.

25. Kenney C, Paxton JH. Intraosseous catheters. Emergent vascular access: Springer; 2021. p. 133–75.

26. Baadh AS, Singh A, Choi A, Baadh PK, Katz DS, Harcke HT. Intraosseous vascular access in radiology: review of clinical status. AJR Am J Roentgenol. 2016;207(2):241–7. https://doi.org/10.2214/AJR.15.15784. Epub 2016 May 10.
27. Teleflex. Arrow® EZ-IO® Intraosseous vascular access system for military use; 2022. https://www.teleflex.com/usa/en/product-areas/military-federal/intraosseous-access/ez-io-system-for-military-use/index.html
28. PerSys Medical. Vascular Access: Meet the NIO—Next-Generation IO™; 2018. https://persysmedical.com/products/vascular-access/
29. Van Loon FHJ, Buise MP, Claassen JJF, Dierick-van Daele ATM, Bouwman ARA. Comparison of ultrasound guidance with palpation and direct visualisation for peripheral vein cannulation in adult patients: a systematic review and meta-analysis. Br J Anaesth. 2018;121(2):358–66. https://doi.org/10.1016/j.bja.2018.04.047. Epub 2018 Jul 2.
30. Lapostolle F, Catineau J, Garrigue B, Monmarteau V, Houssaye T, Vecci I, Tréoux V, Hospital B, Crocheton N, Adnet F. Prospective evaluation of peripheral venous access difficulty in emergency care. Intensive Care Med. 2007;33(8):1452–7. https://doi.org/10.1007/s00134-007-0634-y. Epub 2007 Jun 7.
31. Minville V, Pianezza A, Asehnoune K, Cabardis S, Smail N. Prehospital intravenous line placement assessment in the French emergency system: a prospective study. Eur J Anaesthesiol. 2006;23(7):594–7. https://doi.org/10.1017/S0265021506000202. Epub 2006 Mar 1.
32. Slovis CM, Herr EW, Londorf D, Little TD, Alexander BR, Guthmann RJ. Success rates for initiation of intravenous therapy en route by prehospital care providers. Am J Emerg Med. 1990;8(4):305–7. https://doi.org/10.1016/0735-6757(90)90080-j.
33. Chreiman KM, Dumas RP, Seamon MJ, Kim PK, Reilly PM, Kaplan LJ, Christie JD, Holena DN. The intraosseous have it: a prospective observational study of vascular access success rates in patients in extremis using video review. J Trauma Acute Care Surg. 2018;84(4):558–63. https://doi.org/10.1097/TA.0000000000001795.
34. Bansal R, Agarwal SK, Tiwari SC, Dash SC. A prospective randomized study to compare ultrasound-guided with nonultrasound-guided double lumen internal jugular catheter insertion as a temporary hemodialysis access. Ren Fail. 2005;27(5):561–4. https://doi.org/10.1080/08860220500199084.
35. Milling TJ Jr, Rose J, Briggs WM, Birkhahn R, Gaeta TJ, Bove JJ, Melniker LA. Randomized, controlled clinical trial of point-of-care limited ultrasonography assistance of central venous cannulation: the third sonography outcomes assessment program (SOAP-3) trial. Crit Care Med. 2005;33(8):1764–9. https://doi.org/10.1097/01.ccm.0000171533.92856.e5.
36. Lowther A. Intraosseous access and adults in the emergency department. Nurs Stand. 2011;25(48):35–8. https://doi.org/10.7748/ns2011.08.25.48.35.c8647.
37. DeBoer S, Seaver M, Morissette C. Intraosseous infusion: not just for kids anymore. Emerg. Med Serv. 2005;34(3):54, 56–63; quiz 119.
38. Davidoff J, Fowler R, Gordon D, Klein G, Kovar J, Lozano M, Potkya J, Racht E, Saussy J, Swanson E, Yamada R, Miller L. Clinical evaluation of a novel intraosseous device for adults: prospective, 250-patient, multi-center trial. JEMS. 2005;30(10):20–3.
39. Gerritse BM, Scheffer GJ, Draaisma JM. Prehospital intraosseus access with the bone injection gun by a helicopter-transported emergency medical team. J Trauma. 2009;66(6):1739–41. https://doi.org/10.1097/TA.0b013e3181a3930b.
40. Horwood B, Adams J, Tiffany B, Pollack C, Adams B, Scalzi R, et al. Prehospital use of a sternal intraosseous infusion device. Ann Emerg Med. 1999;4(34):S65–6.
41. Kenichi K, Kyutaro K, Ryo S, Hideharu T. Comparison of the success rate of intraosseous infusion performed by Japanese paramedics. Resuscitation. 2018;130:e138.
42. Gendron B, Cronin A, Monti J, Brigg A. Military medic performance with employment of a commercial intraosseous infusion device: a randomized, crossover study. Mil Med. 2018;183(5–6):e216–e22.
43. İsmailoğlu EG, Zaybak A, Akarca FK, Kıyan S. The effect of the use of ultrasound in the success of peripheral venous catheterisation. Int Emerg Nurs. 2015;23(2):89–93. https://doi.org/10.1016/j.ienj.2014.07.010. Epub 2014 Aug 15.

44. Lamhaut L, Dagron C, Apriotesei R, Gouvernaire J, Elie C, Marx JS, Télion C, Vivien B, Carli P. Comparison of intravenous and intraosseous access by pre-hospital medical emergency personnel with and without CBRN protective equipment. Resuscitation. 2010;81(1):65–8. https://doi.org/10.1016/j.resuscitation.2009.09.011. Epub 2009 Oct 24.

45. Paxton JH, Knuth TE, Klausner HA. Proximal humerus intraosseous infusion: a preferred emergency venous access. J Trauma. 2009;67(3):606–11. https://doi.org/10.1097/TA.0b013e3181b16f42.

46. Reades R, Studnek JR, Vandeventer S, Garrett J. Intraosseous versus intravenous vascular access during out-of-hospital cardiac arrest: a randomized controlled trial. Ann Emerg Med. 2011;58(6):509–16. https://doi.org/10.1016/j.annemergmed.2011.07.020.

47. Lantos D, Goforth D, editors. Intraosseous needles reduce time to first medication for coding inpatients without intravenous access. Critical Care Nurse; 2015: Amer Assoc Critical Care Nurses 101 Columbia, Aliso Viejo, CA 92656 USA.

48. Leidel BA, Kirchhoff C, Bogner V, Braunstein V, Biberthaler P, Kanz KG. Comparison of intraosseous versus central venous vascular access in adults under resuscitation in the emergency department with inaccessible peripheral veins. Resuscitation. 2012;83(1):40–5. https://doi.org/10.1016/j.resuscitation.2011.08.017. Epub 2011 Sep 3.

49. Brillman JC. Emergency medicine: intraosseous infusion for emergency vascular access. West J Med. 1987;146(5):603.

50. Tobias JD, Ross AK. Intraosseous infusions: a review for the anesthesiologist with a focus on pediatric use. Anesth Analg. 2010;110(2):391–401. https://doi.org/10.1213/ANE.0b013e3181c03c7f. Epub 2009 Nov 6.

51. Tocantins L. Rapid absorption of substances injected into the bone marrow. Proc Soc Exper Biol Med. 1940;45(1):292–6.

52. Montez D, Puga T, Miller L, Saussy J, Davlantes C, Kim S, et al. 133 intraosseous infusions from the proximal humerus reach the heart in less than 3 seconds in human volunteers. Ann Emerg Med. 2015;66(4):S47.

53. Spivey WH. Intraosseous infusions. J Pediatr. 1987;111(5):639–43. https://doi.org/10.1016/s0022-3476(87)80236-6. Erratum in: J Pediatr 1987;111 (6 Pt 1):941.

54. Beaumont LD, Baragchizadeh A, Johnson C, Johnson D. Effects of tibial and humerus intraosseous administration of epinephrine in a cardiac arrest swine model. Am J Disaster Med. 2016;11(4):243–51. https://doi.org/10.5055/ajdm.2016.0246.

55. Burgert J, Gegel B, Loughren M, Ceremuga T, Desai M, Schlicher M, O'Sullivan J, Lewis P, Johnson D. Comparison of tibial intraosseous, sternal intraosseous, and intravenous routes of administration on pharmacokinetics of epinephrine during cardiac arrest: a pilot study. AANA J. 2012;80(4 Suppl):S6–10.

56. Anson JA. Vascular access in resuscitation: is there a role for the intraosseous route? Anesthesiology. 2014;120(4):1015–31. https://doi.org/10.1097/ALN.0000000000000140.

57. Selby IR, James MR. The intraosseous route for induction of anaesthesia. Anaesthesia. 1993;48(11):982–4. https://doi.org/10.1111/j.1365-2044.1993.tb07480.x.

58. Mader TJ, Walterscheid JK, Kellogg AR, Lodding CC. The feasibility of inducing mild therapeutic hypothermia after cardiac resuscitation using iced saline infusion via an intraosseous needle. Resuscitation. 2010;81(1):82–6. https://doi.org/10.1016/j.resuscitation.2009.10.003. Epub 2009 Nov 13.

59. Truhlar A, Skulec R, Rozsival P, Cerny V. Efficient prehospital induction of therapeutic hypothermia via intraosseous infusion. Resuscitation. 2010;81(2):262–3. https://doi.org/10.1016/j.resuscitation.2009.10.029. Epub 2009 Dec 16.

60. Hazinski MF, Nolan JP, Billi JE, Böttiger BW, Bossaert L, de Caen AR, Deakin CD, Drajer S, Eigel B, Hickey RW, Jacobs I, Kleinman ME, Kloeck W, Koster RW, Lim SH, Mancini ME, Montgomery WH, Morley PT, Morrison LJ, Nadkarni VM, O'Connor RE, Okada K, Perlman JM, Sayre MR, Shuster M, Soar J, Sunde K, Travers AH, Wyllie J, Zideman D. Part 1: executive summary: 2010 international consensus on cardiopulmonary resuscitation and emergency cardiovascular care science with treatment recommendations. Circulation. 2010;122(16 Suppl 2):S250–75. https://doi.org/10.1161/CIRCULATIONAHA.110.970897.

61. Neumar RW, Otto CW, Link MS, Kronick SL, Shuster M, Callaway CW, Kudenchuk PJ, Ornato JP, McNally B, Silvers SM, Passman RS, White RD, Hess EP, Tang W, Davis D, Sinz E, Morrison LJ. Part 8: adult advanced cardiovascular life support: 2010 American Heart Association guidelines for cardiopulmonary resuscitation and emergency cardiovascular care. Circulation. 2010;122(18 Suppl 3):S729–67. https://doi.org/10.1161/CIRCULATIONAHA.110.970988. Erratum in: Circulation. 2011;123(6):e236. Erratum in: Circulation 2013 Dec 24;128(25):e480.

62. Baert V, Vilhelm C, Escutnaire J, Nave S, Hugenschmitt D, Chouihed T, Tazarourte K, Javaudin F, Wiel E, El Khoury C, Hubert H, GR-RéAC. Intraosseous versus peripheral intravenous access during out-of-hospital cardiac arrest: a comparison of 30-day survival and neurological outcome in the French National Registry. Cardiovasc Drugs Ther. 2020;34(2):189–97. https://doi.org/10.1007/s10557-020-06952-8.

63. Daya MR, Leroux BG, Dorian P, Rea TD, Newgard CD, Morrison LJ, Lupton JR, Menegazzi JJ, Ornato JP, Sopko G, Christenson J, Idris A, Mody P, Vilke GM, Herdeman C, Barbic D, Kudenchuk PJ. Resuscitation outcomes consortium investigators. Survival after intravenous versus intraosseous amiodarone, lidocaine, or placebo in out-of-hospital shock-refractory cardiac arrest. Circulation. 2020;141(3):188–98. https://doi.org/10.1161/CIRCULATIONAHA.119.042240. Epub 2020 Jan 16.

64. Granfeldt A, Avis SR, Lind PC, Holmberg MJ, Kleinman M, Maconochie I, Hsu CH, Fernanda de Almeida M, Wang TL, Neumar RW, Andersen LW. Intravenous vs. intraosseous administration of drugs during cardiac arrest: a systematic review. Resuscitation. 2020;149:150–7. https://doi.org/10.1016/j.resuscitation.2020.02.025. Epub 2020 Mar 3.

65. Feinstein BA, Stubbs BA, Rea T, Kudenchuk PJ. Intraosseous compared to intravenous drug resuscitation in out-of-hospital cardiac arrest. Resuscitation. 2017;117:91–6. https://doi.org/10.1016/j.resuscitation.2017.06.014. Epub 2017 Jun 16.

66. Hamam MS, Klausner HA, France J, Tang A, Swor RA, Paxton JH, O'Neil BJ, Brent C, Neumar RW, Dunne RB, Reddi S, Miller JB. Prehospital tibial intraosseous drug administration is associated with reduced survival following out of hospital cardiac arrest: a study for the CARES Surveillance Group. Resuscitation. 2021;167:261–6. https://doi.org/10.1016/j.resuscitation.2021.06.016. Epub 2021 Jul 5.

67. Kawano T, Grunau B, Scheuermeyer FX, Gibo K, Fordyce CB, Lin S, Stenstrom R, Schlamp R, Jenneson S, Christenson J. Intraosseous vascular access is associated with lower survival and neurologic recovery among patients with out-of-hospital cardiac arrest. Ann Emerg Med. 2018;71(5):588–96. https://doi.org/10.1016/j.annemergmed.2017.11.015. Epub 2018 Jan 6.

68. Mody P, Brown SP, Kudenchuk PJ, Chan PS, Khera R, Ayers C, Pandey A, Kern KB, de Lemos JA, Link MS, Idris AH. Intraosseous versus intravenous access in patients with out-of-hospital cardiac arrest: insights from the resuscitation outcomes consortium continuous chest compression trial. Resuscitation. 2019;134:69–75. https://doi.org/10.1016/j.resuscitation.2018.10.031. Epub 2018 Nov 1.

69. Nguyen L, Suarez S, Daniels J, Sanchez C, Landry K, Redfield C. Effect of intravenous versus intraosseous access in prehospital cardiac arrest. Air Med J. 2019;38(3):147–9.

70. Zhang Y, Zhu J, Liu Z, Gu L, Zhang W, Zhan H, Hu C, Liao J, Xiong Y, Idris AH. Intravenous versus intraosseous adrenaline administration in out-of-hospital cardiac arrest: a retrospective cohort study. Resuscitation. 2020;149:209–16. https://doi.org/10.1016/j.resuscitation.2020.01.009. Epub 2020 Jan 23.

71. Nolan JP, Deakin CD, Ji C, Gates S, Rosser A, Lall R, Perkins GD. Intraosseous versus intravenous administration of adrenaline in patients with out-of-hospital cardiac arrest: a secondary analysis of the PARAMEDIC2 placebo-controlled trial. Intensive Care Med. 2020;46(5):954–62. https://doi.org/10.1007/s00134-019-05920-7. Epub 2020 Jan 30.

72. Hsieh YL, Wu MC, Wolfshohl J, d'Etienne J, Huang CH, Lu TC, Huang EP, Chou EH, Wang CH, Chen WJ. Intraosseous versus intravenous vascular access during cardiopulmonary resuscitation for out-of-hospital cardiac arrest: a systematic review and meta-analysis of observational studies. Scand J Trauma Resusc Emerg Med. 2021;29(1):44. https://doi.org/10.1186/s13049-021-00858-6.

73. Clemency B, Tanaka K, May P, Innes J, Zagroba S, Blaszak J, Hostler D, Cooney D, McGee K, Lindstrom H. Intravenous vs. intraosseous access and return of spontaneous circulation during out of hospital cardiac arrest. Am J Emerg Med. 2017;35(2):222–6. https://doi.org/10.1016/j.ajem.2016.10.052. Epub 2016 Oct 24.

74. Mac Kinnon KA. Intraosseous vascular use at signature healthcare Brockton hospital department of emergency services. J Emerg Nurs. 2009;35(5):425–8. https://doi.org/10.1016/j.jen.2009.01.016. Epub 2009 Mar 27.

75. Zuercher M, Kern KB, Na SH, Hilwig RW, Ummenhofer W, Ewy GA. Early administration of epinephrine improves good neurological outcome at 24 hours in a porcine model of prolonged, untreated ventricular fibrillation. Am Heart Assoc; 2012.

76. Friedman FD. Intraosseous adenosine for the termination of supraventricular tachycardia in an infant. Ann Emerg Med. 1996;28(3):356–8.

77. Langley DM, Moran M. Intraosseous needles: they're not just for kids anymore. J Emerg Nurs. 2008;34(4):318–9. https://doi.org/10.1016/j.jen.2007.07.005. Epub 2008 Mar 7.

78. Davis J, Bates L. Rapid sequence induction via an intraosseous needle. J Intensive Care Soc. 2016;17(2):178–9. https://doi.org/10.1177/1751143715614845. Epub 2016 May 1.

79. Joseph G, Tobias JD. The use of intraosseous infusions in the operating room. J Clin Anesth. 2008;20(6):469–73. https://doi.org/10.1016/j.jclinane.2008.04.014.

80. Guy J, Haley K, Zuspan SJ. Use of intraosseous infusion in the pediatric trauma patient. J Pediatr Surg. 1993;28(2):158–61. https://doi.org/10.1016/s0022-3468(05)80263-5.

81. Hicks MA, Tyagi A. Magnesium sulfate. StatPearls [Internet]: StatPearls Publishing; 2022.

82. Weiser G, Poppa E, Katz Y, Bahouth H, Shavit I. Intraosseous blood transfusion in infants with traumatic hemorrhagic shock. Am J Emerg Med. 2013;31(3):640.e3–4. https://doi.org/10.1016/j.ajem.2012.10.036. Epub 2013 Feb 4.

83. Rosetti VA, Thompson BM, Miller J, Mateer JR, Aprahamian C. Intraosseous infusion: an alternative route of pediatric intravascular access. Ann Emerg Med. 1985;14(9):885–8. https://doi.org/10.1016/s0196-0644(85)80639-9.

84. Tarrow CAB, Turkel H, Thompson CMS. Infusions via the bone marrow and biopsy of the bone and bone marrow. J Am Soc Anesthesiol. 1952;13:501.

85. Kelsall AW. Resuscitation with intraosseous lines in neonatal units. Arch Dis Child. 1993;68(3):324–5. https://doi.org/10.1136/adc.68.3_spec_no.324.

86. Goldstein B, Doody D, Briggs S. Emergency intraosseous infusion in severely burned children. Pediatr Emerg Care. 1990;6(3):195–7. https://doi.org/10.1097/00006565-199009000-00008.

87. Glaeser PW, Hellmich TR, Szewczuga D, Losek JD, Smith DS. Five-year experience in prehospital intraosseous infusions in children and adults. Ann Emerg Med. 1993;22(7):1119–24. https://doi.org/10.1016/s0196-0644(05)80975-8.

88. Vidal R, Kissoon N, Gayle M. Compartment syndrome following intraosseous infusion. Pediatrics. 1993;91(6):1201–2.

89. Valdés M, Araujo P, de Andrés C, Sastre E, Martin T. Intraosseous administration of thrombolysis in out-of-hospital massive pulmonary thromboembolism. Emerg Med J. 2010;27(8):641–4. https://doi.org/10.1136/emj.2009.086223. Epub 2010 Jun 3.

90. Northey LC, Shiraev T, Omari A. Salvage intraosseous thrombolysis and extracorporeal membrane oxygenation for massive pulmonary embolism. J Emerg Trauma Shock. 2015;8(1):55–7. https://doi.org/10.4103/0974-2700.145395.

91. Trauma ACoSCo. ATLS®: advanced trauma life support student course manual; 2018.

92. Hodge D 3rd, Delgado-Paredes C, Fleisher G. Intraosseous infusion flow rates in hypovolemic "pediatric" dogs. Ann Emerg Med. 1987;16(3):305–7. https://doi.org/10.1016/s0196-0644(87)80176-2.

93. Iserson KV. Intraosseous infusions in adults. J Emerg Med. 1989;7(6):587–91. https://doi.org/10.1016/0736-4679(89)90002-4.

94. Bjerkvig CK, Fosse TK, Apelseth TO, Sivertsen J, Braathen H, Eliassen HS, Guttormsen AB, Cap AP, Strandenes G. Emergency sternal intraosseous access for warm fresh whole blood transfusion in damage control resuscitation. J Trauma Acute Care Surg. 2018;84(6S Suppl 1):S120–4. https://doi.org/10.1097/TA.0000000000001850.

95. Burgert JM, Mozer J, Williams T, Gegel BT, Johnson S, Bentley M, Johnson A. Effects of intraosseous transfusion of whole blood on hemolysis and transfusion time in a swine model of hemorrhagic shock: a pilot study. AANA J. 2014;82(3):198–202.

96. Harris M, Balog R, Devries G. What is the evidence of utility for intraosseous blood transfusion in damage-control resuscitation? J Trauma Acute Care Surg. 2013;75(5):904–6. https://doi.org/10.1097/TA.0b013e3182a85f71.

97. Plewa MC, King RW, Fenn-Buderer N, Gretzinger K, Renuart D, Cruz R. Hematologic safety of intraosseous blood transfusion in a swine model of pediatric hemorrhagic hypovolemia. Acad Emerg Med. 1995;2(9):799–809. https://doi.org/10.1111/j.1553-2712.1995.tb03275.x.

98. Tyler JA, Perkins Z, De'Ath HD. Intraosseous access in the resuscitation of trauma patients: a literature review. Eur J Trauma Emerg Surg. 2021;47(1):47–55. https://doi.org/10.1007/s00068-020-01327-y. Epub 2020 Feb 20.

99. Lewis P, Wright C. Saving the critically injured trauma patient: a retrospective analysis of 1000 uses of intraosseous access. Emerg Med J. 2015;32(6):463–7. https://doi.org/10.1136/emermed-2014-203588. Epub 2014 Jun 30.

100. Hulsebos H, Bernard J. Consider autotransfusion in the field. Mil Med. 2016;181(8):e945–7. https://doi.org/10.7205/MILMED-D-15-00046.

101. Boysen SR, Pang JM, Mikler JR, Knight CG, Semple HA, Caulkett NA. Comparison of tranexamic acid plasma concentrations when administered via intraosseous and intravenous routes. Am J Emerg Med. 2017;35(2):227–33. https://doi.org/10.1016/j.ajem.2016.10.054. Epub 2016 Oct 26.

102. Lallemand MS, Moe DM, McClellan JM, Loughren M, Marko S, Eckert MJ, Martin MJ. No intravenous access, no problem: intraosseous administration of tranexamic acid is as effective as intravenous in a porcine hemorrhage model. J Trauma Acute Care Surg. 2018;84(2):379–85. https://doi.org/10.1097/TA.0000000000001741.

103. Wang J, Fang Y, Ramesh S, Zakaria A, Putman MT, Dinescu D, Paik J, Geocadin RG, Tahsili-Fahadan P, Altaweel LR. Intraosseous administration of 23.4% NaCl for treatment of intracranial hypertension. Neurocrit Care. 2019;30(2):364–71. https://doi.org/10.1007/s12028-018-0637-2.

104. Brophy GM, Bell R, Claassen J, Alldredge B, Bleck TP, Glauser T, Laroche SM, Riviello JJ Jr, Shutter L, Sperling MR, Treiman DM, Vespa PM, Neurocritical Care Society Status Epilepticus Guideline Writing Committee. Guidelines for the evaluation and management of status epilepticus. Neurocrit Care. 2012;17(1):3–23. https://doi.org/10.1007/s12028-012-9695-z.

105. Glauser T, Shinnar S, Gloss D, Alldredge B, Arya R, Bainbridge J, Bare M, Bleck T, Dodson WE, Garrity L, Jagoda A, Lowenstein D, Pellock J, Riviello J, Sloan E, Treiman DM. Evidence-based guideline: treatment of convulsive status epilepticus in children and adults: report of the guideline Committee of the American Epilepsy Society. Epilepsy Curr. 2016;16(1):48–61. https://doi.org/10.5698/1535-7597-16.1.48.

106. Jim KF, Lathers CM, Farris VL, Pratt LF, Spivey WH. Suppression of pentylenetetrazol-elicited seizure activity by intraosseous lorazepam in pigs. Epilepsia. 1989;30(4):480–6. https://doi.org/10.1111/j.1528-1157.1989.tb05329.x.

107. Dalziel SR, Borland ML, Furyk J, Bonisch M, Neutze J, Donath S, Francis KL, Sharpe C, Harvey AS, Davidson A, Craig S, Phillips N, George S, Rao A, Cheng N, Zhang M, Kochar A, Brabyn C, Oakley E, Babl FE, PREDICT research network. Levetiracetam versus phenytoin for second-line treatment of convulsive status epilepticus in children (ConSEPT): an open-label, multicentre, randomised controlled trial. Lancet. 2019;393(10186):2135–45. https://doi.org/10.1016/S0140-6736(19)30722-6. Epub 2019 Apr 17.

108. Biesterveld BE, O'Connell R, Kemp MT, Wakam GK, Williams AM, Pai MP, Alam HB. Validation of intraosseous delivery of valproic acid in a swine model of polytrauma. Trauma Surg Acute Care Open. 2021;6(1):e000683. https://doi.org/10.1136/tsaco-2021-000683.

109. Fill K, MacGregor J, Victor A, Raziuddin A. The case files: how low can you go? Emergency Medicine News. 2016;38(12C):10.1097.

110. Kedia N. Treatment of severe diabetic hypoglycemia with glucagon: an underutilized therapeutic approach. Diabetes Metab Syndr Obes. 2011;4:337.
111. Maskell KF, Ferguson NM, Bain J, Wills BK. Survival after cardiac arrest: ECMO rescue therapy after amlodipine and metoprolol overdose. Cardiovasc Toxicol. 2017;17(2):223–5. https://doi.org/10.1007/s12012-016-9362-2.
112. Elliott A, Dubé PA, Cossette-Côté A, Patakfalvi L, Villeneuve E, Morris M, Gosselin S. Intraosseous administration of antidotes—a systematic review. Clin Toxicol (Phila). 2017;55(10):1025–54. https://doi.org/10.1080/15563650.2017.1337122. Epub 2017 Jun 23.
113. Hiller K, Jarrod MM, Franke HA, Degan J, Boyer LV, Fox FM. Scorpion antivenom administered by alternative infusions. Ann Emerg Med. 2010;56(3):309–10. https://doi.org/10.1016/j.annemergmed.2010.04.007.
114. Murray DB, Eddleston M, Thomas S, Jefferson RD, Thompson A, Dunn M, Vidler DS, Clutton RE, Blain PG. Rapid and complete bioavailability of antidotes for organophosphorus nerve agent and cyanide poisoning in minipigs after intraosseous administration. Ann Emerg Med. 2012;60(4):424–30. https://doi.org/10.1016/j.annemergmed.2012.05.013. Epub 2012 Jun 26.
115. Dev SP, Stefan RA, Saun T, Lee S. Videos in clinical medicine. Insertion of an intraosseous needle in adults. N Engl J Med. 2014;370(24):e35. https://doi.org/10.1056/NEJMvcm1211371.
116. Harcke HT, Crawley G, Mabry R, Mazuchowski E. Placement of tibial intraosseous infusion devices. Mil Med. 2011;176(7):824–7. https://doi.org/10.7205/milmed-d-10-00271.
117. Ackert L, Boysen SR, Schiller T. A pilot study comparing bone marrow aspirates and venous blood for emergency point-of-care blood parameters in healthy dogs. J Vet Emerg Crit Care (San Antonio). 2019;29(4):399–406. https://doi.org/10.1111/vec.12858. Epub 2019 Jun 21.
118. Grisham J, Hastings C. Bone marrow aspirate as an accessible and reliable source for critical laboratory studies. Ann Emerg Med. 1991;20(10):1121–4. https://doi.org/10.1016/s0196-0644(05)81388-5.
119. Miller LJ, Philbeck TE, Montez D, Spadaccini CJ. A new study of intraosseous blood for laboratory analysis. Arch Pathol Lab Med. 2010;134(9):1253–60. https://doi.org/10.5858/2009-0381-OA.1.
120. Strandberg G, Larsson A, Lipcsey M, Eriksson M. Comparison of intraosseous, arterial, and venous blood sampling for laboratory analysis in hemorrhagic shock. Clin Lab. 2019;65(7) https://doi.org/10.7754/Clin.Lab.2019.181214.
121. Ummenhofer W, Frei FJ, Urwyler A, Drewe J. Are laboratory values in bone marrow aspirate predictable for venous blood in paediatric patients? Resuscitation. 1994;27(2):123–8. https://doi.org/10.1016/0300-9572(94)90004-3.
122. Orlowski JP, Porembka DT, Gallagher JM, Van Lente F. The bone marrow as a source of laboratory studies. Ann Emerg Med. 1989;18(12):1348–51. https://doi.org/10.1016/s0196-0644(89)80274-4.
123. Greco SC, Talcott MR, LaRegina MC, Eisenbeis PE. Use of intraosseous blood for repeated hematologic and biochemical analyses in healthy pigs. Am J Vet Res. 2001;62(1):43–7. https://doi.org/10.2460/ajvr.2001.62.43.
124. Eriksson M, Strandberg G, Lipcsey M, Larsson A. Evaluation of intraosseous sampling for measurements of alanine aminotransferase, alkaline phosphatase, aspartate aminotransferase, creatinine kinase, gamma-glutamyl transferase and lactate dehydrogenase. Scand J Clin Lab Invest. 2016;76(8):597–600.
125. Montez DF, Puga T, Miller L, Garcia M, Davlantes C, Saussy J, et al. Intraosseous and venous blood lactate levels correlate; PT/INR do not. Acad Emerg Med. 2014;21(5):1.
126. Jousi M, Saikko S, Nurmi J. Intraosseous blood samples for point-of-care analysis: agreement between intraosseous and arterial analyses. Scand J Trauma Resusc Emerg Med. 2017;25(1):92. https://doi.org/10.1186/s13049-017-0435-4.
127. Johnson L, Kissoon N, Fiallos M, Abdelmoneim T, Murphy S. Use of intraosseous blood to assess blood chemistries and hemoglobin during cardiopulmonary resuscitation with drug infusions. Crit Care Med. 1999;27(6):1147–52. https://doi.org/10.1097/00003246-199906000-00039.

128. Abdelmoneim T, Kissoon N, Johnson L, Fiallos M, Murphy S. Acid-base status of blood from intraosseous and mixed venous sites during prolonged cardiopulmonary resuscitation and drug infusions. Crit Care Med. 1999;27(9):1923–8. https://doi.org/10.1097/00003246-199909000-00034.

129. Kissoon N, Peterson R, Murphy S, Gayle M, Ceithaml E, Harwood-Nuss A. Comparison of pH and carbon dioxide tension values of central venous and intraosseous blood during changes in cardiac output. Crit Care Med. 1994;22(6):1010–5. https://doi.org/10.1097/00003246-199406000-00021.

130. Kissoon N, Rosenberg H, Gloor J, Vidal R. Comparison of the acid-base status of blood obtained from intraosseous and central venous sites during steady- and low-flow states. Crit Care Med. 1993;21(11):1765–9. https://doi.org/10.1097/00003246-199311000-00028.

131. Brickman KR, Krupp K, Rega P, Alexander J, Guinness M. Typing and screening of blood from intraosseous access. Ann Emerg Med. 1992;21(4):414–7. https://doi.org/10.1016/s0196-0644(05)82661-7.

132. Greaves I, Evans G, Boyle A. Intraosseous infusions in the adult. Trauma. 1999;1(4):291–9.

133. Krähling H, Masthoff M, Schwindt W, Stracke CP, Schindler P. Intraosseous contrast administration for emergency stroke CT. Neuroradiology. 2021;63(6):967–70. https://doi.org/10.1007/s00234-021-02642-w. Epub 2021 Jan 18.

134. Cohen J, Duncan L, Triner W, Rea J, Siskin G, King C. Comparison of computed tomography image quality using intravenous vs. intraosseous contrast administration in swine. J Emerg Med. 2015;49(5):771–7. https://doi.org/10.1016/j.jemermed.2014.06.036. Epub 2015 Jun 10.

135. Knuth TE, Paxton JH, Myers D. Intraosseous injection of iodinated computed tomography contrast agent in an adult blunt trauma patient. Ann Emerg Med. 2011;57(4):382–6. https://doi.org/10.1016/j.annemergmed.2010.09.025. Epub 2010 Dec 15.

136. Ahrens KL, Reeder SB, Keevil JG, Tupesis JP. Successful computed tomography angiogram through tibial intraosseous access: a case report. J Emerg Med. 2013;45(2):182–5. https://doi.org/10.1016/j.jemermed.2012.11.091. Epub 2013 May 29.

137. Lottenberg L, Lovato L, Bloch S, Puga T, Philbeck T. 1075: the proximal humerus may be a vialbe site for contrast injection using a power infuser for CT exam. Crit Care Med. 2014;42(12):A1619.

138. Plancade D, Nadaud J, Lapierre M, Fétissof H, Schaeffer E, Mellati N, Millot I, Landy C. Feasibility of a thoraco-abdominal CT with injection of iodinated contrast agent on sternal intraosseous catheter in an emergency department. Ann Fr Anesth Reanim. 2012;31(12):e283–4. https://doi.org/10.1016/j.annfar.2012.10.009. Epub 2012 Nov 16.

139. Schindler P, Helfen A, Wildgruber M, Heindel W, Schülke C, Masthoff M. Intraosseous contrast administration for emergency computed tomography: a case-control study. PLoS One. 2019;14(5):e0217629. https://doi.org/10.1371/journal.pone.0217629.

140. Grossman VA. Hot topics: CT contrast and intraosseous lines: friends or enemies? J Radiol Nurs. 2013;1(32):41–4.

141. Stewart FC, Kain ZN. Intraosseous infusion: elective use in pediatric anesthesia. Anesth Analg. 1992;75(4):626–9. https://doi.org/10.1213/00000539-199210000-00029.

142. Anson JA, Sinz EH, Swick JT. The versatility of intraosseous vascular access in perioperative medicine: a case series. J Clin Anesth. 2015;27(1):63–7. https://doi.org/10.1016/j.jclinane.2014.10.002. Epub 2014 Dec 26.

143. Waisman M, Roffman M, Bursztein S, Heifetz M. Intraosseous regional anesthesia as an alternative to intravenous regional anesthesia. J Trauma. 1995;39(6):1153–6. https://doi.org/10.1097/00005373-199512000-00025.

144. Yen K, Riegert A, Gorelick MH. Derivation of the DIVA score: a clinical prediction rule for the identification of children with difficult intravenous access. Pediatr Emerg Care. 2008;24(3):143–7. https://doi.org/10.1097/PEC.0b013e3181666f32.

145. Angles E, Robin F, Moal B, Roy M, Sesay M, Ouattara A, Biais M, Roullet S, Saillour-Glénisson F, Nouette-Gaulain K. Pre-operative peripheral intravenous cannula insertion failure at the first attempt in adults: development of the VENSCORE predictive scale and

identification of risk factors. J Clin Anesth. 2021;75:110435. https://doi.org/10.1016/j.jclinane.2021.110435. Epub 2021 Jul 22.

146. Walsh G. Difficult peripheral venous access: recognizing and managing the patient at risk. JAVA. 2008;13(4):198–203.

147. Rosetti V, Thompson V, Aprahamian C. Difficulty and delay in intravascular access in pediatric arrests (abstract). Ann Emerg Med. 1984;13:406.

148. Bosomworth NJ. The occasional intraosseous infusion. Can J Rural Med. 2008;13(2):80–3.

149. Topjian AA, Raymond TT, Atkins D, Chan M, Duff JP, Joyner BL Jr, Lasa JJ, Lavonas EJ, Levy A, Mahgoub M, Meckler GD, Roberts KE, Sutton RM, Schexnayder SM. Pediatric Basic and Advanced Life Support Collaborators. Part 4: pediatric basic and advanced life support: 2020 American Heart Association guidelines for cardiopulmonary resuscitation and emergency cardiovascular care. Circulation. 2020;142(16_suppl_2):S469–523. https://doi.org/10.1161/CIR.0000000000000901. Epub 2020 Oct 21.

150. de Caen AR, Berg MD, Chameides L, Gooden CK, Hickey RW, Scott HF, Sutton RM, Tijssen JA, Topjian A, van der Jagt ÉW, Schexnayder SM, Samson RA. Part 12: pediatric advanced life support: 2015 American Heart Association guidelines update for cardiopulmonary resuscitation and emergency cardiovascular care. Circulation. 2015;132(18 Suppl 2):S526–42. https://doi.org/10.1161/CIR.0000000000000266.

151. Maconochie IK, Aickin R, Hazinski MF, Atkins DL, Bingham R, Couto TB, Guerguerian AM, Nadkarni VM, Ng KC, Nuthall GA, Ong GYK, Reis AG, Schexnayder SM, Scholefield BR, Tijssen JA, Nolan JP, Morley PT, Van de Voorde P, Zaritsky AL, de Caen AR, Pediatric Life Support Collaborators. Pediatric life support: 2020 international consensus on cardiopulmonary resuscitation and emergency cardiovascular care science with treatment recommendations. Circulation. 2020;142(16_suppl_1):S140–84. https://doi.org/10.1161/CIR.0000000000000894. Epub 2020 Oct 21.

152. Kanter RK, Zimmerman JJ, Strauss RH, Stoeckel KA. Pediatric emergency intravenous access. Evaluation of a protocol. Am J Dis Child. 1986;140(2):132–4. https://doi.org/10.1001/archpedi.1986.02140160050030.

153. Haas NA. Clinical review: vascular access for fluid infusion in children. Crit Care. 2004;8(6):478–84. https://doi.org/10.1186/cc2880. Epub 2004 Jun 3.

154. Iserson KV, Criss EA. Pediatric venous cutdowns: utility in emergency situations. Pediatr Emerg Care. 1986;2(4):231–4. https://doi.org/10.1097/00006565-198612000-00006.

155. Abe KK, Blum GT, Yamamoto LG. Intraosseous is faster and easier than umbilical venous catheterization in newborn emergency vascular access models. Am J Emerg Med. 2000;18(2):126–9. https://doi.org/10.1016/s0735-6757(00)90001-9.

156. Engle WA. Intraosseous access for administration of medications in neonates. Clin Perinatol. 2006;33(1):161–8, ix. https://doi.org/10.1016/j.clp.2005.11.006.

157. Pifko EL, Price A, Busch C, Smith C, Jiang Y, Dobson J, Tuuri R. Observational review of paediatric intraosseous needle placement in the paediatric emergency department. J Paediatr Child Health. 2018;54(5):546–50. https://doi.org/10.1111/jpc.13773. Epub 2017 Nov 10.

158. Maxien D, Wirth S, Peschel O, Sterzik A, Kirchhoff S, Kreimeier U, Reiser MF, Mück FG. Intraosseous needles in pediatric cadavers: rate of malposition. Resuscitation. 2019;145:1–7. https://doi.org/10.1016/j.resuscitation.2019.09.028. Epub 2019 Oct 1.

159. Nijssen-Jordan C. Emergency department utilization and success rates for intraosseous infusion in pediatric resuscitations. CJEM. 2000;2(1):10–4. https://doi.org/10.1017/s1481803500004334.

160. Oksan D, Ayfer K. Powered intraosseous device (EZ-IO) for critically ill patients. Indian Pediatr. 2013;50(7):689–91. https://doi.org/10.1007/s13312-013-0192-z. Epub 2012 Dec 5.

161. Banerjee S, Singhi SC, Singh S, Singh M. The intraosseous route is a suitable alternative to intravenous route for fluid resuscitation in severely dehydrated children. Indian Pediatr. 1994;31(12):1511–20.

162. Jawad N, Brown K, Sebire N, Arthurs O. Accuracy of paediatric intraosseous needle placement from post mortem imaging. J Forens Radiol Imaging. 2016;4:63–9.

163. Myers LA, Arteaga GM, Kolb LJ, Lohse CM, Russi CS. Prehospital peripheral intravenous vascular access success rates in children. Prehosp Emerg Care. 2013;17(4):425–8. https://doi.org/10.3109/10903127.2013.818180. Epub 2013 Aug 16.

164. Fidancı İ, Güleryüz OD, Yenice ÖD. Successful intraosseous adenosine administration in a newborn infant with supraventricular tachycardia. Turk J Pediatr. 2020;62(6):1064–8. https://doi.org/10.24953/turkjped.2020.06.019.

165. Alawi KA, Morrison GC, Fraser DD, Al-Farsi S, Collier C, Kornecki A. Insulin infusion via an intraosseous needle in diabetic ketoacidosis. Anaesth Intensive Care. 2008;36(1):110–2. https://doi.org/10.1177/0310057X0803600120.

166. Fields JM, Piela NE, Au AK, Ku BS. Risk factors associated with difficult venous access in adult ED patients. Am J Emerg Med. 2014;32(10):1179–82. https://doi.org/10.1016/j.ajem.2014.07.008. Epub 2014 Jul 30.

167. Phillips L, Brown L, Campbell T, Miller J, Proehl J, Youngberg B. Recommendations for the use of intraosseous vascular access for emergent and nonemergent situations in various health care settings: a consensus paper. Crit Care Nurse. 2010;30(6):e1–7. https://doi.org/10.4037/ccn2010632.

168. Kehrl T, Becker BA, Simmons DE, Broderick EK, Jones RA. Intraosseous access in the obese patient: assessing the need for extended needle length. Am J Emerg Med. 2016;34(9):1831–4. https://doi.org/10.1016/j.ajem.2016.06.055. Epub 2016 Jun 15.

169. Petitpas F, Guenezan J, Vendeuvre T, Scepi M, Oriot D, Mimoz O. Use of intra-osseous access in adults: a systematic review. Crit Care. 2016;20:102. https://doi.org/10.1186/s13054-016-1277-6.

170. LaRocco BG, Wang HE. Intraosseous infusion. Prehosp Emerg Care. 2003;7(2):280–5. https://doi.org/10.1080/10903120390936950.

171. Brickman K, Rega P, Choo M, Guinness M. Comparison of serum phenobarbital levels after single versus multiple attempts at intraosseous infusion. Ann Emerg Med. 1990;19(1):31–3. https://doi.org/10.1016/s0196-0644(05)82136-5.

172. Cotte J, Prunet B, d'Aranda E, Asencio Y, Kaiser E. Un syndrome des loges secondaire à la pose d'un cathéter intra-osseux [A compartment syndrome secondary to intraosseous infusion]. Ann Fr Anesth Reanim. 2011;30(1):90–1. https://doi.org/10.1016/j.annfar.2010.05.038. French. Epub 2010 Nov 30.

173. Burke T, Kehl DK. Intraosseous infusion in infants. Case report of a complication. J Bone Joint Surg Am. 1993;75(3):428–9. https://doi.org/10.2106/00004623-199303000-00015.

174. Arakawa J, Woelber E, Working Z, Meeker J, Friess D. Complications of intraosseous access: two case reports from a single center. JBJS Case Connect. 2021;11(2) https://doi.org/10.2106/JBJS.CC.19.00382.

175. Nutbeam T, Fergusson A. Intraosseous access in osteogenesis imperfecta (IO in OI). Resuscitation. 2009;80(12):1442–3. https://doi.org/10.1016/j.resuscitation.2009.08.016. Epub 2009 Oct 4.

176. Frascone R, Kaye K, Dries D, Solem L. Successful placement of an adult sternal intraosseous line through burned skin. J Burn Care Rehabil. 2003;24(5):306–8. https://doi.org/10.1097/01.BCR.0000085875.68085.6B.

Intraosseous Access Site Selection

4

Katherine Quibell and Julia Yip

Introduction

The intraosseous (IO) space, including the medullary cavity in the diaphysis of the bone and the cancellous bone in the epiphysis and metaphysis, offers an alternate route to securing rapid, definitive vascular access in an emergent setting [1]. In particular, this space can function as a "non-collapsible" route for emergent vascular access in the event of peripheral venous collapse [1–3].

Infusion of medication and fluids through the intramedullary space has been performed clinically in humans since the 1930s but gained popularity during World War II, as it offered a safer venue for intravenous access with lower rates of infection than cannulation of peripheral veins using steel needles [3]. The advent of plastic cannulae and improved methods for direct venous cannulation ushered in a rapid decline in the use of IO access, resulting in very few reports of IO infusion provided in the English-language literature during the 1960s and 1970s [3].

Although intraosseous infusion became more popular for the resuscitation of pediatric subjects during the 1980s, the manually driven catheters of that era were of limited utility in cannulating the relatively more dense bones of adults [2, 3]. The 1990s witnessed the development of many automatic and semiautomatic IO devices, which truly revolutionized the use of IO cannulation in the treatment of adults, although site selection remained relatively restricted in clinical practice to the proximal and distal tibia in children. The appearance of devices intended for use at the sternum and manubrium improved care for adults, but would not see use in the care of pediatric subjects.

K. Quibell (✉)
Western University of Health Sciences, Pomona, CA, USA
e-mail: katherine.quibell@westernu.edu

J. Yip
Department of Emergency Medicine, Wayne State University School of Medicine, Detroit, MI, USA
e-mail: gg1367@wayne.edu

The Iraq War was instrumental in facilitating wider use of intraosseous access first abroad and then later in civilian medicine; additionally, the challenges of caring for soldiers on the battlefield forced creativity and a reimagining of practical intraosseous insertion sites. The result was a broader, yet still incomplete, understanding of the efficacy of various IO cannulation sites. During the 2000s, it became clear that more central (i.e., proximal humeral and femoral) IO insertion sites may offer advantages over distal sites, especially in regard to fluid flow rates. Today, clinicians have access to nearly a century of clinical data describing a vast array of potential IO cannulation sites, each with its own history of clinical use and risk-benefit profile.

Given the abundance of cannulation sites that have been successfully used and reported in the existing medical literature, an examination of site-specific advantages, disadvantages, and other considerations may allow the practitioner to make a more informed decision when selecting an IO cannulation site for their own unique patient and clinical situation. General considerations when selecting the optimal site include patient age, relative anticipated flow rate of the cannulation site, accessibility of the site, site-specific complication risks, and devices available for use. In this chapter, we will begin with a discussion of the most commonly used IO insertion sites, with particular attention to those site characteristics of particular importance to the clinician. These common infusion sites (in order of decreasing frequency as reported in the medical literature) include the proximal tibia, proximal humerus, sternum/manubrium, distal femur, and distal tibia. We will also discuss a number of less commonly used sites, including the clavicle, calcaneus, iliac crest, distal radius, and distal ulna. Along the way, we will discuss some of the historical factors that have shaped the clinical use of these insertion sites over the last century.

Common Cannulation Sites

Sternum

Although the proximal tibia was the first infusion site to be explored in animal models circa 1916, the sternum was the site selected for the earliest IO cannulations used in the medical management of human subjects [2]. During the 1920s, sternal trephination for bone marrow sampling became an established technique for the diagnosis of various hematological disorders. This led to the first IO infusions in human subjects at the sternum during the 1930s [2].

Early experimentation with intraosseous cannulation focused primarily on achieving access at bones rich in red bone marrow, which was thought to be critical to successful infusion. The sternum was the focus of early studies in adults due to its high red marrow content and easy accessibility as a relatively superficial flat bone [4, 5]. Anatomically, the sternum is located at the center of the upper chest and is divided into three sections: the trapezoid-shaped **manubrium** (most superiorly), the **body** of the sternum (i.e., gladiolus), and the triangular-shaped **xiphoid process** (inferiorly). The manubrium and the body of the sternum are separated by the **angle of Louis** (i.e., sternal angle), which is often palpable externally. The xiphoid process is not a viable IO infusion site, as it is largely cartilaginous in children and calcifies in human subjects by the age of 40 years. Early clinical studies suggested that the optimal sternal body puncture site is **midline at the body of the sternum, 3 cm inferior to the manubriosternal junction** [5]. This site is at the level of the second intercostal space, which is optimal because it is far (2–3 cm) from the great vessels of the chest; more inferior sternal body sites (e.g., at the level of the third or fourth intercostal space) are considered at high risk as they overly the pericardium and heart. Meanwhile, the ideal manubrial puncture site is at the sternal **midline, 1–2 cm superior to the manubriosternal junction** [4, 6, 7]. Although the manubrium contains more yellow (i.e., fatty) marrow than the body of the sternum in adults, this site remains hematopoietically active with adequate venous drainage to permit IO infusion. Due to its greater distance from the heart and great vessels, **cannulation of the manubrium is considered to be safer than cannulation of the body of the sternum**.

While these three structures are generally considered to be a single bone, the medullary cavities of the sternal body and the manubrium rarely communicate. Consequently, both sites can receive medullary infusates simultaneously [8, 9]. These medullary spaces drain almost directly to the central venous system via the internal thoracic and subclavian veins [10]. This proximity to the central circulation facilitates more rapid volume infusion when compared to more distant sites, including the proximal humerus and proximal tibia [4, 10–12]. As illustrated in Fig. 4.1, modern IO devices typically cannulate a site on the manubrium of the sternum,

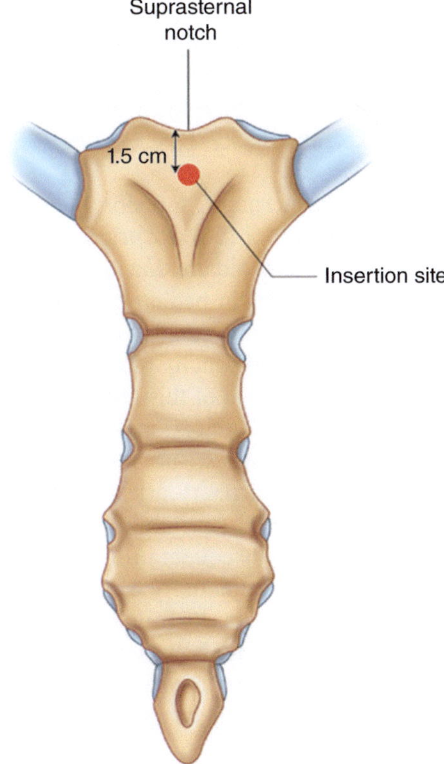

Fig. 4.1 The manubrial intraosseous insertion site (indicated by a red dot), located 1.5 cm below the suprasternal notch in the upper half of the manubrium. *(Image courtesy of Springer Nature. © 2021. All rights reserved* [2]*)*

approximately 1.5 cm below the **suprasternal notch** [2, 4, 6, 7]. This notch (sometimes referred to as the "jugular" notch) is located at the most superior aspect of the manubrium and is readily identifiable in most adults at the anterior midline of the chest centered between the two clavicles.

The sternal insertion site was commonly employed during the 1940s, including military applications, and especially in cases of extremity injury [2]. However, sternal infusion has never been commonly endorsed for pediatric subjects due to concerns about the potential for injury to the heart and other intrathoracic structures [2]. While through-and-through sternal perforation is rarely seen with IO cannulation, it remains a theoretical risk of this insertion site. Some providers may also be concerned about the potential for sternal IO catheter placement to disrupt external chest compressions during cardiopulmonary resuscitation (CPR) following cardiac arrest [2]. Consequently, the proximal tibial site has emerged over the last 40 years as a preferred site, and the sternal site remains relatively underutilized by modern providers [2, 10, 13].

In addition to its potential for dual cannulation and high fluid flow rates, other advantages of the sternal IO site include its easy accessibility (i.e., relative lack of subcutaneous fat, ready identification of the suprasternal notch) and relatively thin bony cortex facilitating entry into the marrow space [4, 5, 10]. This site has been shown to be easily identifiable, with evidence of high rates of successful cannulation by trainees and EMS personnel working in the prehospital setting [10]. Though some practitioners may choose to briefly pause CPR chest compressions during sternal IO catheter placement, the use of automatic or semiautomatic mechanical IO cannulation devices enables rapid and precise placement so as to minimize interruptions [4, 10]. Devices currently available for sternal IO infusion include the FAST-1® (First Access for Shock and Trauma) (Teleflex, Inc.), which is available for the civilian market, and the EZ-IO® TALON (Teleflex, Inc.), which is exclusively sold to the military.

Currently, sternal IO infusion is only FDA approved for adults and children aged 12 years and older [10]. Restrictions on the use of sternal IO catheters in patients less than 12 years old are due to a theoretically higher risk of complications related to size differences in pediatric anatomy compared to adults, including damage to retrosternal structures and lower flow rates due to a smaller reservoir of red marrow [10]. However, the paucity of clinical data on sternal IO infusion in children makes any valid assessment of this potential increased risk implausible.

One unique complication with sternal IO infusion is the potential for injury to retrosternal structures, including the pericardium, wall of the right atrium and right ventricle, coronary arteries, and great vessels. If an IO cannula is inserted too deeply into the sternum, it could theoretically lacerate one or more of these structures, and subsequent infusion of fluids through the catheter could exacerbate this problem by potentially creating an iatrogenic retrosternal or pericardial effusion. For this reason, **a failed sternal IO attempt should reasonably suggest that the provider look elsewhere for a suitable IO cannulation site**, as perforation of the deep sternal cortex could introduce a channel for subsequent extravasation of fluids or medications into the retrosternal space [14]. Other complications, such as the risk of dislodgement or subsequent infection, are shared with other IO sites; no data exist to suggest that sternal IO catheters are associated with any increased risk of these complications when compared to other IO sites. In fact, the sternal site may offer less opportunity for line entanglement or dislodgement due to its central location on the patient [10]. Absolute contraindications to sternal IO infusion include suspected unhealed sternal fracture or history of surgical sternotomy [15].

Proximal Tibia

The proximal tibia was highlighted as the optimal site for infants and children <5 years old relatively early in the history of intraosseous cannulation, based upon laboratory studies in dogs with results extrapolated to young children [14]. Researchers in the 1940s postulated that since red marrow in the tibia and femur begins its transition to yellow marrow at 5–7 years of age, these locations should not be used after this age [14]. Of course, such theories have subsequently been debunked by decades of clinical evidence. In fact, the proximal tibial IO insertion site remains the most studied and reported in the literature to date.

The ideal proximal tibia IO cannulation site has traditionally been defined as located **1 cm medial and 2 cm inferior to the tibial tuberosity**. If providers have difficulty identifying the tibial tuberosity on obese patients or very small children, they can alternatively use the patella (which may be more easily palpated) as an external landmark. In this case, the ideal insertion site in adult subjects would be 3–4 cm (approximately 2 fingerbreadths) below the inferior margin of the patella. One common mistake made by emergency care providers (and even some instructors on IO device insertion) is to assume that centimeters are equivalent to finger breadths, so that a measurement of 2 cm becomes two fingerbreadths. This is erroneous, and this mistake should be avoided. Given that the average width of an adult human's index finger is 16–20 mm, two finger widths by an adult emergency care provider more closely approximate a distance of 3.2–4.0 cm. **Providers are encouraged to use centimeters (not fingerbreadths) to determine insertion site**, as this error can lead to significant overestimation of distances, especially among pediatric patients [16, 17]. One study predicated upon posthumous radiographic data has suggested that operators should measure the distance from the tibial tuberosity using the width of the *patient's* finger as a guide, to better match the relative proportions of infants and young children [17]. Although this guidance has not been extensively studied or validated, it is likely that the optimal distance from the tibial tuberosity is not the same for adults as it is for small children or infants. More distal placement of the IO catheter relative to the subject's tibial length may result in increased risk of complications due to the smaller diameter of the marrow cavity at the mid-shaft. This could increase the risk of bony fracture, through-and-through penetration, or low infusion flow rates. An illustration of the relevant tibial anatomy, including the optimal insertion site in adult subjects (indicated by the red dot), is provided in Fig. 4.2.

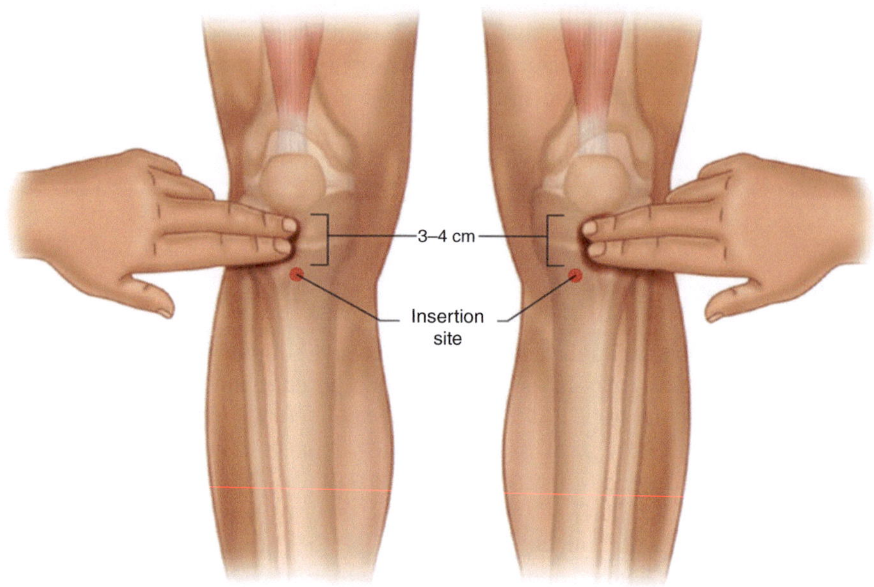

Fig. 4.2 Proximal tibial intraosseous catheter insertion site in adult subjects. *(Image courtesy of Springer Nature. © 2021. All rights reserved* [2]*)*

Figure 4.2 also demonstrates the close proximity of the proximal tibial site to important anatomic structures, including the patella (i.e., knee cap), tibial tuberosity, and knee joint space. Early proponents of IO infusion at the proximal tibia appropriately identified the potential for injury to the **epiphyseal growth plate** in children <17 years old and consequently recommended that IO catheters should be inserted at an angle away from the plate to avoid this theoretical complication. Under austere conditions, especially when using a manual IO catheter designed for adult subjects, this may have been appropriate guidance for the times. However, modern insertion techniques do not include this guidance, and the current recommendation is for insertion **perpendicular to the cortex of the bone**, not at an angle. In fact, angled insertion may actually place the catheter at increased risk of dislodgement due to the effects of gravity and patient movement on the cannula hub. With proper cannulation site identification and insertion technique, this theoretical risk of growth plate injury is greatly minimized, and **no reports of growth plate injury have yet been reported** despite multiple radiographic studies and long-term observational studies in children who received proximal tibial IO infusion [2].

Familiarity with the site, in combination with its relative ease of identification using external anatomic landmarks, makes the proximal tibial site the most popular and most consistently used IO insertion site for most providers. In fact, **first-attempt placement success rate at the proximal tibia site has been shown to be consistently higher than for the proximal humerus site among inexperienced providers** [18]. But this modest increase in catheter placement success must be balanced with substantially lower fluid infusion rates than the sternum or proximal humerus [19, 20]. These lower gravity-driven flow rates may be augmented using higher infusion pressures (e.g., pressure bag, syringe injection), although it remains unknown whether increased infusion pressures can adequately move fluids and medications from distal sites such as the proximal tibia into the central circulation in states of hypotension or cardiac arrest with external chest compressions. Given that CPR generates only very low systemic blood pressure (i.e., one-third of normal intravascular pressures), **shorter distances between the target bone and the central circulation should be favored over longer distances**. Given that IO cannulation is generally reserved for critically ill patients, many of whom are in cardiac arrest, the distal tibia site may perhaps be less clinically useful than its popularity would suggest. Unfortunately, very few studies have compared real-world performance for proximal tibial IO infusion to more central insertion sites such as the proximal humerus, sternum, or clavicle.

Contraindications to the placement of a proximal tibia IO catheter are similar to those associated with other sites, including inability to correctly identify the proper insertion site, bony fracture at or proximal to the target bone, evidence of skin or soft tissue infection at the site, and extremity amputation distal to the site [15]. Additionally, infusion through the peripheral veins of the lower extremity (whether by indirect intraosseous or direct intravenous access) is not generally recommended in hypovolemic states due to likely poor perfusion of the extremity. Complications at the distal tibial site are very well represented in the literature due to its relative popularity, including bone fracture (generally in infants), fluid extravasation, osteomyelitis, compartment syndrome, and limb ischemia [15, 21, 22].

Although the vast majority of the clinical evidence for the use of intraosseous infusion in humans has been accumulated at the proximal tibial site, it remains to be seen whether this site is an optimal (or even preferred) IO infusion site. In cases where a small volume of medication must be administered emergently in a patient with adequate lower extremity perfusion, this site likely performs adequately. However, lingering concerns about the adequacy of venous return from the lower extremities associated with low-flow physiological conditions have led some clinicians to prefer the proximal humerus site. It is likely that a true comparison of the physiological effects of proximal tibial and proximal humeral infusion will only be possible after a critical mass of providers gain experience and comfort with humeral IO infusion.

Distal Femur

The distal femur has been considered by some clinicians to be the site of choice for infants and children less than 5 years old as early as the 1940s and has been used extensively in the pediatric population [3, 4, 14, 22–24]. Its utility appears to be more limited in adults, presumably due to the density of the femur bone, excessive depth of soft tissue overlying the insertion site, and concerns about potential injury to the quadriceps muscles and tendons. However, recent advances in IO device technology, combined with increasing concerns about the use of more distal IO infusion sites, have led to speculation about the potential for increased use of this insertion site among adult subjects.

The recommended femoral IO cannulation site in adults is **2–3 cm proximal to the superior aspect of the patella (or external condyle of the femur) at the long axis midline of the femur** [4, 25]. In infants and children, the recommended cannulation site is **just proximal to the patella (1 cm maximum), approximately 1 cm medial to the midline of the longitudinal axis of the femur** [23]. The rationale for this recommendation to move slightly medial to the midline of the bone seems to be to avoid injury to the quadriceps tendon, a precaution that may be feasible in very small children. In adults, of course, the tendon is much too wide to avoid penetrating. But in children, who have more narrow femurs, this migration to a more medial insertion site may also expose a wider aspect of the distal femur.

Traditionally, some authors have suggested that the catheter should be inserted 10°–30° away from the joint space to reduce the risk of growth plate injuries [25]. However, similar advice was traditionally given for the proximal tibial IO insertion site, and this is no longer commonly recommended when using modern IO devices. Rather, IO cannulae should be inserted perpendicular to the cortex of the bone. In any event, **particular care should be taken to avoid overly distal placement of the catheter**, which could result in injury to the growth plate, patella, or synovial cavity [14]. When attempting to place a distal femoral IO catheter in children, it is important to remember that an angle perpendicular to the bony surface may not also be perpendicular to the stretcher. External rotation of the lower extremity so that the foot is pointing 45° from the plane of the stretcher may help to expose the proper insertion site and facilitate proper placement. With all patients (adult or pediatric), it is important to place the knee in full extension before inserting the catheter, as flexion of the knee during placement will distort the soft tissues and potentially cause additional injury to the tendons and other structures when the knee is subsequently extended.

An illustration of the relevant anatomical structures, including the recommended distal femoral insertion site, is provided in Fig. 4.3. Although the IO catheter in this figure has been rotated medially to allow visualization of the insertion site, the proper angle of insertion is perpendicular to the flat surface of the femoral bone.

The femur generally has the largest medullary cavity of any long bone, providing the largest possible target for an IO cannula. One recent study evaluating success rates for physicians, nurses, and paramedics attempting distal femoral IO catheter placement suggests that operators with a wide range of clinical experience can maintain good control of the depth of penetration and insertion with this approach [24]. In one large study of adult cardiac arrest victims receiving IO catheter placement, the rate of dislodgement was shown to be lower (10%) for femoral IO catheters than for proximal humeral or proximal tibial catheters (both approximately 15%), possibly due to increased density of the femoral cortex in weight-bearing adults [26]. Although limited data are available, complications relating to this insertion site are likely similar to those associated with the use of the proximal humerus or proximal tibia.

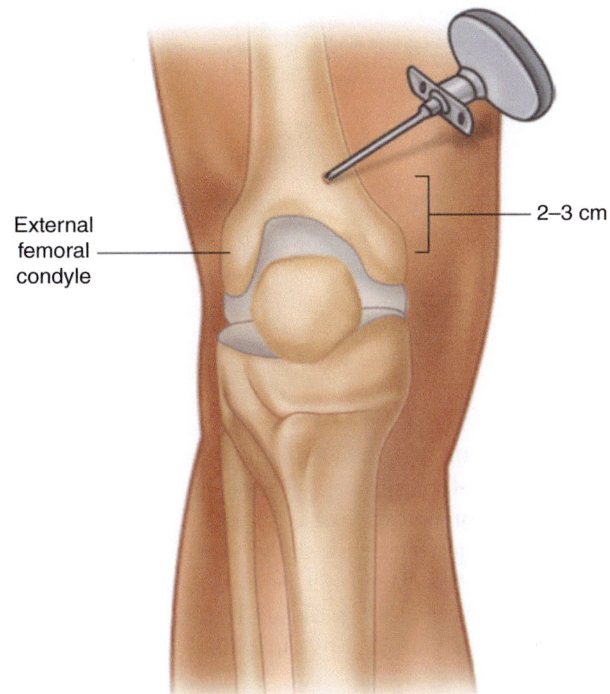

Fig. 4.3 Distal femur intraosseous insertion site (indicated by the red dot), shown in relation to the patella and external femoral condyle. *(Image courtesy of Springer Nature. © 2021. All rights reserved [2])*

Distal Tibia

Given the historic popularity of the proximal tibia as an IO insertion site, the distal tibia has been recommended by some authors as an alternative tibial insertion site. It is currently unknown to what degree venous drainage fields from the proximal tibia and the distal tibia overlap, but it is likely that substances infused into the distal tibia are collected by smaller and more peripheral tributaries than those substances infused via the proximal tibial site. This suggests that the distal tibia may be an inferior option when compared to more proximal sites, but it could be considered when other options are not available.

External landmarks for distal tibial IO cannulation are often easily identifiable, although patients with lower extremity edema or ankle swelling from any cause should probably not be treated with this approach, due to increased risk of soft tissue compression from the catheter hub and/or risk of adjacent venous injury that could worsen local swelling. The recommended insertion site for adult subjects is **2 finger widths (2–3 cm) proximal to the medial malleolus** [18, 27]. In small children (e.g., <40 kg), the recommended insertion site is located 1 finger width (1–2 cm) proximal to the medial malleolus. The provider should notice that the bone is flat at this location, and the catheter should be inserted perpendicular to the surface of the bone. Care should be taken to avoid vascular structures, especially the **greater saphenous vein**, which typically courses just anterior to the insertion site.

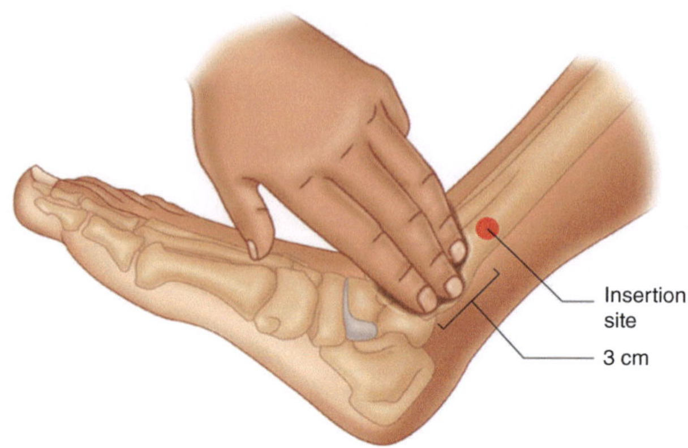

Fig. 4.4 Distal tibial intraosseous insertion site. *(Image courtesy of Springer Nature. © 2021. All rights reserved* [2])

The relevant distal tibial anatomy, including recommended insertion site, is provided in Fig. 4.4.

Studies comparing flow rates through access points at the proximal and distal tibia IO infusion sites have shown significantly faster flow at the proximal site when compared to the distal tibia, both with and without the use of pressure bags [27]. However, flow rates at the distal tibia have generally not been well characterized, as this site is rarely utilized by clinicians.

Proximal Humerus

While the sternal, proximal tibia, femoral (and to a lesser degree distal tibial) IO infusion sites were all described extensively in the early IO literature, infusion via the proximal humerus is a relatively modern approach to this time-honored technique. Anecdotal reports of proximal humeral IO infusion can be found in the medical literature from the mid-2000s, initially in the military arena as a result of overseas conflicts in the Middle East. The use of this site by military personnel in treating victims of blast injuries, often with multiple limb amputations and in a state of hemorrhagic shock, quickly demonstrated its utility in the civilian world for the rapid infusion of fluids, blood products, and medications [15]. Use of this site likely arose out of situational convenience. As injured troops were being removed from casualty scenes in the backs of helicopters, they were often seated, leaning against the helicopter door, with an attendant at their side, where the proximal humerus was easily accessible and not covered by protective gear, unlike the sternal site [15].

During the late 2000s, civilian clinician researchers began to investigate the optimal insertion site, which was ultimately found to be at the anterior aspect of the greater tuberosity of the humerus [15, 16]. It is important to note that this insertion site is not at the "humeral head," despite multiple colloquial references in the medical literature, as the humeral head is actually a point of articulation within the shoulder joint. The recommended insertion site is at the **center of the greater tubercle of the humerus, 1 cm above the surgical neck of the humerus** [15, 18]. This target lies just lateral to the bicipital groove, which contains the biceps brachii tendon and should be avoided. The provider should be able to palpate this groove in most patients, reducing the risk of injury to this tendon with IO catheter insertion. Some manufacturers have suggested that the elbow should be flexed, with the hand placed over the umbilicus during insertion. This maneuver may be helpful in that it internally rotates the humerus to shield the bicipital groove and may enhance exposure to the proper insertion site. However, in the setting of cardiac arrest, an equivalent (and more practical) maneuver would be to extend the elbow and place the hand under the patient's lower back to keep the arm in a secured position during placement.

Although the medullary cavity at the proximal humerus insertion site is quite large, the angle of insertion can be challenging for inexperienced providers and **improper insertion angle is likely a common (and under-recognized) cause of proximal humeral IO catheter failure**. Identifying the proper insertion site on the bone is only half of the guidance needed to ensure proper placement—the angle of insertion is equally important. Some manufacturers endorse a three-dimensional insertion angle in which the needle tip is directed **45° posteriorly from the coronal plane and 45° inferiorly from the axial plane** of the patient. This equates in most subjects to aiming the catheter tip at the inferior angle of the contralateral scapula. As with other IO catheter insertion sites, finding an angle perpendicular to the flat surface of the bone is ideal, but it can be difficult to palpate the direction of this surface in patients with excessive soft tissue depth due to subcutaneous fat or substantial muscle mass.

An illustration of the relevant proximal humerus anatomy, including the recommended insertion site, is provided in Fig. 4.5.

The proximal humerus insertion site is not currently recommended for patients weighing <40 kg, and this site is **not generally used in pediatric subjects** due to concern about excessive insertion depths causing injury to deep structures within or adjacent to the shoulder joint [4]. Excessive depth is not usually a concern with

Fig. 4.5 Proximal humerus anatomy, showing angle of insertion and recommended insertion site. *(Image courtesy of Springer Nature. © 2021. All rights reserved [2])*

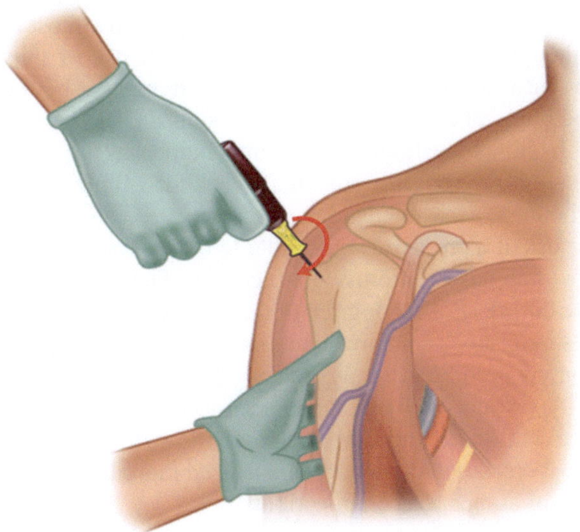

adult subjects, but inadequate depth of insertion is another common cause of IO device failure at this site [4]. Although no reliable guidelines have been established to predict the length of catheter needed to cannulate the proximal humerus site, a 45 mm length cannula is generally preferred at this site, due to the high rate of dislodgement (up to one-third of cases) seen with shorter length devices [4]. Whatever length of cannula is used, optimal placement will result in the catheter flange or hub resting gently at or slightly above the skin surface.

Excessive force or other causes of over-insertion can indent the skin and soft tissues, which produces backward force on the catheter and likely contributes to rapid catheter dislodgement. Researchers have found greater first-attempt success rates and fewer incidences of extravasation with use of a 45 mm catheter when compared to a 25 mm catheter in adult subjects [18]. Excessive arm movement is also known to increase the risk of dislodgement, including raising the patient's arm above their head to facilitate computed tomography (CT) scanning [4].

Recent data suggest that the proximal humerus site may offer a higher infusion rate than the proximal tibia, likely due to a combination of lower intramedullary pressure and closer proximity to the central circulation with enhanced venous drainage [20, 28]. However, first-attempt success rates tend to be higher for proximal tibial IO insertion than for the humeral site, likely due to greater provider familiarity with the insertion technique and difficulties in identifying anatomic landmarks in select patients [28, 29].

Measures have been taken to examine the effects of body mass index (BMI) on first-time humeral IO cannulation success rates, with at least one study showing a slightly higher (though not statistically significant) time to identifying landmarks using ultrasound in patients with higher BMI [28]. In this same study, investigators found that **patients with higher BMIs had landmarks that were still palpable and relatively superficial** [28]. This study also demonstrated the potential use of ultrasound visualization to more consistently identify humeral landmarks without significantly increasing catheter placement times [28].

Use of the proximal humerus site has been almost exclusively reported in adults, although one group did report successful use of this site in a 6-year-old female patient who failed multiple other IO attempts at both proximal tibias, distal femur, and bilateral anterior superior iliac spines [30].

In adults, the humeral site offers numerous advantages, including a fairly central location proximal to potentially wounded limbs, a rapid flow rate, and relatively prominent anatomic landmarks. Flow rates can also be significantly increased with the use of a pressure bag, similar to other favored sites [20]. In fact, the humeral IO flow rate has been proven sufficient to facilitate IO infusion of parenteral contrast dye during a CT angiogram of the chest/abdomen/pelvis in a morbidly obese patient in septic shock, with resultant images comparable to CTs obtained with dye injection via peripheral venous routes [29].

At present, the humeral IO insertion site appears to be safe, effective, and associated with improved flow rates over more distal infusion sites [4]. However, as this site increases in popularity and is used more frequently, additional reports may surface of associated complications.

Less Common Sites

Using the general principles of infusion into the intraosseous space but inspired by less-than-ideal clinical circumstances, clinician-researchers have explored a variety of novel IO insertion sites that are not currently well studied. These include the clavicle, calcaneus, iliac crest, distal radius, and distal ulna. Although these IO infusion sites are just beginning to be explored, they show limited clinical application thus far.

Clavicle

Authors as far back as 1940 have referenced the clavicle as a possible site for intraosseous vascular access, although little research has been done to validate its use [5, 24, 31]. Clinician-researchers postulated that it could be a viable point of access in the event of lower extremity, pelvic, or abdominal trauma, providing an alternate route for near-immediate access to the superior vena cava [19]. It was also thought to be particularly relevant in patients without an available distal access point undergoing cardiopulmonary resuscitation, making the sternum less optimal [19].

The largest study to date assessing clavicular access was published in 1994, reporting 29 adult cases of clavicular cannulation using a manual IO catheter [19]. The authors noted only two instances of failed cannulation, attributed to failure of the manual catheter to penetrate the bony cortex [19]. No significant complications were reported, and flow rate through the clavicle site was found to be comparable to subclavian venous infusion [19]. However, other intraosseous access sites (i.e., the anterior superior iliac spine and proximal tibia) offered faster infusion rates in the same study [19].

The reported site of clavicle cannulation is **just lateral to the sternoclavicular joint, at the horizontal midline of the clavicle** [19]. Although it is classified as a long bone, the clavicle has no marrow cavity. Rather, it is composed of spongy (cancellous) bone with a shell of compact bone. Nonetheless, this spongy bone appears to function similarly to a medullary cavity in its capacity to absorb and transport infusates. An illustration of the relevant clavicle anatomy, including reported IO insertion site, is provided in Fig. 4.6.

In theory, the clavicle could offer the same flow advantages as the sternal or proximal humeral sites, with the additional benefit of being distant from the site of chest compressions. The clavicle is also relatively superficial and readily palpable on most (even very obese) patients. Although no automatic or semiautomatic IO devices have been studied (or reported to have been used clinically) at the clavicular site, manual cannulation appears to be associated with a high first-attempt placement success rate [19]. Additionally, the clavicle offers a potential way to circumvent the theoretical risks of fat or bone marrow emboli with IO infusion [19].

Drawbacks of the clavicle as an IO access point include limited knowledge of possible difficulties that may arise with its use, its close proximity to large vascular

Fig. 4.6 Clavicle intraosseous insertion site, including relevant anatomic structures. *(Image courtesy of Springer Nature. © 2021. All rights reserved [2])*

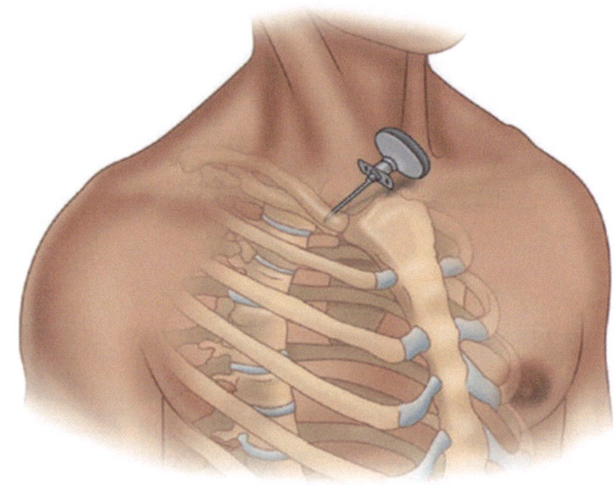

structures (i.e., the subclavian vein and artery), and a thicker bony cortex when compared to the sternum, likely necessitating the use of a thicker and/or harder catheter [19]. These factors may increase the risk of injury to surrounding structures during insertion, including damage to the subclavian vessels or pneumothorax. Use in pediatric patients has not been reported, and therefore its utility in the pediatric population is unknown. Furthermore, no major manufacturers currently endorse the use of their devices at this location.

Calcaneus

The first clinical use of the calcaneus as a point of intraosseous access was reported in 1998, in the treatment of a 3-year-old male with vascular collapse due to meningococcal septicemia [31]. The calcaneus site was selected after multiple previous failed attempts at proximal tibial resulted in multiple bent needles but no successful cannulation. In this case, calcaneus access was successful and proved sufficient for fluid resuscitation, with a flow rate comparable to that expected of a proximal tibia infusion [31]. The authors reported no complications [31].

This case report prompted further investigation into the utility of the calcaneus (as well as other cancellous bones) as an intraosseous access point, refuting the historical assumption that the presence of red marrow was a requirement for successful IO infusion [32]. Subsequent cadaver studies and case reports have confirmed that **the calcaneus may be a viable alternative to more traditional medullary IO infusion sites** [32, 33]. While it is unlikely that IO infusion into cancellous bones will ever replace traditional intramedullary infusion, emergency care providers in the hospital or prehospital setting should consider cancellous bone infusion when the cannulation of traditional bony targets is found to be either unsuccessful or impractical [32].

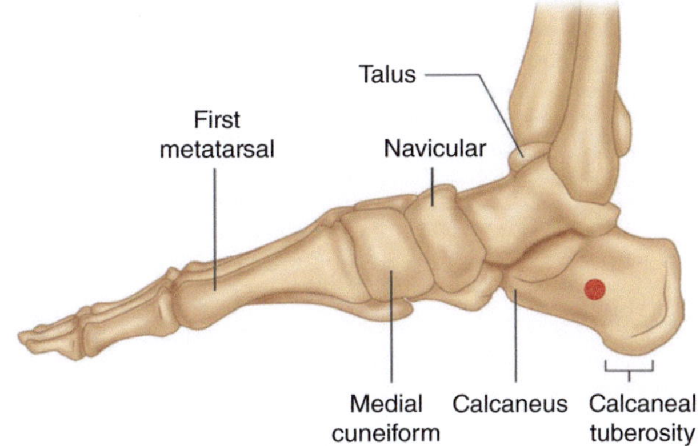

Fig. 4.7 Calcaneus intraosseous insertion site (indicated by the red dot), including relevant anatomy. *(Image courtesy of Springer Nature. © 2021. All rights reserved* [2]*)*

The reported site of calcaneal IO insertion is at the **anterior aspect of the medial process of the calcaneal tuberosity,** corresponding to a location 2 cm from the calcaneal tuberosity on a line between the calcaneal tuberosity and the medial prominence of the first metatarsal [33]. Sufficient care should be taken to avoid the epiphyseal plate posteriorly and the posterior tibial vessels anterosuperiorly [4, 31]. An illustration of the relevant calcaneal anatomy including insertion site is provided in Fig. 4.7.

Iliac Bone

The anterior iliac crest is a common site for intraosseous bone marrow biopsy for the diagnosis of bone marrow disease but has only rarely been used as a means of obtaining emergent vascular access [34, 35]. The **anterior superior iliac spine (ASIS)** is a bony projection of the iliac bone of the pelvis that provides attachment for the inguinal ligament and sartorius muscle. It is the most anterior portion of the iliac crest and is therefore important as an external landmark to aid in iliac IO cannulation. Although various insertion sites have been proposed, one common insertion site appears to be **one-fourth the distance from the ASIS to the posterior superior iliac spine, with the needle angled toward the lower extremity and at an angle of 45° from the long axis of the body** [7]. An illustration of the relevant iliac crest anatomy including insertion site (identified by a red dot) is provided in Fig. 4.8.

At present, iliac IO infusion has been suggested as an alternative technique for patients who have injuries to all four extremities or other contraindications to more commonly used IO infusion sites [35]. One military group has reported the use of iliac IO infusion to treat hemorrhagic shock in the setting of severe trauma with multiple limb amputations [35]. Another study in cardiac arrest victims compared iliac IO infusion at the ASIS to proximal tibial infusion and the clavicle. This comparison study used a manual IO needle, with no reference to the depth of insertion required for any of the sites. However, using a standardized cannula at all sites, they found that the mean infusion flow rate at 80 cm gravity infusion pressure via the

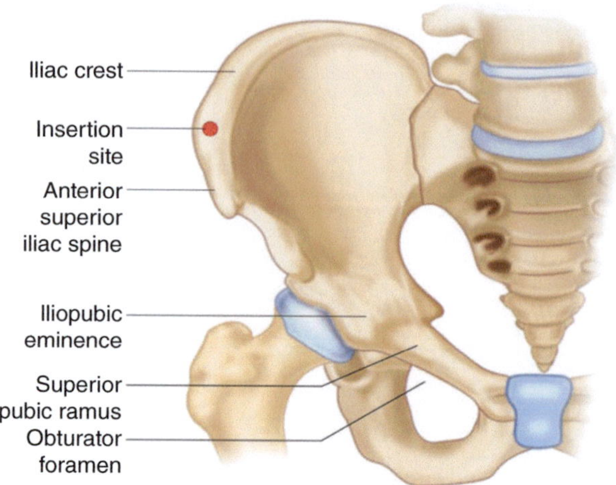

Fig. 4.8 Iliac crest intraosseous insertion site, including reported IO insertion site. *(Image courtesy of Springer Nature. © 2021. All rights reserved* [2])

ASIS (32.2 ± 4.5 mL/kg/h) was higher than subclavian vein infusion (15.2 ± 1.5 mL/kg/h) or IO infusion via the proximal tibia (18.9 ± 1.3 mL/kg/h) or the clavicle (11.9 ± 0.7 mL/kg/h) [19]. This finding is perhaps not surprising considering that the iliac bone is the largest bone in the pelvis and likely provides a large potential reservoir for infusates with exceedingly good venous drainage.

Although various commercial biopsy needles are available for bone marrow extraction at the iliac bone, these catheters tend to be longer (e.g., 68–152 mm) than the IO cannulae commonly used for emergent vascular access (e.g., 25 mm, 45 mm) [36, 37]. The optimal cannula length for iliac bone IO infusion remains unclear, although it seems likely that a 45 mm or 68 mm cannula may be adequate for cannulation of the ASIS in adult subjects. At present, no commercially available IO devices have been endorsed for use in obtaining emergent vascular access at the iliac crest.

Advantages offered by this location include easy identification of bony landmarks, a more central location on the body (which may prevent tangling of lines when the patient is moved), close proximity to the central venous circulation, and potentially higher flow rates than other IO infusion sites [35]. Clearly, use of this site should be avoided in the case of blunt trauma with suspected pelvic fracture [4]. Clinicians may also be concerned about the risk for complete (i.e., through-and-through) penetration through the iliac crest with resultant injury to the deep circumflex iliac artery or other adjacent pelvic structures, although such complications have not yet been reported and are deemed to be unlikely [7, 33].

Radius and Ulna

Given the significant interest in proximal humerus IO infusion that has emerged over the last few decades, it is not surprising that other sites on the upper extremity are currently being considered as well. The most promising of these appear to be the

Fig. 4.9 Distal radius intraosseous catheter insertion site and relevant anatomy. *(Image courtesy of Springer Nature. © 2021. All rights reserved* [2]*)*

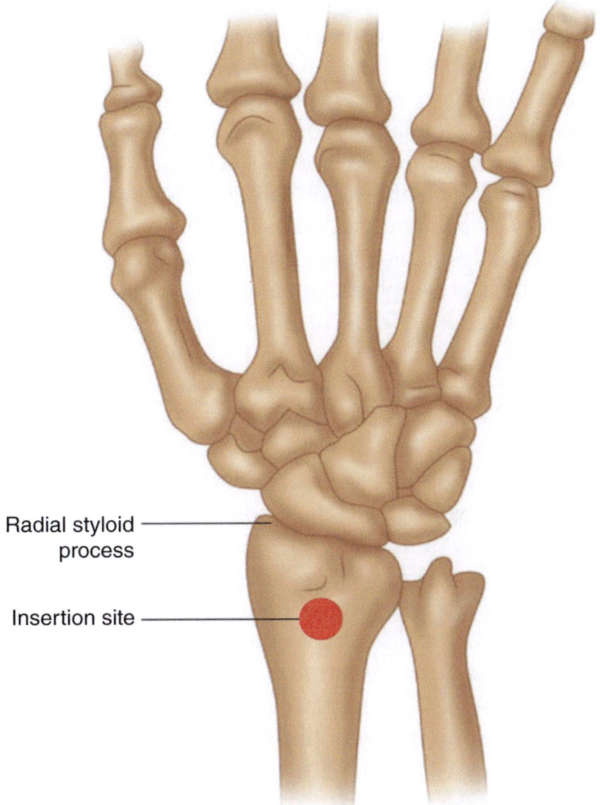

distal radius and distal ulna, as these insertion sites are relatively superficial and may be closer to the central venous circulation than lower extremity sites [38, 39]. Both bones possess a medullary space and are rich with collateral circulation [32, 38]. The proposed insertion site for radial IO infusion is at the **posterior distal metaphysis of the radius, opposite to the radial pulse area** [40]. The recommended depth of IO cannula insertion at the radial styloid is 10–15 mm [40]. An illustration of the relevant distal radius anatomy, including insertion site (identified as a red dot), is provided in Fig. 4.9.

Data on the use of IO infusion at the distal radius and distal ulna remain extremely limited. One study conducted in 1995 in a canine model suggested that the distal radial metaphysis and the distal ulnar metaphysis may be optimal IO infusion sites [39]; a subsequent trial by the same group involving 12 patients undergoing orthopedic surgery reported 100% success at cannulation with no observed complications [40]. Another cadaveric study of the radial site enrolling only two subjects (i.e., four radial IO insertions) showed that half of the attempted radial IO infusions were unsuccessful due to reflux of the contrast agent back through the insertion site around the sides of the catheter [32].

Although IO cannulation of the distal radius has been described, **experimental or clinical use of the distal ulna site remains theoretical**. These sites have not yet received much attention beyond preclinical studies, and clinicians may be hesitant to use them due to concerns about the potential for neurovascular injury (e.g., radial/ulnar arteries, radial/ulnar nerves), injury to the wrist joint, or complications relating to extravasation and infection. The radius and ulna may also be more difficult to immobilize than the more central insertion sites, especially in awake patients. Despite these limitations, bolus IO infusion of fluids at the radius or ulna may serve to potentially engorge more proximal veins of the upper extremity, facilitating subsequent direct peripheral or central venous cannulation, although such techniques remain unreported in the medical literature.

General Considerations

Intraosseous vascular access is clearly a valuable technique for the resuscitation of critically ill patients, and the modern emergency care provider is able to select from a wide variety of insertion sites and devices. However, each of these sites is associated with its own specific advantages and disadvantages. Thus, a systematic approach to IO catheter insertion site selection may be of use.

Once the provider has determined that IO catheter placement is clinically indicated, it is important to consider which insertion sites will facilitate optimal management of the patient. The provider should consider **which IO devices are available in their immediate environment**, recognizing that certain devices may be designed for use at a specific site. For example, in the civilian arena, the FAST-1® (First Access for Shock and Trauma) (Teleflex, Inc.) device is indicated only for sternal IO infusion and is the only civilian device currently marketed for this infusion site. While manually placed catheters may be used at any site, **automatic spring-driven devices may be preferred in larger bones** with less risk of iatrogenic fracture or over-penetration. Cannulation of delicate bones may require semiautomatic devices, which allow greater user control over catheter direction and force during the insertion attempt. Thus, the availability of specific IO devices may exert considerable influence over a provider's site selection.

Providers should also consider which sites they have significant experience with, as **the probability of successful placement is likely to be improved at sites familiar to the user**. When forced to decide between multiple sites with a similar risk-benefit profile, providers should prioritize those sites that they are most competent to access. Once they have exhausted familiar sites, it may be appropriate to consider other sites that are more unfamiliar.

High-volume fluid boluses may require pressurized infusion (e.g., pressure bag, syringe injection), as well as a high capacity for infusate within the medullary space. Although reports of flow rates available at different sites vary, it is generally known that under the same infusion pressure, **larger target bones (e.g., proximal humerus, femur, iliac crest) and bones closer to the chest (e.g., sternum, clavicle) are associated with higher rates of flow** than smaller and more distal targets. That said, more distal targets (e.g., proximal tibia, distal tibia, radius, ulna) may be more than adequate to permit medication infusion or even small boluses in patients with uncompromised systemic blood pressures.

Prevention of dislodgement is of paramount importance to successful use of the IO technique, as IO line failure can lead to a wide variety of therapeutic mishaps, including failure of medication infusion, extravasation, and compartment syndrome, among others. For this reason, the clinician should consider how well the IO catheter can be stabilized during subsequent care and transport and avoid the placement of lines in locations that increase the likelihood of dislodgement. Target sites such as the distal femur, proximal tibia, sternum, and clavicle are not likely to be affected by patient movement; more distal sites may be at greater risk of accidental (or intentional) dislodgement by an awake (and potentially agitated) patient. Immobilization of the insertion site should be considered whenever possible. For example, excessive movement of the shoulder (including lifting the arm above the head for CT imaging studies) will greatly increase the chance of proximal humeral IO catheter dislodgement.

Absolute or relative contraindications to IO catheter placement at specific sites should also be considered, and providers should be familiar with such restrictions before attempting placement. In patients with known or suspected trauma, great care should be taken to identify any fractured bones or large hematomas suggesting that indirect venous access at or distal to the injury site may be suboptimal. Significant swelling of the soft tissues overlying a proposed insertion site may suggest poor venous circulation, occult trauma, or other pathology that may complicate therapy. Evidence of previous orthopedic surgery, such as scars at or near a proposed insertion site, may rule out certain sites as well. Patient anatomy is another important consideration, as proper identification of external anatomic landmarks is essential to proper IO device insertion. **Any deformity of the surrounding anatomy or excessive soft tissue making proper landmark identification impossible should be considered to be a contraindication to selection of the proposed target bone**.

When an initial IO cannulation attempt fails, providers should attempt to determine whether or not the bone has been perforated during the failed attempt. It is **currently recommended that IO cannulation not be performed on the same target bone more than once**, as holes in the bony cortex from previous failed attempts may provide an outlet for extravasation of infusate delivered via the successfully placed IO device. Various time frames have been suggested (e.g., 24–48 h) after which time subsequent IO placement in the same bone may be attempted, but these recommendations are anecdotal and no clinical evidence exists to support them.

Conclusion

Modern emergency care providers have a wide variety of options to consider when selecting an optimal IO insertion site for their patient. While all IO infusion sites share certain characteristics common to this technique, each site has its own specific advantages and disadvantages. Providers should consider multiple factors when selecting an insertion site, including site-specific, patient-specific, and device-specific factors. Although the proximal tibial site is among the oldest and best characterized, use of this site may be suboptimal due to its distance from the central circulation. The proximal humerus site appears to be an optimal IO site for patients with hemodynamic instability, but many providers appear to be unfamiliar with this technique and it has only recently become the subject of significant study. The sternal site is readily accessible and has a favorable clinical profile, but its use is limited by the inability to use most commercially available IO devices at this site. The distal femur site is currently available for pediatric indications, but is not well studied in adult patients. The distal tibial site is mentioned occasionally in clinical reports, but appears to be very uncommonly used other than extreme circumstances when other sites are not available. Recent reports of infusion via flat cancellous bones such as the clavicle and the calcaneus have suggested that a discrete medullary cavity may not be required to facilitate IO infusion. Some sites, including the clavicle, iliac crest, distal radius, and distal ulna, have been used clinically but remain poorly described in the medical literature. As the vast majority of IO device deployments reported in the medical literature have been completed at the proximal tibial site, further study is needed to determine whether the efficacy and safety profiles of IO infusion at these other sites are comparable.

Key Concepts

- The proximal tibial, distal femoral, and sternal IO infusion sites were historically the first cannulation sites utilized by clinician-scientists. Since then, many other IO infusion sites have been described in the medical literature, each with its own distinct advantages and disadvantages.
- The identification of an optimal IO catheter insertion site is dependent upon many factors, including the patient's age and medical condition, accessibility of the proposed site, evidence of orthopedic injury or prior surgery, ability to identify external landmarks, and provider experience with the site.
- The proximal tibia is the most common IO infusion target, but the distal location of this site limits its utility in the setting of compromised blood flow to the lower extremities, as seen with profound hypotension or while receiving external chest compressions.
- The highest IO flow rates have been shown to be associated with the iliac, sternal, and proximal humerus infusion sites. Of these, the proximal humerus appears to be the best studied.

References

1. Burgert JM. A primer on intraosseous access: history, clinical considerations, and current devices. Am J Disaster Med. 2016;11(3):167–73.
2. Kenney C, Paxton JH. Chapter 7. Intraosseous catheters. In: Paxton JH, editor. Emergent vascular access: a guide for healthcare professionals. Basel, Switzerland: Springer Nature; 2021. p. 133–75.
3. Jaimovich DG, Kecskes S. Intraosseous infusion: a re-discovered procedure as an alternative for pediatric vascular access. Indian J Pediatr. 1991;58:329–34.
4. Paxton JH. Intraosseous vascular access: a review. Trauma. 2012;14(3):195–232.
5. Tocantins LM, O'Neill JF. Infusion of blood and other fluids into the circulation via the bone marrow. Proc Soc Exp Biol Med. 1940;45:782–3.
6. Bailey H. Bone marrow as a site for the reception of infusions, transfusion, and anaesthetic agents: a review of the present position. Br Med J. 1944;1:181–2.
7. Tarrow AB, Turkel H, Thompson MS. Infusions via the bone marrow and biopsy of the bone and bone marrow. Anesthesiology. 1952;13(5):501–9.
8. Tocantins LM, O'Neill JF, Jones HW. Infusions of blood and other fluids via the bone marrow. JAMA. 1941;117(15):1229–34.
9. Tocantins LM, O'Neill JF, Price AH. Infusions of blood and other fluids via the bone marrow in traumatic shock and other forms of peripheral circulatory failure. Ann Surg. 1941;114:1085–92.
10. Laney JA, Friedman J, Fisher AD. Sternal intraosseous devices: review of the literature. West J Emerg Med. 2021;22(3):690–5.
11. Hoskins SL, Kramer GC, Stephens CT, Zachariah BS. Efficacy of epinephrine delivery via the intraosseous humeral head route during CPR. Circulation. 2006;114(18):1204.
12. Miller L, Kramer GC, Bolleter S. Rescue access made easy: intraosseous infusion, once limited to use on children, is now becoming a reliable access site for adults. JEMS. 2005:8–19.
13. Bewick VJ, Mersh RJ. Intraosseous cannulation in children. Anaesth Intensive Care Med. 2020;21(12):630–3.
14. Tocantins LM, O'Neill JF. Complications of intra-osseous therapy. AnnSurg. 1945;122(2):266–77.
15. Rush S, D'Amore J, Boccio E. A review of the evolution of intraosseous access in tactical settings and a feasibility study of a human cadaver model for a humeral head approach. Mil Med. 2014;179(8):24–8.
16. Hopp AC, Long JR, Fox MG, Flug JA. Iatrogenic humeral anatomic neck fracture after intraosseous vascular access. Skel Radiol. 2020;49:1481–5.
17. Capobianco S, Weiss M, Schraner T, Stimec J, Neuhaus K, Neuhaus D. Checking the basis of intraosseous access: radiological study on tibial dimensions in the pediatric population. Ped Anesthesia. 2020;30:1116–23.
18. Petitpas F, Guenezan J, Vendeuvre T, Scepi M, Oriot D, Mimoz O. Use of intra-osseous access in adults: a systematic review. Crit Care. 2016;20:102–10.
19. Iwama H, Katsumi A, Shinohara K, Kawamae K, Ohtomo Y, Akama Y, Tase C, Okuaki A. Clavicular approach to intraosseous infusion in adults. Fukushima J Med Sci. 1994;40(1):1–8.
20. Ong MEH, Chan YH, Oh JJ, Ngo AS. An observational, prospective study comparing tibial and humeral intraosseous access using the EZ-IO. Am J Emerg Med. 2009;27(1):8–15.
21. Palazzolo A, Akers KG, Paxton JH. Complications of intraosseous catheterization in adult patients: a review of the literature. Curr Emerg Hosp Med Rep. 2023;11:35–48. https://doi.org/10.1007/s40138-023-00261-8.
22. Bouhamdan J, Polsinelli G, Akers KG, Paxton JH. A systematic review of complications from pediatric intraosseous cannulation. Curr Emerg Hosp Med Rep. 2022;10:116–24. https://doi.org/10.1007/s40138-022-00256-x.
23. Eifinger F, Scaal M, Wehrle L, Maushake S, Fuchs Z, Koerber F. Finding alternative sites for intraosseous infusions in newborns. Resuscitation. 2021;163:57–63.

24. Truemper EJ, Beamer CL, Miller LJ, Montez DF, Puga TA, Bolleter S, Philbeck TE. Distal femur site is a viable option for IO vascular access in pediatric patients. Ann Emerg Med. 2012;60(4S):S90.
25. Fiser DH. Intraosseous infusion. N Engl J Med. 1990;322(22):1579–81.
26. Rayas EG, Winckler C, Bolleter S, Stringfellow M, Miramontes D, Shumaker J, Lewis A, Wampler D. Distal femur versus humeral or tibial IO, access in adult out of hospital cardiac resuscitation. Resuscitation. 2022;170:11–6.
27. Tan BKK, Chong S, Koh ZX, Ong MEH. EZ-IO in the ED: an observational, prospective study comparing flow rates with proximal and distal tibia intraosseous access in adults. Am J Emerg Med. 2012;30:1602–6.
28. Bustamante S, Bajracharya GR, Cheruku S, Leung S, Mao G, Singh A, Mamoun N. Point-of-care ultrasound to identify landmarks of the proximal humerus: potential use for intraosseous vascular access. J Ultrasound Med. 2021;40(4):725–30.
29. Budach NM, Niehues SM. CT angiography of the chest and abdomen in an emergency patient via humeral intraosseous access. Emerg Radiol. 2017;24:105–8.
30. Ozturk G, Balaban B, Kendirli T. Is humerus a good choice for intraosseous access during fluid resuscitation in a child with severe septic shock? Turk Arch Pediatr. 2022;57(2):237–8.
31. McCarthy G, Buss P. The calcaneum as a site for intraosseous infusion. J Accid Emerg Med. 1998;15:421.
32. McCarthy G, O'Donnell C, O'Brien M. Successful intraosseous infusion in the critically ill patient does not require a medullary cavity. Resuscitation. 2003;56:183–6.
33. Clem M, Tierney P. Intraosseous infusions via the calcaneus. Resuscitation. 2004;62:107–12.
34. Lavis M. Pre-hospital adult intraosseous infusion. Pre-hosp Immed Care. 1999;3:89–92.
35. Fulghum G, Gravano B, Foudriat A, Rush S, Paladino L. Prehospital iliac crest intraosseous whole blood infusion. J Spec Oper Med. 2021;21(4):90–3.
36. Reed LJ, Raghupathy R, Strakhan M, Philbeck TE, Kim MY, Battini R, Hussain Z, Abdullah S, Schweber S, Bala K, Pacello T. The OnControl bone marrow biopsy technique is superior to the standard manual technique for hematologists-in-training: a prospective, randomized comparison. Hematol Rep. 2011;3(3):e21. https://doi.org/10.4081/hr.2011.e21. Epub 2011 Oct 25.
37. Paxton JH, Knuth TE, Klausner HA. Proximal humerus intraosseous infusion: a preferred emergency venous access. J Trauma. 2009;67(3):606–11. https://doi.org/10.1097/TA.0b013e3181b16f42.
38. Matthew MK, Hausman MR. Surgical approaches from the angiosomal perspective. Chapter 9. In: Slutsky DJ, Osterman AL, editors. Fractures and injuries of the distal radius and carpus: the cutting edge. Philadelphia: Saunders; 2009. p. 103–23.
39. Waisman M, Roffman M, Bursztein S, Heifetz M. Intraosseous regional anesthesia as an alternative to intravenous regional anesthesia. J Trauma. 1995;39(6):1153–6. https://doi.org/10.1097/00005373-199512000-00025.
40. Waisman M, Waisman D. Bone marrow infusion in adults. J Trauma. 1997;42(2):288–93.

Manual Intraosseous Devices

5

David Greiver, Sarah Chung, and James H. Paxton

Introduction

Manual intraosseous (IO) catheters greatly predated modern automatic and semiautomatic devices and were the only means of accessing the bone marrow space for the first 60 years of clinical use for this technique. Although they have been largely supplanted by newer technologies, manual catheters continue to be valued in austere environments due to their portability and versatility of use. This chapter describes the history of manual IO infusion devices, including more recent additions to the field.

On the most basic level, a manual IO catheter consists of a **handle** to guide insertion (removed after successful placement), a surgical steel **cannula** used for infusion, a sharpened **stylet** (i.e., obturator) to facilitate penetration of the bone and prevent blockage of the cannula during insertion, and a **hub connector** to allow attachment of infusion tubing to the cannula. While early models were often made of surgical steel and reusable, modern manual IO catheters are invariably disposable single-use devices.

Manual IO Devices

In the earliest days of IO vascular access, providers utilized existing needle devices to access the intramedullary space, primarily stainless steel hypodermic needles and lumbar puncture needles. One of the first devices designed specifically for IO access was the Witts sternal puncture needle, introduced by British hematologist **John**

D. Greiver (✉) · S. Chung · J. H. Paxton
Department of Emergency Medicine, Wayne State University School of Medicine, Detroit, MI, USA
e-mail: david.greiver@wayne.edu; sarah.chung2@med.wayne.edu; james.paxton@wayne.edu

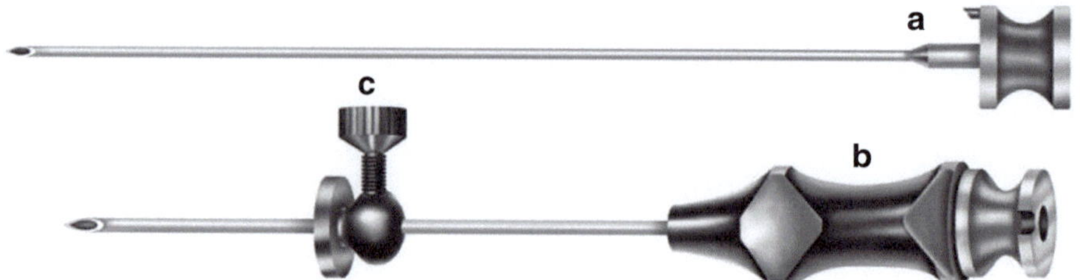

Fig. 5.1 Witts lumbar puncture needle, including internal stylet (**a**), infusion needle (**b**), and adjustable guard (**c**) [1]

Leslie Witts at St. Bartholomew's Hospital (London) during the mid-1930s [1]. Lumbar puncture needles had been in use since the 1890s to access cerebrospinal fluid within the subarachnoid space [2], and catheters like the Witts needle were modeled on their design. The Witts needle included an internal stylet, infusion needle, and adjustable guard (Fig. 5.1). The adjustable guard was considered to be an essential and distinguishing feature of the device, as it helped to prevent over-insertion of the device [1].

As the procedure became more common, providers began experimenting with modification of existing needle types and even developed their own manual IO devices. Device improvements were generally intended to make the procedure safer and more successful; consequently, the use of standard hypodermic needles gradually fell out of favor as it was felt to increase the risk of sternal perforation and other complications [3].

American physician Leandro Tocantins was one of the first clinician-researchers to report his own design of an intraosseous infusion catheter [4]. Tocantins' three-part device, initially used for sternal infusion, consisted of a 15-gauge needle surrounding an 18-gauge hollow trephine needle with beveled stylet. After the device was inserted into the sternum, the stylet was removed and bone marrow was aspirated through the 18-gauge trephine needle, which was also subsequently removed. The remaining 15-gauge outer needle was then used to infuse fluids or medication via a customized infusion apparatus [4]. Using this system (Fig. 5.2), blood or other fluids were "pulled" into the syringe through a two-way stopper and then subsequently "pushed" forward into the patient under syringe pressure.

Tocantins' dual-needle design was endorsed by the anesthesiologist Emmanuel Papper, who was a vocal advocate for the use of IO infusions during World War II [5]. This needle was ultimately adopted by the US National Research Council and became standard issue for American combat medics throughout World War II [6].

Inspired by Tocantins' needle design, Henry Turkel and Frank Bethell developed their own "new and simple instrument for administration of fluids through the bone marrow," first reported in 1944 [7, 8]. The Turkel device similarly employed two (14 gauge outer, 17 gauge inner) needles, each with its own internal stylet. The outer needle featured a hub which could be connected to infusion tubing. A slot in the outer needle was aligned with a projection on the side of the stylet, ensuring that the

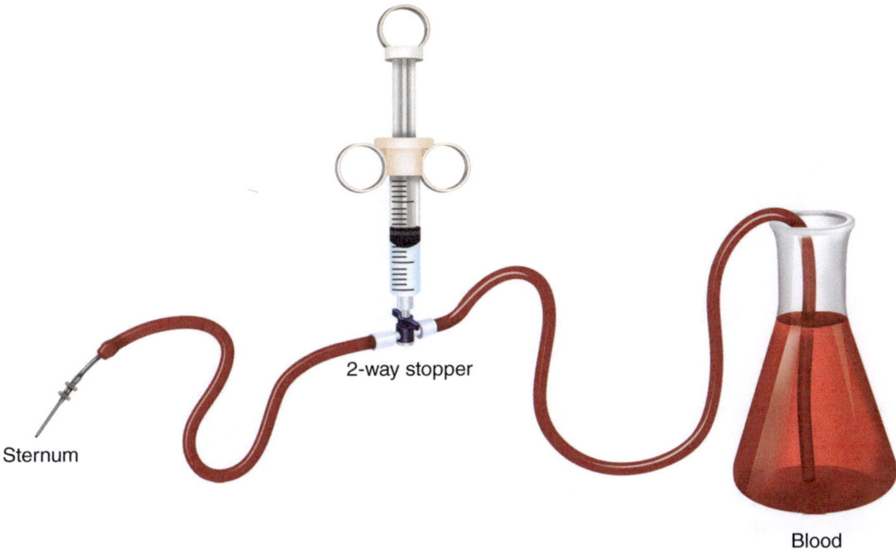

Fig. 5.2 Tocantins' push-pull system for IO infusion [4]

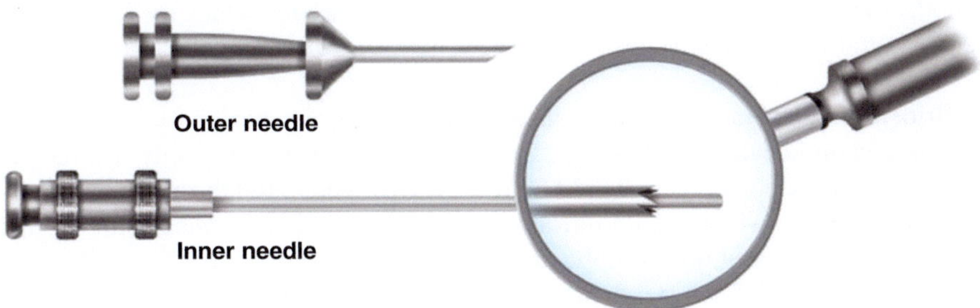

Fig. 5.3 The Turkel Trephine Instrument [8]

point of the needle would remain aligned with the stylet tip during insertion. Once the outer needle and stylet were introduced, the stylet was removed and the inner (cutting) needle with its own stylet was inserted inside the outer needle cannula. The inner needle tip projected 6 mm past the end of the outer needle, with four sharp sawlike cutting teeth at its tip. The inner surface of this tip was cone-shaped, intended to trap bony material from the anterior lamella of the sternum, which would be retained within the inner needle upon removal. Thus, the Turkel needle permitted both bone marrow sampling and subsequent IO infusion. Of note, the stylet of the inner needle was made to be slightly longer than the shaft, reducing the risk that the cutting tip would be bent with insertion. The Turkel system also included a "right-angle observation tube," supplying a low-profile attachment between the infusion tubing and the outer needle (Fig. 5.3).

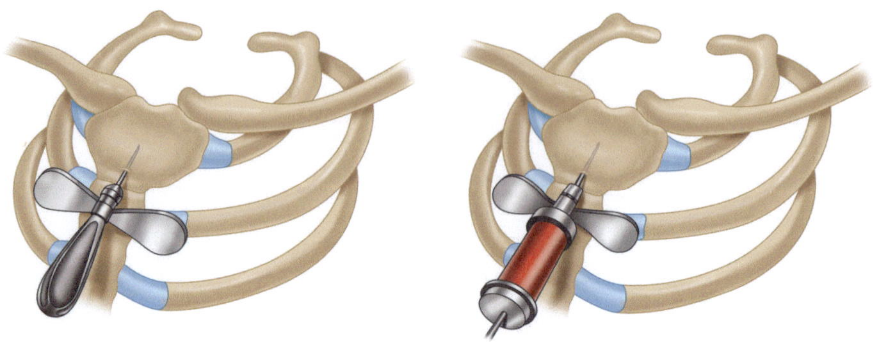

Fig. 5.4 Bailey's winged catheter design [9]

Turkel and Bethell believed that the use of their catheter would reduce the risk of certain complications attributable to "uncontrollable force," including over-penetration of the needle into the mediastinum and shattering of the anterior lamella, producing bony fragments that might occlude the needle, promote clot formation, and compromise flow. Their design was also expected to reduce the risk of needle dislodgement, as the inner needle created a pilot hole through which the larger outer needle could be gently advanced without excessive rocking or manipulation of the device [7].

British surgeon Hamilton Bailey also introduced his own design for a manual IO sternal puncture device in 1944 (Fig. 5.4). Bailey claimed that the only real danger of sternal intraosseous access would be if the device punctured through both plates of the manubrium which would introduce fluid into the superior mediastinum, and he had reportedly seen this complication occur in his own practice. To combat this danger, Bailey modified a standard 15-gauge Witts needle to add "wings" designed to limit the needle's depth of penetration. Bailey felt that this device provided a "foolproof" way to safely access the sternal bone marrow cavity [9]. After placement, the wings were taped to the patient's chest to further secure the device [9].

While the manual IO devices used by Bailey, Tocantins, and Turkel were designed for use at the sternum in adult patients, several physicians at the time were skeptical of sternal punctures, especially among pediatric patients. These concerns were fueled by anecdotal reports of death attributed to sternal puncture, including two adult deaths reported from India in 1947 [10]. In the first case, a guarded needle was used by an experienced physician to perform the procedure. However, the patient immediately went into shock upon needle insertion and was declared dead 3 min later. Autopsy revealed a miniscule puncture through the posterior plate of the sternum, producing a 3/4 in. laceration on the right ventricle, which was determined to be the cause of the patient's death. The patient in the second case died under similar circumstances after the needle punctured the posterior plate of the sternum producing a 7/8 in. laceration to the right ventricle. In both cases, the needle length was believed to be too short to have reached the right ventricle under normal

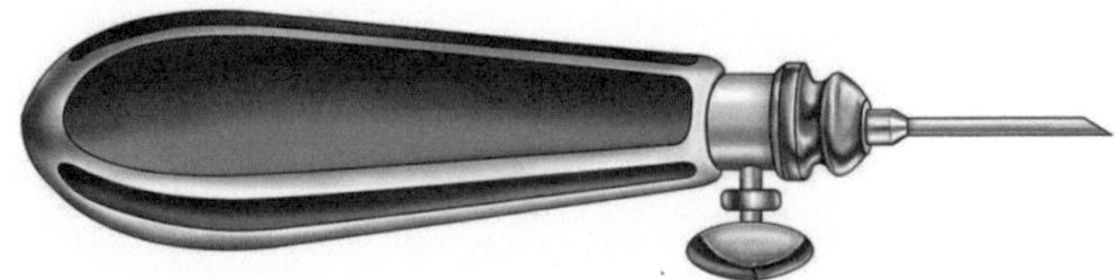

Fig. 5.5 The Gimson needle [12]

circumstances. However, it was concluded that the patients held their breath in response to the anxiety induced by the sternal puncture, which increased CO_2 tension on the heart, resulting in an outward expansion of the ventricles into the needle tip [10]. The report of these two deaths, as well as a handful of other anecdotal reports, further inspired clinicians to seek out a safer site for manual IO device insertion.

Gerhard Behr, a British pathologist, was among those who argued for a proximal tibial site of infusion in children. However, Behr found that sustained pressure from the wings of Bailey's catheter caused excess pressure on the delicate skin of pediatric subjects. After 2 days of insertion, one of his pediatric patients developed skin necrosis in the area under the wings. Such experiences led Behr to propose the use of a "naked" needle (i.e., without wings) at the proximal tibial site, which he found to be sufficiently stable without exerting undue pressure on the patient's skin [11].

As the proximal tibial IO infusion site began to gain traction among pediatric subjects, new manual IO devices continued to appear. British pediatrician Janet Gimson proposed her own design for an IO catheter for tibial IO access in pediatric patients (Fig. 5.5). Gimson's device consisted of a lighter needle, with four different options of needle length: 1/4 in. for premature infants and neonates, as well as 3/8, 1/2, and 5/8 in. lengths for children 5 years or older. The Gimson device was composed of a single needle with a stylet, as well as an immovable flange which limited movement of the needle once the device had been inserted into the bone. Its adapter was set at a right angle to reduce kinking and excessive pull on the attached tubing [12].

The earliest IO devices were also used as bone marrow biopsy needles, developed primarily by hematologists for use with bone marrow aspiration. The most popular of these sternal IO biopsy needles during the 1930s appears to have been the Klima-Rosegger needle developed circa 1935 and the Salah needle, both of which featured an adjustable guard to prevent over-penetration [13]. These needles are depicted in Fig. 5.6.

The therapeutic use of IO infusion to treat non-hematological disorders fell out of favor in the 1950s, leading to a relative lull in English-language reports of novel manual IO devices during the decades that followed. But with the resurgence of interest in IO infusion during the mid-1980s, new catheter designs began to appear again.

In 1971, Iranian hematologist Khosrow Jamshidi patented a new needle specifically designed for bone marrow biopsy [14]. This needle was unique in that its interior was tapered distally towards a non-serrated cutting end, allowing a precisely cut bone specimen to enter the needle easily while minimizing damage to the surrounding soft tissues and preventing occlusion of the needle (Fig. 5.7).

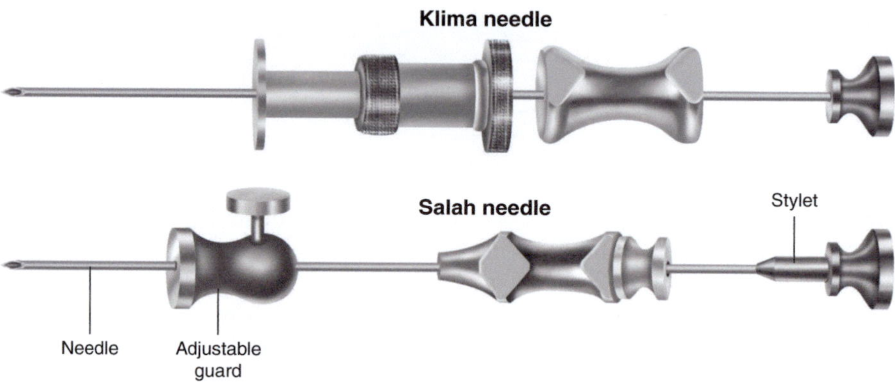

Fig. 5.6 Klima and Salah needles [13]

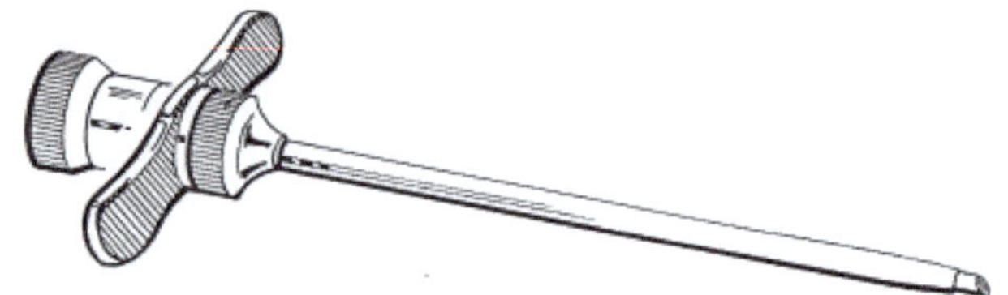

Fig. 5.7 Jamshidi™ needle for iliac crest biopsy. *(Image courtesy of Becton, Dickson and Company. © 2023 Becton, Dickson and Company. All rights reserved)*

The Jamshidi™ needle is currently available in two versions from Becton, Dickinson and Company (Franklin Lakes, NJ): the original Jamshidi™ and the T-handle model (Fig. 5.8). The original device featured a razor-sharp bevel tip and a tapered distal tip, ranging in diameter from 8 to 13 gauge and in length from 50 to 152 mm. The T-handle Jamshidi™ is of similar length but contains a two-piece T-handle which provides additional tactile feedback and increased control, as well as a trocar-tapered stylet point and triple-crown cannula tip. This modified design is reported to result in superior cortical penetration, with 25% less force required for insertion compared to the original model.

In 1986, Kenneth Iserson and Elizabeth Criss compared ease of IO insertion on pediatric cadaver legs using standard metal needles, standard bone marrow biopsy needles, and 13-gauge Jamshidi™ needle. They found that the Jamshidi™ needle was the easiest to insert and was consistently placed successfully on the first attempt. Also, unlike the other needles, the Jamshidi™ needle never bent or became plugged during attempted insertions [15]. These advantages led to rapid acceptance of the Jamshidi™ needle by both emergency and pediatric clinicians during the 1980s [16].

The modern Jamshidi™ needle typically used for sternal IO infusion is disposable and much shorter than the model used for iliac crest biopsy. The Illinois lancet tip modification, introduced in 1988 with the Monoject® Illinois Needle (Sherwood Medical, St. Louis, Missouri), was later incorporated into the Jamshidi™ Illinois needle (Becton, Dickinson and Company, Franklin Lakes, NJ) (Fig. 5.9). The blue

Fig. 5.8 Original
Jamshidi™ (left) and
T-handle Jamshidi™
disposable IO catheters,
indicated for biopsy at the
iliac crest *(Images courtesy
of Becton, Dickson and
Company. © 2023 Becton,
Dickson and Company. All
rights reserved)*

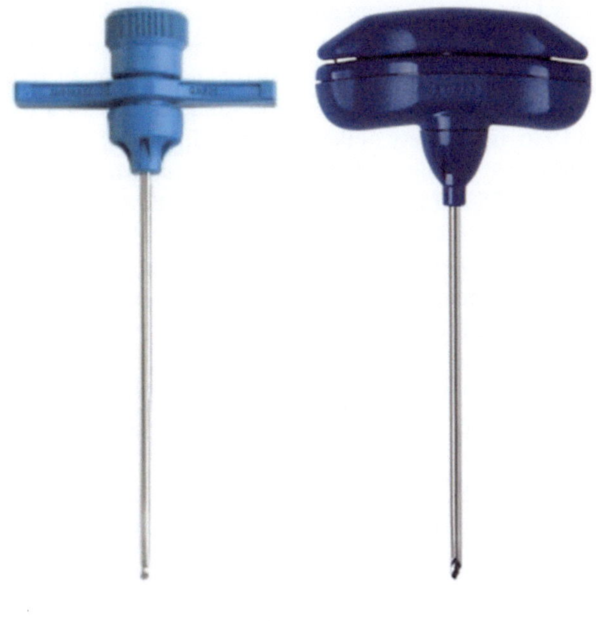

Fig. 5.9 Jamshidi™
modified Illinois
disposable needle,
indicated for sternal or
pediatric use *(Image
courtesy of Becton,
Dickson and Company. ©
2023 Becton, Dickson and
Company. All rights
reserved)*

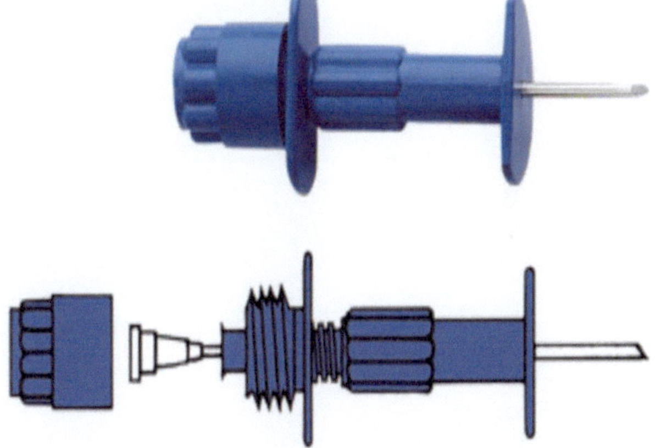

plastic hub of this needle sticks out about 2 inches from the surface of the skin after insertion, which is felt by some users to increase the risk of accidental dislodgement.

The Monoject™ Illinois Sternal-Iliac Needle (Cardinal Health, Dublin, Ohio) is 16 gauge in diameter with a lancet tip and an adjustable depth guard, permitting a range of insertion depths from 5 to 48 mm. The device also features a locking nut allowing for precise control over the depth of insertion and is marketed for both sternal and iliac crest insertion. This needle also has two versions: original and T-handle. The original model was available in two sizes: 18 gauge (with an adjustable length of 14–38 mm) and 15 gauge (24–48 mm). It has an adjustable depth guard for patient safety and a sharp lancet point for bone penetration. The T-handle model is also available in 15- and 18-gauge versions. This needle features a depth stop that is recommended for sternal use but can be removed for iliac crest insertion.

Cook Medical (Bloomington, Indiana) released the Cook intraosseous catheter in 1986, in a variety of designs, including a 45° trocar, 35° lancet, or pencil point tip. The Cook needle is currently available in a range of gauges (14–18 gauge) and lengths (25–40 mm). There have been three versions of this needle: the standard model, the Dieckmann modification, and the Sussmane-Raszynski design. The Cook IO catheter with Dieckmann™ modification includes two opposing side ports positioned near the distal tip of the catheter to ensure proper flow even when the tip is obstructed (Fig. 5.10).

The Sussmane-Raszynski design included a brass hub and base plate, a stylet with a trocar bevel (45° angle), and a cannula shaft with a fine needle screw design to prevent dislodgement of the needle cannula (Fig. 5.11).

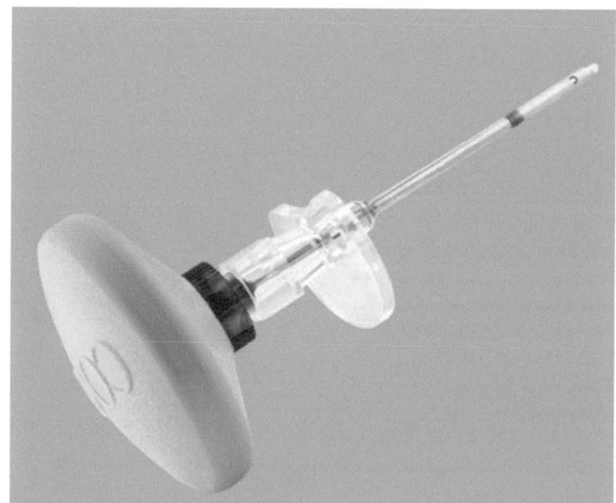

Fig. 5.10 Cook manual IO needle with Dieckmann™ modification *(Image courtesy of Cook Medical. © 2023 Cook Medical. All rights reserved)*

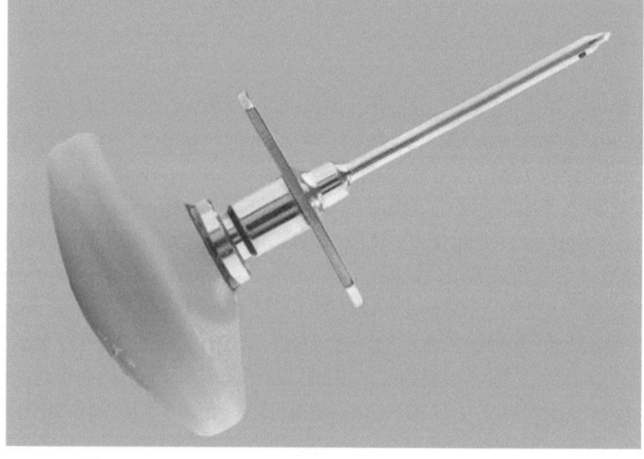

Fig. 5.11 Sussmane-Raszynski™ needle. *(Image courtesy of Cook Medical. © 2023 Cook Medical. All rights reserved)*

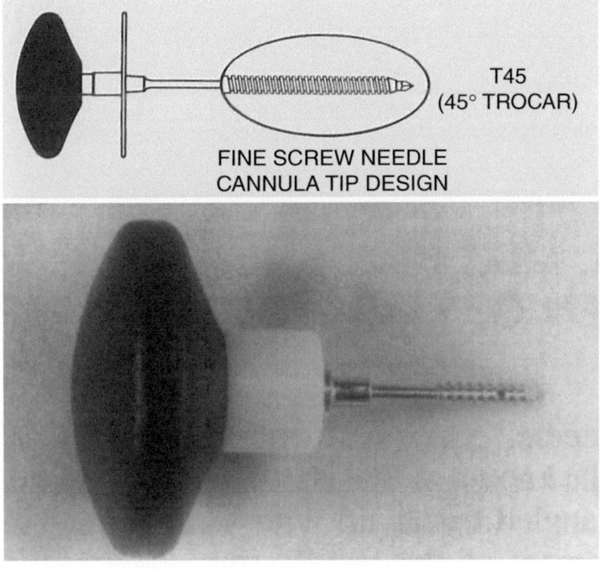

Fig. 5.12 Sur-Fast™ needle. *(Images courtesy of Cook Medical. © 2023 Cook Medical. All rights reserved)*

In 1998, a study by Brunhild Halm and Loren Yamamoto compared the efficacy of the Jamshidi vs. the Dieckmann Modified Cook Needle for IO infusion. The study reported that the Jamshidi needle took less time to insert and was easier to use than the Dieckmann [17].

The Sur-Fast™ needle was patented by Cook in 1996, featuring an angled trocar tip and screw threading along the length of the cannula to facilitate advancement of the needle through clockwise rotation (Fig. 5.12). However, a scalpel skin incision was recommended before accessing the bone, which complicated the insertion process. The needle's screw design allowed for an easy removal through a counter-clockwise rotation of the device [18]. One study completed in 2000 found the Sur-Fast™ to be more difficult to use and no more effective than a standard Jamshidi™ needle for obtaining IO vascular access [19]. This device is no longer commercially available.

The FAST-1® (First Access for Shock and Trauma) intraosseous infusion system, originally introduced by Pyng Medical (Vancouver, Canada) in 1998, was the first new sternal IO catheter to appear on the market in over a decade (Fig. 5.13). Pyng Medical led the early development of adult IO catheters during the 1990s. In its earliest days, Pyng had considered licensing the Sternal Access Vascular Entry (SAVE) manual IO infusion device from the US Army and University of California, which featured a self-tapping screw and stabilization features to prevent over-advancement. Ultimately, they found that a novel approach was needed, leading to the development of the FAST-1® system.

The FAST-1® device is placed manually, inserted by continuous manual pressure (approximately 8.5 kg of force) on the sternum with an array of ten stabilizer needles and a central infusion catheter [20]. The FAST-1® contains a target patch, intended to facilitate proper insertion at a site 1.5 cm below the sternal

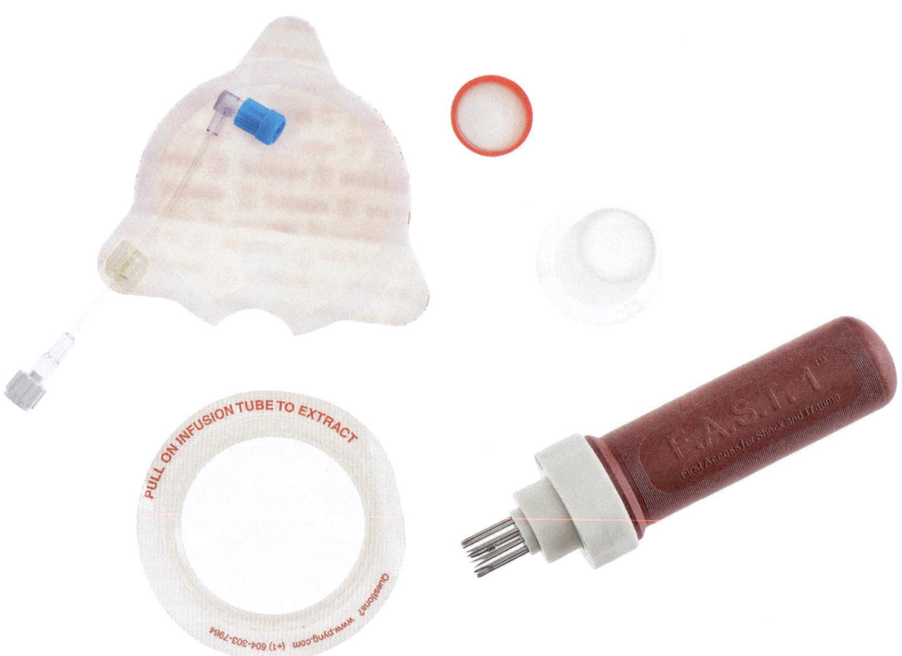

Fig. 5.13 The FAST-1® intraosseous system. *(Image courtesy of Teleflex Incorporated. © 2023 Teleflex Incorporated. All rights reserved)*

notch. The unit's introducer complex contains a "bone cluster" of stabilizing needles, which form a circle around the central infusion tip. This bone cluster of needles is pressed firmly against the manubrium, triggering the release of a spring-loaded inner needle with metal tip attached to a flexible infusion tube. This infusion tip advances exactly 5 mm beyond the stabilizing needles, positioning it firmly in the bone marrow. The remainder of the device is then withdrawn, leaving only the inner infusion needle and its associated tubing. The earliest version of the FAST-1® device required a separate threaded tip removal tool [18], but this extraction device is no longer required or suggested for removal of the device. This device has been extremely popular in the US military, with Army combat medics receiving training on use of the FAST-1® in the battlefield [21]. One early clinical report on the first 50 uses of this device demonstrated a 78% first-attempt placement success rate, with no complications noted on up to 2-month follow-up [22].

The FAST-Responder® (Fig. 5.14) introduced by Pyng Medical in 2014, the FAST Tactical®, and the FastX® were short-lived variants of the FAST-1® device that were ultimately phased out after Teleflex acquired Pyng in 2017. The FAST-Responder® incorporated an integral adhesive insertion template, which was intended to add stability to the device. As a result, fewer stabilizing needles were required. Also, the FAST-R could be removed without the need for a removal tool [23].

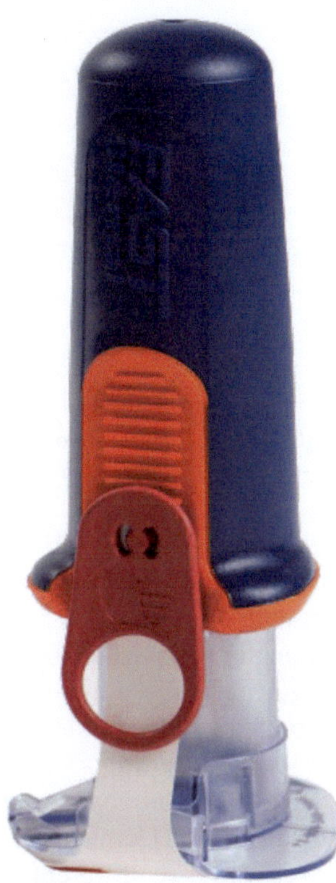

Fig. 5.14 The FAST-Responder®. *(Image courtesy of Teleflex Incorporated. © 2023 Teleflex Incorporated. All rights reserved)*

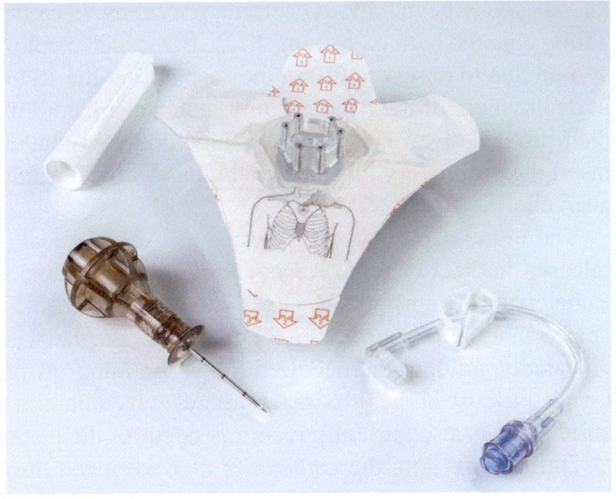

Fig. 5.15 The TALON™ device. *(Image courtesy of Teleflex Incorporated. © 2023 Teleflex Incorporated. All rights reserved)*

In 2013, Vidacare launched its Tactically Advanced Lifesaving Intraosseous Needle (TALON™) device (Fig. 5.15), a manually inserted alternative to the EZ-IO® line. As a manually inserted device, the TALON™ was FDA cleared for sternal

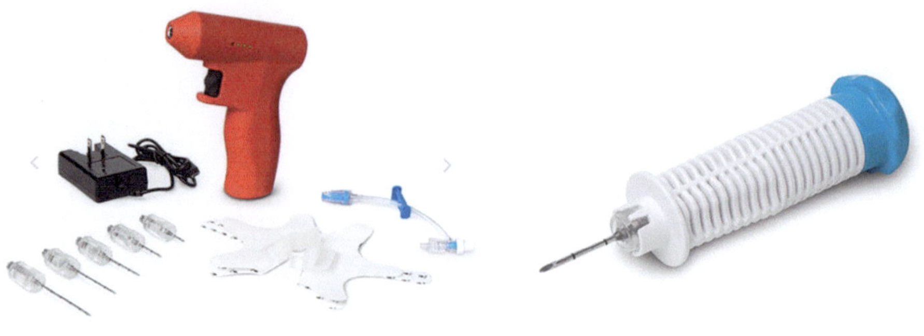

Fig. 5.16 The BD™ Intraosseous Powered Driver (left) and manual driver (right). *(Images courtesy of Becton, Dickson and Company. © 2023 Becton, Dickson and Company. All rights reserved)*

insertion (unlike the drill-assisted EZ-IO®) allowing providers in austere military environments more versatility in site selection. This catheter is 15 gauge in diameter, with a length of 38.5 mm. A similar product, the Manual EZ-IO® catheter, was originally released in 2005 featuring 25 mm and 15 mm lengths, but the device was lengthened to 38.5 mm in 2019. Unlike the TALON™, which is more expensive and marketed strictly to the military for clinical use, the manual EZ-IO® is not cleared for sternal insertion.

The BD™ Intraosseous Powered Driver (Fig. 5.16) was introduced by Becton, Dickinson and Company (Franklin Lakes, NJ) in 2020, including a battery-powered driver and five different lengths of IO catheter (15, 25, 35, 45, and 55 mm). According to the manufacturer, the driver can be recharged to last 12× longer than the non-rechargeable EZ-IO® driver, providing 70 catheter insertions at 10 s each on a fully charged battery. In June 2022, BD issued a voluntary recall notice for this IO system due to observed difficulties separating the stylet from the IO needle, failure in deployment of the needle safety mechanism, and difficulties separating the needle from the driver. This system did include a manual driver, which could be used to insert the proprietary IO catheters by hand when the battery-powered driver was not available.

The Intraosseous Access System by SAM Medical (SAM IO) is a newer device, released in 2021. The IO Access System kit contains a driver; 15, 25, and 45 mm catheters; an extension set; and a safety cap (Fig. 5.17). The driver is a handheld device that creates a rotational spin of the needle when its trigger is compressed repeatedly, guiding the needle through the bone. At present, this device is recommended for use at the proximal humerus, proximal tibia, and distal tibia in adults or children. It is also currently recommended for the distal femur of pediatric patients.

During insertion, the catheter is first advanced through the skin and other soft tissues of the patient until the catheter tip contacts the bone surface. Once the needle reaches cortical bone, the trigger is compressed repeatedly while applying a gentle

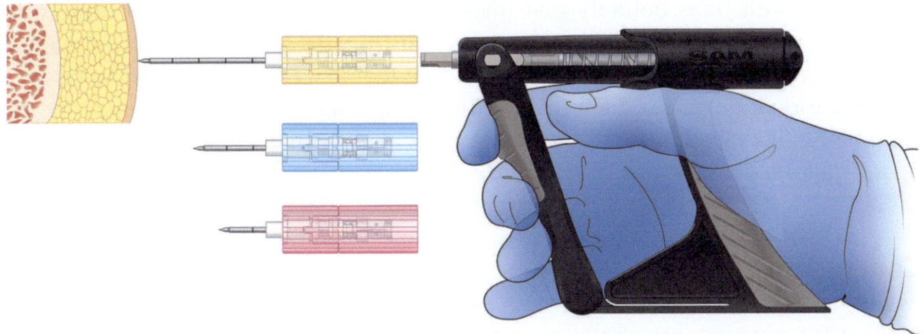

Fig. 5.17 SAM IO® Intraosseous system. *(Images courtesy of SAM Medical. © 2023 SAM Medical. All rights reserved)*

steady downward pressure to achieve entry into the marrow space. The mechanical rotation of the needle should be the primary mechanism to penetrate the bone, rather than the force of the downward pressure. A sudden release of tension indicates entry into the medullary space, at which point the stylet is removed along with the driver. The stabilizing adhesive device is then placed around the catheter, the cannula is connected to the extension tubing, and infusion is initiated. This system also includes an adapter facilitating the insertion of EZ-IO® catheters with the SAM manual driver.

General Considerations

Manual IO catheters were once the standard of care for IO infusions, but have been largely supplanted by modern automatic and semiautomatic devices. The primary advantages of manual IO devices are their portability and lack of reliance upon battery-operated drivers or other adjunct technology. Manual IO catheters are the "go-to" IO line for emergency care providers operating in the most austere of environments, including military personnel. That said, these catheters are most useful for adult patients when used at the sternal insertion site, as the sternum consists of a relatively soft bony cortex with minimal overlying soft tissue. These catheters are also highly effective for pediatric resuscitation, as they allow precise control over the depth of insertion and do not appear to be associated with a significant risk of bony fracture or other complications due to excessive force of insertion or over-penetration of the target bone.

In the more dense bones of adult subjects, manual IO catheters appear to be sub-optimal. Modern providers appear to prefer automatic or semiautomatic IO devices over manual devices in the treatment of adult subjects and possibly among pediatric subjects as well. It is unlikely that manually inserted IO devices will ever completely disappear from the market, but it is clear from the relative absence of manual IO catheter reports in the modern IO literature that newer technologies are favored over traditional devices. Many manual IO devices have been discontinued by the major IO catheter manufacturers, presumably due to increased competition from nonmanual IO devices.

Conclusion

Manual IO catheters have been used for most of the last century to cannulate the softer bones of adult subjects (e.g., sternum) and the commonly accessed bones of pediatric subjects (e.g., distal femur, proximal tibia, distal tibia). While it is unlikely that manually driven IO catheters will ever regain their once prominent position in the realm of intraosseous infusion, they will likely remain an important part of the armamentarium of emergency care providers in the most austere environments, including military applications.

Key Concepts
- The earliest manual IO infusion devices were modeled upon previously available vascular access devices, including steel peripheral intravenous access needles and lumbar puncture needles.
- The earliest manual IO devices relied entirely upon direct manual force to push the sharpened tip of the catheter through the cortical bone and into the medullary space. This technique was ideal for softer bones, such as those seen with pediatric patients and at the adult sternum, but made cannulating denser bones quite challenging.
- Over the last century, many different manual IO devices have been developed with myriad design variations intended to facilitate placement and infusion. Production of most novel catheter designs has been discontinued, leaving only a few traditional designs available for clinical use by the modern provider.
- Modern manual IO catheters feature stronger steel cannulae, larger handles, and other technological improvements intended to increase user control over the insertion process and to facilitate device deployment at sites with thicker bony cortices.
- The primary advantages of manual IO devices are their portability and ability to be used under austere conditions that may make the use of automatic or semiautomatic devices less desirable.

References

1. Napier LE, Gupta PC. Sternum puncture: the findings in normal Indians. Ind Med Gaz. 1938;73(1):1–7.
2. Calthorpe N. The history of spinal needles: getting to the point. Anaesthesia. 2004;59(12):1231–41. https://doi.org/10.1111/j.1365-2044.2004.03976.x.

3. Turkel H. Deaths following sternal puncture. AMA Arch Surg. 1956;73(1):183–4. https://doi. org/10.1001/archsurg.1956.01280010185025.
4. Tocantins LM, O'Neill JF, Price AH. Infusions of blood and other fluids via the bone marrow in traumatic shock and other forms of peripheral circulatory failure. Ann Surg. 1941;114(6):1085–92. https://doi.org/10.1097/00000658-194112000-00015.
5. Papper EM, Rovenstine EA. Utility of marrow cavity of sternum for paternal fluid therapy. War Med. 1942;2:277–83.
6. Paxton JH. Intraosseous vascular access: a review. Trauma. 2012;14(3):195–232.
7. Turkel H, Bethell FH. A new and simple instrument for administration of fluids through bone marrow. War Med. 1944;5:222–5.
8. Tarrow AB, Turkel H, Thompson MS. Infusions via the bone marrow and biopsy of the bone and bone marrow. Anesthesiology. 1952;13(5):501–9. https://doi.org/10.109 7/00000542195209000-00007.
9. Bailey H. Bone marrow as a site for the reception of infusions, transfusions, and anesthetic agents. Br Med J. 1944;1:181–2.
10. Bardhan PN. A medical misadventure—death from sternal puncture. Ind Med Gaz. 1947;82(8):459–61.
11. Behr G. Bone-marrow infusions. Br Med J. 1944;1(4338):305.
12. Gimson JD. Bone-marrow transfusion in infants and children. Introducing a specially designed needle. Br Med J. 1944;1(4352):748–9.
13. Klima R, Rosegger H. Zur methodik der diagnostschen sternalpunktion. Klinische Woechenschrift [German]. 1935;14:541–2.
14. Jamshidi K, Windschitl HE, Swaim WR. A new biopsy needle for bone marrow. Eur J Haematol. 1971;8(1):69–71.
15. Iserson KV, Criss E. Intraosseous infusions: a usable technique. Am J Emerg Med. 1986;4(6):540–2. https://doi.org/10.1016/S0735-6757(86)80014-6.
16. Shaltot A, Michell PA, Betts JA, Darby AJ, Gishen P. Jamshidi needle biopsy of bone lesions. Clin Radiol. 1982;33(2):193–6. https://doi.org/10.1016/s0009-9260(82)80061-5.
17. Halm B, Yamamoto LG. Comparing ease of intraosseous needle placement: Jamshidi versus cook. Am J Emerg Med. 1998;16(4):420–1. https://doi.org/10.1016/s0735-6757(98)90146-2.
18. Calkins MD, Fitzgerald G, Bentley TB, Burris D. Intraosseous infusion devices: a comparison for potential use in special operations. J Trauma. 2000;48(6):1068–74. https://doi. org/10.1097/00005373-200006000-00012.
19. Jun H, Haruyama AZ, Chang KS, Yamamoto LG. Comparison of a new screw-tipped intraosseous needle versus a standard bone marrow aspiration needle for infusion. Am J Emerg Med. 2000;18(2):135–9. https://doi.org/10.1016/s0735-6757(00)90003-2.
20. Johnson DL, Findlay J, Macnab AJ, Susak L. Cadaver testing to validate design criteria of an adult intraosseous infusion system. Mil Med. 2005;170(3):251–7. https://doi.org/10.7205/ milmed.170.3.251.
21. Gendron B, Cronin A, Monti J, Brigg A. Military medic performance with employment of a commercial intraosseous infusion device: a randomized, crossover study. Mil Med. 2018;183(5–6):e216–22. https://doi.org/10.1093/milmed/usx078.
22. Macnab A, Christenson J, Findlay J, Horwood B, Johnson D, Jones L, et al. A new system for sternal intraosseous infusion in adults. Prehosp Emerg Care. 2000;4(2):173–7.
23. Burgert JM. A primer on intraosseous access: history, clinical considerations, and current devices. Am J Disaster Med. 2016;11(3):167–73. https://doi.org/10.5055/ajdm.2016.0236.

Automatic and Semiautomatic Devices

6

Parker J. Marsh and James H. Paxton

Introduction

Over the last few decades, manually inserted intraosseous (IO) catheters have been largely supplanted by mechanically assisted insertion devices. Unlike manual IO trocars, which depend upon the provider pushing or twisting the trocar through the soft tissues and into the bony cortex of the target bone, automatic and semiautomatic devices **utilize force derived from springs** (in the case of automatic devices) or **internal motors** (with semiautomatic devices) to drive the trocar into position. The advent of these devices has allowed IO devices to be more easily inserted in the harder, more dense bones of adult subjects. In many ways, the development of these technologies has reinvigorated the use of IO devices for critically ill patients, especially adults and larger children. Despite these advances, the Advanced Trauma Life Support (ATLS) guidelines state that the IO route should only be used in adults after three unsuccessful peripheral intravenous (PIV) access attempts or 2 min of failed attempted PIV insertions [1].

For the purposes of this chapter, we have defined **automatic** intraosseous devices as those devices that **do not require additional direction by the provider after the insertion mechanism is triggered**. It is understood that these devices still require significant user interaction to place and situate the device properly prior to deployment, in addition to constant firm pressure to avoid recoil and resultant misplacement. **Automatic** devices are typically driven into the bone by a tension-loaded spring, which is released when the trigger is activated. Once triggered, the trocar is automatically delivered into position through the bony cortex without the need for additional effort on the part of the provider. These devices are designed to deliver a

P. J. Marsh (✉) · J. H. Paxton
Department of Emergency Medicine, Wayne State University School of Medicine, Detroit, MI, USA
e-mail: parker.marsh@med.wayne.edu; james.paxton@wayne.edu

© The Author(s), under exclusive license to Springer Nature Switzerland AG 2024
J. H. Paxton (ed.), *Intraosseous Vascular Access*,
https://doi.org/10.1007/978-3-031-61201-5_6

preset amount of force when triggered, and the amount of force delivered may vary according to the specific model being utilized. In contrast, **semiautomatic** intraosseous devices augment the provider's ability to insert the trocar but still rely upon the provider to provide continuous guidance and direction to the trocar throughout the process of penetrating the soft tissues and bone. These semiautomatic devices typically utilize a motorized driver unit to "drill" the catheter into place, allowing the provider continuous control over the direction and depth of insertion even after the mechanism has been triggered.

This chapter describes the automatic and semiautomatic IO devices currently available to providers, including insight into the historical development of these devices, their relative advantages and disadvantages, and special considerations for their use. We will also discuss likely directions of future use and study for these devices.

Automatic Devices

The Bone Injection Gun (BIG)

The first commercially available automatic intraosseous vascular access device was the Bone Injection Gun (BIG®), developed by WaisMed Medical (West Hempstead, NY) in 1998. This device was initially FDA approved for use at the proximal tibia in adults (in 1998) and children (in 2002), with its indication expanded to include the proximal humerus site for adults in 2006. WaisMed was subsequently acquired by PerSys Medical (founded as Performance Systems (Houston, TX)) in 2014.

The BIG® intraosseous catheter is a single-use, disposable spring-loaded device, available in both 15-gauge (adult) and 18-gauge (pediatric) sizes [2]. The device consists of a safety latch, a housing shaft containing the cannula and tension-loaded spring, and a plastic barrel protecting the catheter (Fig. 6.1). The pediatric BIG® device is recommended for children 0–12 years of age or a tissue depth range of

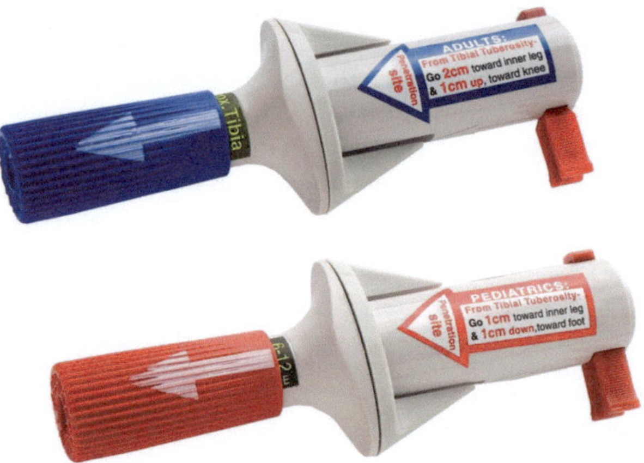

Fig. 6.1 The Bone Injection Gun® (BIG) adult (blue) and pediatric (red) devices. (*Image courtesy of Safeguard Medical. © 2023 Safeguard Medical. All rights reserved*)

0.5–1.5 cm for use at the proximal tibial insertion site. The depth of penetration can be adjusted as needed (according to the patient's age, weight, and tissue thickness) by twisting the barrel in a clockwise direction and similarly retracted by rotating the device in a counterclockwise manner. The depth of insertion is labeled on the barrel. Standard manufacturer-recommended depths are as follows: ages 0–3 years old (0.5–1.0 cm), 3–6 years old (1.0–1.5 cm), and 6–12 years old (1.5 cm) [2].

Placement starts by applying the device perpendicularly to the proposed injection site, keeping the safety latch in place (Fig. 6.2). The safety latch is then pinched and removed from the device once the device has been secured with the nondominant hand. The provider then places the palm of their dominant hand on top of the device, with two fingers surrounding the wings. The spring-loaded deployment mechanism can then be activated. Once the catheter is in place, the internal trocar is gently removed and the red safety latch is used to secure the cannula in place. This device does not require significant pressure to be applied by the user, other than the minimal force needed to keep the device stable and perpendicular to the target bone during the insertion process.

The BIG® is spring loaded rather than battery powered and therefore is a very mobile device (weighing less than 3 ounces) that can be carried without fear of battery depletion or energy source availability [3]. The manufacturer-estimated shelf life of this device is 5 years.

Results from the first clinical trial of the BIG® were reported by Waisman in 1997 [4]. In this study, 76% (38/50) of subjects received device placement at the proximal tibia, while the remainder received infusion at other sites (i.e., medial malleolus, lateral malleolus, distal radius). The authors reported a 100% success rate for device placement, with no observed complications. Further reports in a novice manikin trial reported successful deployment in 91.6% of cases [5].

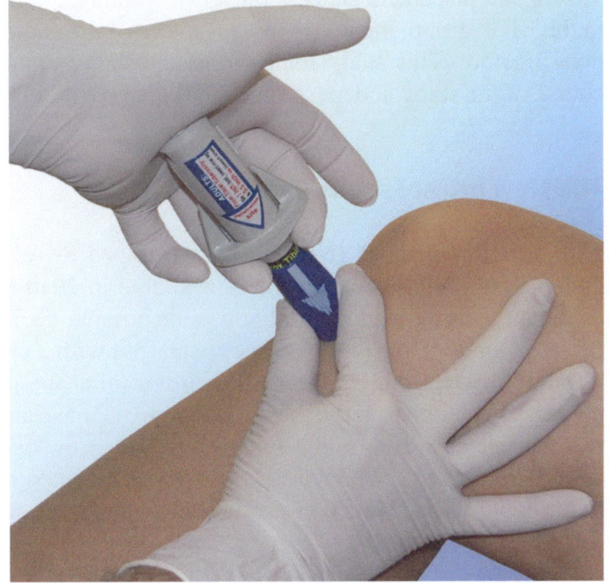

Fig. 6.2 Deployment of the adult Bone Injection Gun (BIG) device at the proximal tibia. *(Image courtesy of Safeguard Medical. © 2023 Safeguard Medical. All rights reserved)*

The BIG® was further studied in a canine model with successful placement in 83% of subjects, with an average time to placement of 22.4 ± 8.2 s [6]. Another study comparing the BIG® to Jamshidi™ manual IO (Baxter Healthcare Corp, Deerfield, Illinois) in a pediatric manikin model found BIG® placement to be significantly faster (11.93 vs. 16.91 s; $p = 0.02$) than use of the manual IO device [7].

But the BIG® does not always perform as favorably against other automatic or semiautomatic devices. Ramirez et al. conducted a prospective crossover study including 40 paramedics comparing the BIG® to the NIO-P™. Successful intraosseous placement was obtained in 95% of cases using the BIG® and 100% of cases using the NIO-P™. The reported T1 (i.e., time from device acquisition to device deployment) was significantly faster with the NIO-P™ than with the BIG® (5.4 ± 3.5 s vs. 3.5 ± 2.5 s; $p = 0.014$). Additionally, the mean T3 time (i.e., time from acquisition to aspiration and tubing connected) was also found to be faster with the NIO-P™ (11.5 ± 2.5 vs. 25 ± 5.5 s; $p < 0.001$) [1].

Leidel et al. studied 40 adults during resuscitation efforts comparing the BIG® and EZ-IO® [8]. They found a first-placement-attempt success rate of 80% with the BIG® and 90% with the EZ-IO®. Additionally, the mean time of the procedure was 2.2 min ± 1.0 for the BIG® versus 1.8 min ± 0.9 for the EZ-IO® [8]. The two most common complications reported in this study were the stylet becoming stuck in the bone and failure to penetrate the cortex of the bone during attempted insertion. These manikin studies were then supplemented by a more robust helicopter emergency medical service (HEMS) retrospective study. The BIG®, EZ-IO®, and two manual IO devices (i.e., FAST1™, Jamshidi™) were compared during adult and pediatric resuscitations. In this study, 70 patients underwent 78 insertion attempts. Rates of first-attempt success were significantly higher in the EZ-IO® group compared to the manual devices and the BIG® ($p < 0.01/p < 0.001$). All three modern devices (BIG®, EZ-IO®, and FAST1™) had comparable complication rates, ease of use scores, and placement success rates [9]. Notably, three mechanical errors occurred in the BIG® group, including two instances of the catheter bending and one case of bone fracture. This study found consistent failure rates from 43 to 50% over the course of the study, independent of the care provider [10].

The New Intraosseous (NIO)

The New Intraosseous (NIO™) was developed by WaisMed Medical (Yokneam, Israel) and was first commercially available in 2014 [2]. The NIO™ device is an automatic (spring-loaded), single-use, disposable device that is available in adult, pediatric, and infant sizes. It comes packaged with a catheter, stylet, and stabilizer. The NIO™ is currently approved for insertion at the proximal tibia and proximal humerus [11]. Importantly, these devices do not have an exposed catheter tip, which enhances device safety and is intended to reduce the risk of needlestick injuries and infections. Once the desired depth has been selected based upon the specific soft tissue depth at the planned insertion site, the device is activated by a twist-to-unlock handle, placed perpendicular to the bone surface, and deployed by activating the spring mechanism. The manufacturer reports a 5-year shelf life for this device.

The NIO Adult™ catheter features a 15-gauge cannula with a penetration depth of 25 mm and effective needle length of 42 mm (Fig. 6.3). The device weighs 3.5 oz. (100 g).

In 2017, Shina and colleagues reported the results of a study analyzing 50 medical students (mean age 21.7 years) without prior knowledge of IO devices comparing attempted IO cannulation of a porcine hind leg using the EZ-IO® and NIO™ devices. They found a success rate of 92% (46/50) for the NIO™ and 88% (44/50) for the EZ-IO®, but the difference was deemed to be statistically insignificant [12]. Reported complications included two NIO™ catheters that were not properly fixed in the bone, resulting in failure of spring release. In one case, the student accidentally removed the NIO™ catheter while attempting to extract the stylet. Finally, the authors reported a single case of inability to attach the syringe to the catheter hub [12]. The authors also reported complications associated with the EZ-IO® device, including three cases of catheter removal during attempted stylet extraction, two cases of inappropriate insertion angle (i.e., not 90 degrees from the bone surface) with failure to penetrate the bone marrow cavity, and one case of inability to remove the stylet.

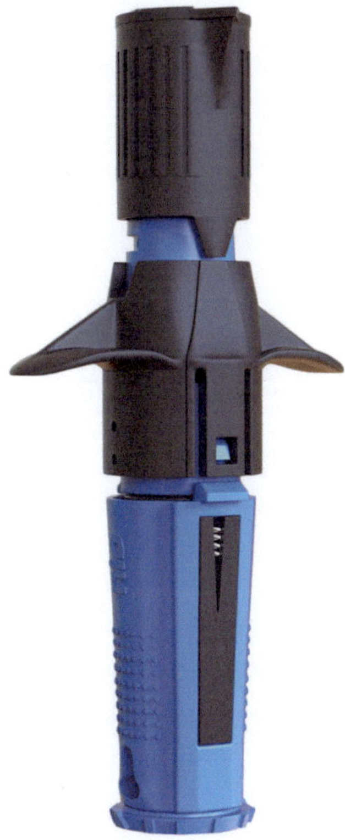

Fig. 6.3 The New Intraosseous (NIO™) adult device. *(Image courtesy of Safeguard Medical. © 2023 Safeguard Medical. All rights reserved)*

Szarpak and colleagues conducted a similar study among paramedics without prior device experience, testing their ability to obtain vascular access during simulated CPR in an adult cadaver model. Thirty-eight paramedics received a 5-min tutorial on the EZ-IO® and NIO™ prior to beginning the study. This study reported a first-attempt placement success rate of 100% for the EZ-IO® and 97.4% for the NIO™, which was not a statistically significant difference. However, median procedure time was significantly shorter for the NIO™ (16.8 s; IQR 15–20.5) than with the EZ-IO® (42 s; IQR 38–53) ($p < 0.001$) [13].

The NIO Pediatric™ (NIO-P™) model is similar to the adult version, but intended for patients 3–12 years of age. The injection depth can be adjusted at the base on the needle stabilizer [14]. The preset depth for this device is 14 mm (for ages 3–9 years). However, by removing the red spacer at the end of the device, the depth can be increased to 18 mm for patients 9–12 years of age or those with increased subcutaneous tissue (Fig. 6.4). The device also includes a marking ("R" for the patient's right leg, and "L" for the left leg) that is to be placed on the prominent aspect of the tibial tuberosity to ensure that the device is deployed medial to this landmark at the proximal tibia site.

Direct venous access can be especially challenging in pediatric subjects, with one study of pediatric cardiovascular arrest patients reporting that 6% (4/66) do not

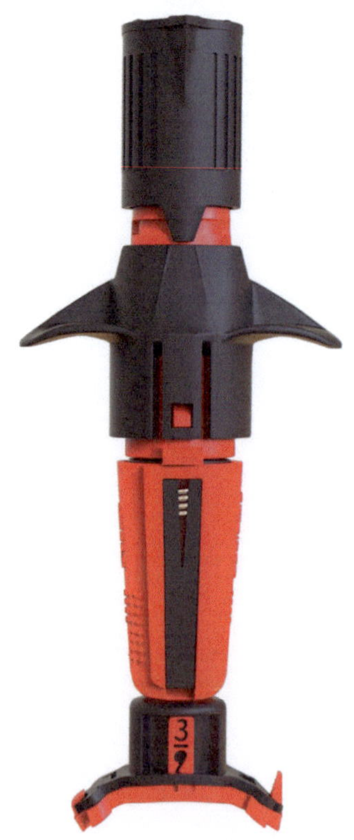

Fig. 6.4 The NIO Pediatric™ device. *(Image courtesy of Safeguard Medical. © 2023 Safeguard Medical. All rights reserved)*

receive PIV access prior to termination of resuscitative efforts and 24% (16/66) require 10 or more minutes to achieve PIV access [15]. Difficulties and delays in establishing direct venous access to treat cardiac arrest have led to a significant interest in the use of IO devices for pediatric resuscitation.

In 2017, Bielski and colleagues reported the results of their study comparing four major IO devices (NIO-P™, EZ-IO®, BIG®, Jamshidi™) used by 87 paramedics on a pediatric manikin model during simulated cardiopulmonary resuscitation. They found that the median time required to obtain IO access was 9 s (IQR, 8–12) for the NIO-P™, 12 s (IQR, 9–16) for BIG®, 13.5 s (IQR, 11–17) for the EZ-IO®, and 15 s (IQR, 13–19) for the Jamshidi™. The mean time required for NIO-P™ insertion (21 s; IQR 18–25) was less than that required for the EZ-IO® (28 s; IQR 22–31) ($p = 0.013$) [16]. The NIO-P™ was also rated easiest to use, followed (in order of ease of use) by the EZ-IO®, BIG®, and Jamshidi™.

Drozd and colleagues performed a similar study using level 2 personal protective equipment (PPE), as was commonly used for the resuscitation of COVID-19 patients during the pandemic [17]. They found a first-attempt placement success rate of 100% for both the NIO-P™ and EZ-IO® while employing PPE, which was significantly higher than the success rates associated with either the Jamshidi™ (80.0%; $p = 0.02$) or PIV access (69.2%; $p < 0.001$). Furthermore, use of the NIO-P™ achieved vascular access faster than use of the EZ-IO®. The time from when the device was removed from packaging to achieving vascular access was 33 ± 4 s with the NIO-P™ compared to 37 ± 6.7 s for the EZ-IO® device ($p < 0.001$). The NIO-P™ was also selected 78.5% of the time and EZ-IO® in 21.5% ($p < 0.001$) based on user preference for their clinical practice over use of the Jamshidi™ or PIV access [13].

The newest version of this device is the NIO Infant™ (NIO-I™), intended for patients 0–3 years of age (Fig. 6.5). This device features a Stepped Needle®, facilitating graduated penetration into the bone marrow to avoid overpenetration [14]. This model also includes a special fixation feature (Fig. 6.6) in the packaging to avoid subsequent dislodgment of the catheter, which is a significant concern in the pediatric population and has been estimated to occur in up to 12% of all IO catheter placements [16].

Fig. 6.5 The NIO Infant™ device. (*Image courtesy of Safeguard Medical. © 2023 Safeguard Medical. All rights reserved*)

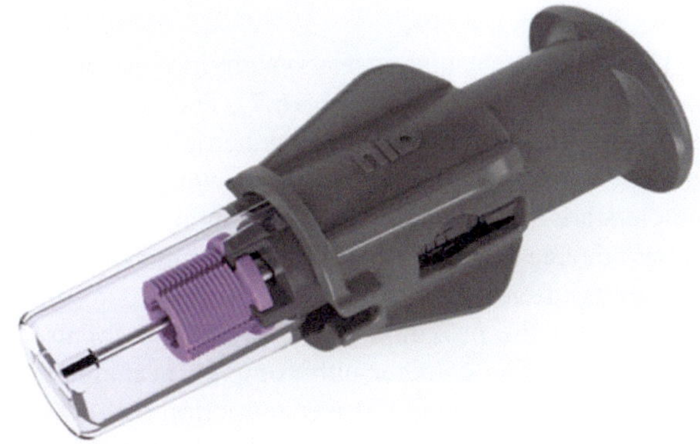

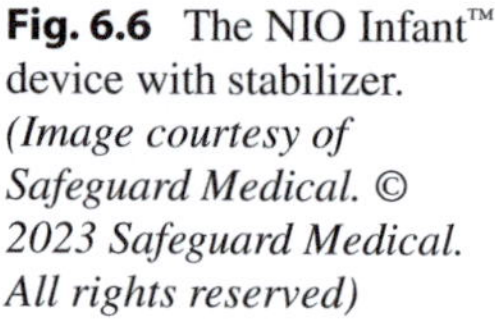

Fig. 6.6 The NIO Infant™ device with stabilizer. *(Image courtesy of Safeguard Medical. © 2023 Safeguard Medical. All rights reserved)*

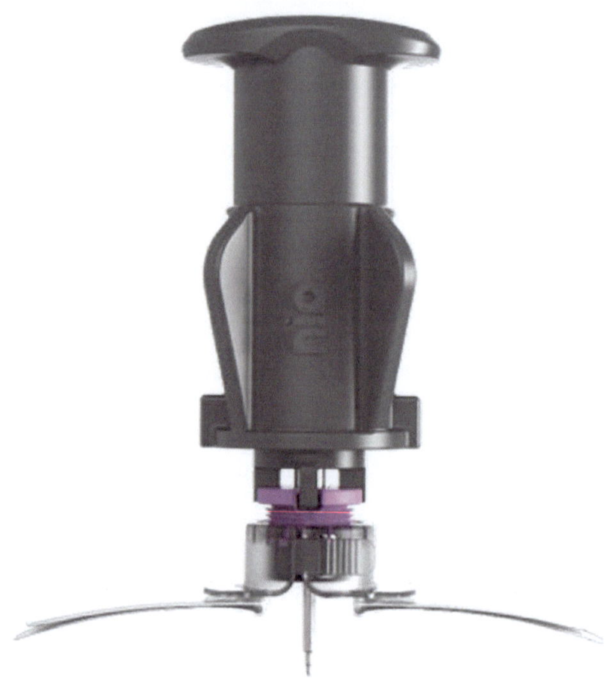

Semiautomatic Devices

The EZ-IO Intraosseous Vascular Access System

The Arrow® EZ-IO® Intraosseous Vascular Access System is an FDA-approved device utilizing a 15-gauge surgical steel catheter inserted by a handheld battery-powered motorized driver. This device was first developed and marketed by Vidacare Corporation (Shavano Park, Texas, USA) in 2004. The technology was subsequently acquired by Teleflex Medical Research (Triangle Park, North Carolina, USA) in 2013 and has since been incorporated into the Teleflex Arrow® line of vascular access products [18, 19].

The EZ-IO® vascular access system includes a powered driver, as well as 45, 25, and 15 mm catheter lengths (Fig. 6.7). The catheter hubs are color coded based upon patient weight and desired tissue penetration depth. The 15 mm catheter has a pink hub (for patients weighing 3–39 kg), while the 25 mm (blue) and 45 mm (yellow) catheters are marketed for patients weighing >39 kg. Like all automatic or semiautomatic devices, this system is not recommended for sternal use. While the 25 mm catheter is often used at the proximal tibial site, the 45 mm catheter is generally preferred for the proximal humeral site and for use at the proximal tibia in very obese adults. The catheter-hub complex is magnetically attached to the drill, for ease of loading and quick driver retraction following placement. Early versions of the EZ-IO® powered driver featured an elongated handle, including the blue-colored

Fig. 6.7 The Arrow®
EZ-IO® Intraosseous
Vascular Access System.
(*Image courtesy of Teleflex,
Incorporated.* © 2023.
*Teleflex Incorporated. All
rights reserved*)

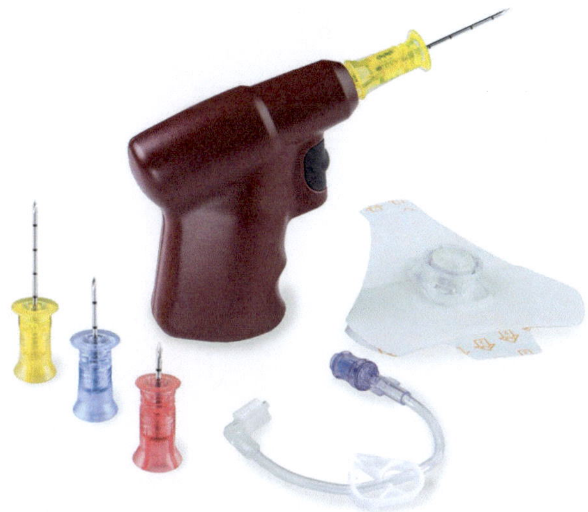

G1 (generation 1) driver (with two D batteries) and the maroon-colored G2 driver with a disposable lithium battery. The modern EZ-IO® G3 driver has a shorter handle but still utilizes a non-rechargeable lithium battery. The G3 driver marketed to civilian providers is red (Fig. 6.7), while the version marketed for military use is black.

The insertion site for the EZ-IO® in the proximal humerus is just superior to the surgical neck of the humerus. Before placing the device at the proximal humerus, the patient's arm should be properly positioned to expose the insertion site on the anterolateral arm and avoid the bicipital groove and biceps tendon, which are located medial to the optimal insertion site on the greater tubercle of the humerus. Arm positioning is achieved with internal rotation and adduction of the arm using one of two methods: (1) placing the patient's hand over the umbilicus with the arm tight to the body or (2) placing the arm tight against the body and pronating the hand so that the thumb is pointing posterior to the patient with the palm facing outward (i.e., away from the patient). If the patient is receiving active chest compressions, it may be necessary to stabilize the arm by placing the hand under the patient's ipsilateral buttock or thigh with the arm against the side of the chest, palm facing down (i.e., palm on the stretcher).

Once the arm is properly positioned, the surgical neck can be identified by first palpating the humeral diaphysis (e.g., shaft) and then moving the provider's hand proximally until the greater tubercle is met. The junction between the diaphysis and the greater tubercle of the humerus is the surgical neck. It may be helpful to imagine the greater tubercle of the humerus as a golf ball sitting on a golf tee. The surgical neck is the top of the golf tee. Once the surgical neck is identified, the correct insertion site is identified on the anterolateral part of the arm approximately 1–2 cm proximal (i.e., superior) to that point, corresponding to the most prominent aspect

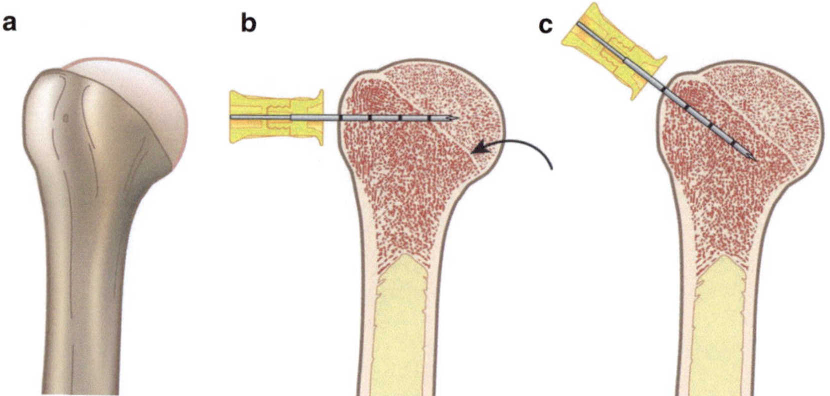

Fig. 6.8 The Arrow® EZ-IO® insertion angle for catheter placement at the proximal humerus site. (**a**) View of the right humeral head. (**b**) Disrupted epiphyseal plate due to improper insertion angle. (**c**) Proper angle of placement into the medullary cavity. (*Image courtesy of Teleflex, Incorporated. © 2023. Teleflex Incorporated. All rights reserved*)

of the greater tubercle. The driver should be advanced posteromedial at a 45° angle to the coronal (frontal) plane, as if aiming toward the contralateral hip. This approach is crucial to avoid advancing the catheter into the epiphyseal plate (Fig. 6.8). Insertion at this angle facilitates placement in an anterior insertion parallel to the epiphyseal plate. The provider should attempt to avoid placement of the catheter tip within the humeral head. This is because the epiphyseal plate (i.e., growth plate) and humeral head are more densely trabeculated and less vascular than the diaphysis, which may lead to slower flow rates and subsequently poor fluid and medication uptake into the systemic vasculature.

The EZ-IO® catheters all feature a series of graduated black lines surrounding the cannula at 10 mm increments, as measured from the catheter tip. In fact, the 45 mm catheter has four such lines, positioned at 10, 20, 30, and 40 mm from the catheter tip. Similarly, the 25 mm catheter has two black lines (at 10 and 20 mm), and the 15 mm catheter has one line (at 10 mm). These lines are intended to allow the provider to visually assess the depth of the target bone prior to initiating the motorized driver and penetrating the bone. It is recommended that the black line closest to the hub (i.e., the 5 mm line) be visible on the cannula after the needle has penetrated through the skin and soft tissues and contacted the cortex but prior to activating the driver. This practice is meant to prevent the user from attempting to place an inappropriately short catheter at the selected insertion site. Once the catheter tip has contacted the bony cortex, and after assuring visibility of at least the most proximal black line, the device is driven forward into the bone by slight manual pressure combined with the rotatory motion of the drill mechanism. The user will feel a sudden loss of resistance once the catheter has fully penetrated the cortex of the bone, indicating that the catheter tip is now inside the medullary cavity. Once this loss of resistance is felt, the user should remove their finger from the driver trigger to cease further forward motion of the catheter tip. The driver is then withdrawn, the stylet is removed (by unscrewing its associated hub from the catheter-associated hub), and an EZ-Stabilizer® dressing is applied to anchor the catheter in place. This stabilizer dressing consists of an adhesive patch surrounding a plastic column that fits around the catheter hub to prevent subsequent movement of the catheter after placement. The EZ-Connect® extension tubing set is then attached via Luer-lock connection to the catheter hub. Bone marrow aspirate and other samples can be directly obtained by using the extension sets or an aspiration syringe to test for successful placement prior to infusing fluids.

The EZ-IO® G3 driver features a battery indicator light to gauge remaining power in the driver device. This indicator light functionality was not available on the system's earlier G1 or G2 models. A solid green light on the battery indicator suggests that the device is fully charged, while a blinking red light indicates that <10% battery life is remaining. The EZ-IO® G3 driver uses lithium batteries with an estimated shelf life of 10 years or 500 insertions, and the driver batteries are not rechargeable. Once the battery has been depleted, the driver can no longer be used and must be discarded. Although early instruction to providers recommended frequent monitoring of the powered driver's battery life to ensure that the device is adequately charged, this is no longer recommended. This is because any depression of the trigger (even to check battery life) will drain battery charge. In the event that a driver battery is found to be depleted, EZ-IO® catheters can still be inserted manually using a separate manual driver.

The EZ-IO® device has been extensively studied, with one Teleflex study reporting that dye injected into a proximal humerus EZ-IO® catheter was shown to reach the right atrium of a healthy subject on fluoroscopy within 2.42 (±0.39) seconds [20].

Dolister and colleagues conducted a clinical experiment recruiting 105 participants who would have otherwise received central venous catheterization for difficult vascular access, but instead received EZ-IO® placement at the proximal tibia, distal tibia, or proximal humerus based upon the provider's clinical judgment. In this study, 94% of IO placements were successful on the first attempt, and the mean time to establish IO access was 103.6 ± 96.2 s [21].

The EZ-IO® system has been shown to be easy to use by a variety of emergency care providers, including those with no experience with IO catheter placement. In 2009, Levitan and colleagues reported the results of a cadaveric study including 42 emergency medicine (EM) attending physicians, 31 EM residents, 13 non-EM physicians, and 13 non-physicians [22]. None of the subjects had previously used an EZ-IO®, and 80.8% had never previously placed an IO catheter. In total, 94% (289/297) of insertions were successful following a 5-min training presentation. The median insertion time was 6 s (IQR 5–8) [22]. Participants subjectively rated the EZ-IO® as faster and easier to use than a central venous catheter and stated that they would use this device in a cardiac arrest scenario [22].

A similar prehospital study on human subjects supported these findings. In 2012, Santos and colleagues reported a study of 58 critically ill patients (mostly adults) who received 60 insertions of the 25 mm EZ-IO® catheter at the proximal tibia, with a 90% placement success rate. The indications for IO cannulation included cardio-respiratory arrest ($n = 36$, 62%), traumatic cardiac arrest ($n = 7$, 12%), major trauma ($n = 7$, 12%), and shock ($n = 3$, 5%) [23].

Kurowski and colleagues compared the EZ-IO®, BIG®, and Jamshidi™ in a manikin study recruiting a total of 107 paramedics. They found that the mean placement time for the BIG® was 2.0 ± 0.7 min compared to 3.1 ± 0.9 min for EZ-IO® and 4.2 ± 1.0 min for the Jamshidi™. First-attempt placement success rates were 82.7% for the EZ-IO®, 91.6% for the BIG®, and 47.7% for the Jamshidi™ [5]. In 2010, Leidel and colleagues reported a first-attempt success rate of 80% with the BIG® and 90% with the EZ-IO®; the mean time required for placement was 2.2 ± 1.0 min for the BIG® versus 1.8 ± 0.9 min with the EZ-IO® [8]. The overall success rate and complications were not significantly different between groups [8].

In 2007, Brenner and colleagues reported the results of a cadaveric study comparing the EZ-IO® to manual IO catheter insertion with a Cook catheter [24]. They found that the EZ-IO® had a higher first-attempt success rate and was considered to be more user friendly with fewer complications [24]. In 2008, a query of the Vidacare Intraosseous Databank was published, reporting on 1199 uses of the EZ-IO® system [25]. This report found a 92% overall placement success rate for the EZ-IO®, with an insertion time of 10 s or less in 84% of providers who achieved first-attempt placement success [25]. In a 2010 report by Sunde and colleagues, including 78 IO insertion attempts on 70 patients, the authors found a 96% placement success rate for the EZ-IO® compared to 56% with the BIG® (56%) [10]. Drozd and colleagues similarly reported a 96% first-attempt success rate for the EZ-IO®, but also found a 94% success rate for the BIG® [17, 26]. The EZ-IO® was further studied by Pasley in a cadaveric model, who reported successful placement and infusion in 81.3% of subjects [27]. These authors reported that increased thickness of the soft tissue overlying the insertion site may contribute to an increased risk of needle dislodgment [27].

One recent randomized simulation study compared placement of the spring-loaded NIO-I™ device to the EZ-IO® 15 mm catheter and the manual Jamshidi™ IO catheter among pediatric residents and specialists [28]. In this study using Cornish hen bones as a model for the neonatal tibia, providers found the EZ-IO® device to be subjectively easier to insert than the other devices, but associated with a significantly lower first-attempt success rate (46.7% vs. 77.4% for NIO-I™ and 80.7% for Jamshidi™). The hen bone model used in this study did not include associated soft tissues, which may have influenced the results. However, the discrepancy between these results and those reported by other studies in the adult model does suggest that the EZ-IO® device may be more difficult to place correctly on the first attempt in neonatal subjects than for older patients.

Given the device's high rate of successful placement by emergency care providers and low rate of reported complication, the manufacturers of the EZ-IO® system have been instrumental in seeking an extended dwell time for the catheter. In 2020, the device received FDA approval for 48-h dwell time (previously 24 h) in patients older than 12 years old when PIV access is unavailable or is unreliable [29, 30]. This extended dwell time was further investigated to identify any complications, and it was determined that there was no evidence of risk of infection, osteomyelitis, or other adverse events by increasing the IO catheter dwell time to 48 h [31].

The BD™ Intraosseous Powered Driver

The BD™ Intraosseous Vascular Access System (Fig. 6.9) is FDA approved for use at the proximal humerus, proximal tibia, and distal tibia in adult and pediatric patients, with an additional indication at the distal femur in children [32]. This system includes a driver and separate battery-charging device, with a single charge lasting approximately 70 insertions at 10 s per attempt. This system uses a four-light system to indicate the level of battery charge. Four solid green lights indicate that the device is fully charged. Four blinking lights indicate a malfunction such as overheating, that the device is too cold, that the driver stalled, or that the trigger is stuck. Three green lights indicate 50–75% battery remaining, while two green lights indicate battery charge of 25–50%, and one green light warns that there is <25% of battery life remaining. Blinking red indicates insufficient battery remaining and that charging is required. Importantly, this driver cannot be used while charging, and it is recommended to recharge the device every 3 months independent of usage.

The BD™ Intraosseous Vascular Access System offers five different catheter lengths: 15, 25, 35, 45, and 55 mm. This may be compared to the EZ-IO® system,

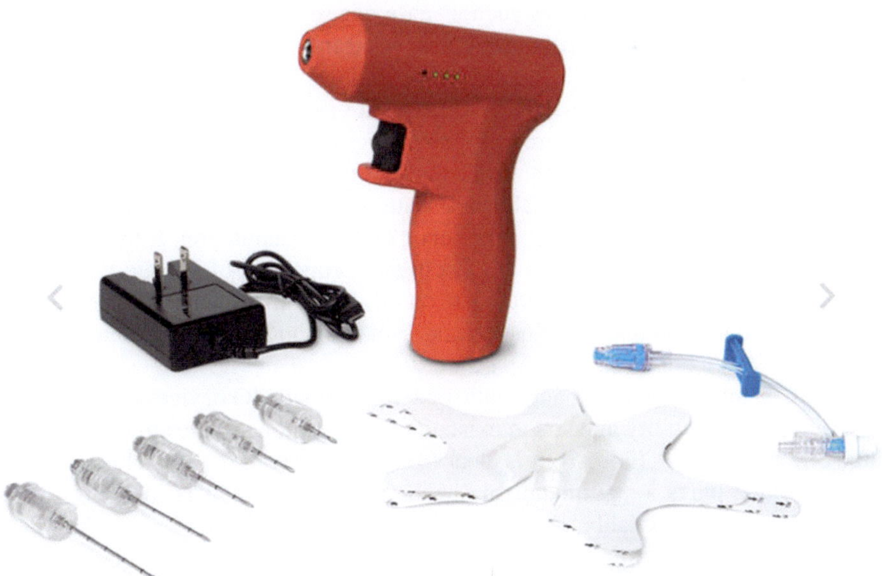

Fig. 6.9 The BD™ Intraosseous Vascular Access System. *(Images courtesy of Becton, Dickson and Company. © 2023 Becton, Dickson and Company. All rights reserved)*

which offers only three different lengths (15, 25, and 45 mm). These catheters are not color coded, but do feature graduated black lines every 10 mm as with the EZ-IO® system [32].

Little and colleagues compared the EZ-IO® with the BD™ Intraosseous Vascular Access System to determine which IO device was preferred among 22 licensed emergency medicine physicians who were trained in IO access [33]. In this study, each provider used both devices on five different adult humerus models for a total of ten insertions and then completed a 27-question survey. The authors found that most participants preferred the BD™ Intraosseous Vascular Access System ($n = 20$; 90.9%; 95% CI: 70.8%, 98.9%; $P = 0.0001$). The main reasons cited for this preference were safety ($n = 12$; 54.5%), snap-securement dressing ($n = 6$; 27.2%), and ease of use ($n = 3$; 13.6%) [33].

Future Directions

The use of automatic and semiautomatic IO devices has seen extraordinary growth since these devices were first introduced to the clinical arena in the late 1990s. The existing data suggest positive outcomes (e.g., high first-attempt placement success rates, ease of use, low complication rates) for automatic and semiautomatic IO catheter placement based upon data from both novice users and medical personnel who have experience inserting IO catheters. Unfortunately, much of the existing medical literature is in the form of cadaver and manikin studies, suggesting that additional clinical data are needed. The existing medical literature focuses predominantly upon provider-centered outcomes such as ease of use and placement success rate, with minimal attention paid to other clinical outcomes or patient-centered criteria [34]. More research is needed to evaluate how patients view IO access and whether they value criteria such as placement success rate as highly as providers do. It is possible that other patient-centered outcomes are more important to patients than these provider-centered outcomes. Since the vast majority of subjects receiving IO access are critically ill and generally insensate or otherwise cognitively impaired, very little data exist on the patient experience with IO cannulation. If the use of IO cannulation is ever to expand to include a higher proportion of sensate and cognitively intact patients, patient-centered data on the desirability of IO access is needed to guide clinicians on the use of this technique in this population of emergency care patients.

Placement success rates for automatic or semiautomatic IO devices are generally high, but great variability appears to exist among the various studies that have compared different devices [34, 35]. It is clear from the review of the available data that device training plays a significant role in the ability of providers to establish IO access quickly and reliably. Additional studies including providers who have received adequate training on multiple IO catheters are needed to elucidate how much of the difference in placement success rates is determined by provider-specific factors, rather than device-specific factors.

Conclusion

Automatic and semiautomatic devices utilize force derived from springs (in the case of automatic devices) or internal motors (with semiautomatic devices) to advance the catheter into its proper position. The introduction of these devices has allowed IO catheters to be placed into the harder, more dense bones of adult subjects. Data obtained by manikin, animal, human cadaveric, and some clinical trials have shown promising outcomes for the use of IO devices in cardiovascular resuscitation efforts and other emergent cases, especially those encountered in military arenas. However, additional research is needed to determine appropriate indications for each of these devices, considering their unique characteristics and indications for use.

Key Concepts

- Automatic IO devices do not require additional guidance or direction from the provider once the insertion mechanism has been triggered. In contrast, semiautomatic devices augment the insertion process but permit the provider to exert continuous control over the direction and depth of insertion throughout the insertion process.
- Automatic and semiautomatic devices have improved first-attempt success rates, reduced mean placement times, and reduced immediate complication rate when compared to manual IO devices.
- Currently available automatic and semiautomatic IO infusion devices appear to be easy to use with a high placement success rate, even among novice providers.
- The EZ-IO® and NIO™ appear to be the most widely used mechanical IO devices in both the hospital and prehospital settings, with higher first-attempt success rates and shorter mean placement times than other devices.
- The existing medical literature on IO devices focuses primarily upon provider-centered outcomes such as perceived ease of placement and rate of successful placement. Additional research is needed to assess other important clinical and patient-centered outcomes.

References

1. Garau Ramirez J, Truszewski Z, Drozd A. Comparison of two intraosseous access devices employed during simulated cardiopulmonary resuscitation. A prospective, randomized, cross-over, manikin study. Disaster Emerg Med J. 2016;1(1):24–9.
2. Bone injectio gun—pediatric [internet]. Persys Medical; 2009. https://persysmedical.com/products/vascular-access/bone-injection-gun-pediatric/. Accessed 4 June 2022.
3. Astasio-Picado Á, Cobos-Moreno P, Gómez-Martín B, Zabala-Baños MDC, Aranda-Martín C. Clinical management of intraosseous access in adults in critical situations for health professionals. Healthcare (Basel). 2022;10(2):367. https://doi.org/10.3390/healthcare10020367.
4. Waisman M, Waisman D. Bone marrow infusion in adults. J Trauma. 1997;42(2):288–93.
5. Kurowski A, Timler D, Evrin T, et al. Comparison of 3 different intraosseous access devices for adult during resuscitation. Randomized crossover manikin study. Am J Emerg Med. 2014;32(12):1490–3.

6. Olsen D, Packer BE, Perrett J, et al. Evaluation of the bone injection gun as a method for intraosseous cannula placement for fluid therapy in adult dogs. Vet Surg. 2002;31(6):533–40.
7. Spriggs NM, White LJ, Martin SW, Brawley D, Chambers RM. Comparison of two intraosseous infusion techniques in an EMT training program. Acad Emerg Med. 2000;7(10):1168.
8. Leidel BA, Kirchhoff C, Braunstein V, et al. Comparison of two intraosseous access devices in adult patients under resuscitation in the emergency department: a prospective, randomized study. Resuscitation. 2010;81(8):994–9.
9. Hartholt KA, van Lieshout EM, Thies WC, et al. Intraosseous devices: a randomized controlled trial comparing three intraosseous devices. Prehosp Emerg Care. 2010;14(1):6–13.
10. Sunde GA, Heradstveit BE, Vikenes BH, Heltne JK. Emergency intraosseous access in a helicopter emergency medical service: a retrospective study. Scand J Trauma Resusc Emerg Med. 2010;18:52. https://doi.org/10.1186/1757-7241-18-52.
11. NIO™ adult: proximity to the bone. YouTube: PerSys Medical; 2017. https://www.youtube.com/watch?v=PzdAROAsovc. Accessed 4 June 2022.
12. Shina A, Baruch EN, Shlaifer A, et al. Comparison of two intraosseous devices: the NIO versus the EZ-IO by novice users—a randomized cross over trial. Prehosp Emerg Care. 2017;21(3):315–21.
13. Szarpak L, Truszewski Z, Smereka J, et al. Ability of paramedics to perform intraosseous access. A randomized cadaver study comparing EZ-IO® and NIO® devices. Resuscitation. 2016;104:e5–6.
14. Nio™ infant training—deploying [internet]. Youtube: PerSys Medical; 2020 https://www.youtube.com/watch?v=XaZhbSDIKLg.
15. Rossetti V, Thompson BM, Aprahamian C, et al. Difficulty and delay in intravascular access in pediatric arrests. Ann Emerg Med. 1984;13(5):406.
16. Bielski K, Szarpak L, Smereka J, et al. Comparison of four different intraosseous access devices during simulated pediatric resuscitation. A randomized crossover manikin trial. Eur J Pediatr. 2017;176(7):865–71.
17. Drozd A, Smereka J, Pruc M, et al. Comparison of intravascular access methods applied by nurses wearing personal protective equipment in simulated COVID-19 resuscitation: a randomized crossover simulation trial. Am J Emerg Med. 2021;49:189–94.
18. Teleflex to incorporate the vidacare EZ-IO® intraosseous vascular access system at SCCM [press release]. Teleflex Incorporated, 01/08/2014.
19. Paxton JH, Knuth TE, Klausner HA. Proximal humerus intraosseous infusion: a preferred emergency venous access. J Trauma. 2009;67(3):606–11.
20. Montez DF, Puga T, Miller L, et al. 133 intraosseous infusions from the proximal humerus reach the heart in less than 3 seconds in human volunteers. Ann Emerg Med. 2015;66(4, Supplement):S47.
21. Dolister M, Miller S, Borron S, et al. Intraosseous vascular access is safe, effective and costs less than central venous catheters for patients in the hospital setting. J Vasc Access. 2013;14(3):216–24.
22. Levitan RM, Bortle CD, Snyder TA, et al. Use of a battery-operated needle driver for intraosseous access by novice users: skill acquisition with cadavers. Ann Emerg Med. 2009;54(5):692–4.
23. Santos D, Carron PN, Yersin B, et al. EZ-IO® intraosseous device implementation in a prehospital emergency service: a prospective study and review of the literature. Resuscitation. 2013;84(4):440–5.
24. Brenner T, Bernhard M, Helm M, et al. Comparison of two intraosseous infusion systems for adult emergency medical use. Resuscitation. 2008;78(3):314–9.
25. Fowler RL, Pierce A, Nazeer S, et al. 362: 1,199 case series: powered intraosseous insertion provides safe and effective vascular access for emergency patients. Ann Emerg Med. 2008;52(4, Supplement):S152.
26. Dolister M, Miller ST, Borron S, et al. 393 intraosseous vascular access can be used safely and effectively, and at a lower cost than central venous catheters, for pediatric and adult patients in the hospital setting. Ann Emerg Med. 2011;58(4):S311.

27. Pasley J, Miller CH, DuBose JJ, et al. Intraosseous infusion rates under high pressure: a cadaveric comparison of anatomic sites. J Trauma Acute Care Surg. 2015;78(2):295–9.
28. Keller A, Boukai A, Feldman O, Diamand R, Shavit I. Comparison of three intraosseous access devices for resuscitation of term neonates: a randomised simulation study. Arch Dis Child Fetal Neonatal Ed. 2022;107(3):289–92. https://doi.org/10.1136/archdischild-2021-321988. Epub 2021.
29. Sou V, McManus C, Mifflin N, et al. A clinical pathway for the management of difficult venous access. BMC Nurs. 2017;16(1):64.
30. Overbaugh R, Davlantes C, Miller L, et al. Intraosseous vascular access catheter appears safe during extended dwell: a preliminary report. Ann Emerg Med. 2015;66(4):s5–6.
31. Philbeck TE, Puga TA, Montez DF, et al. Intraosseous vascular access using the EZ-IO can be safely maintained in the adult proximal humerus and proximal tibia for up to 48 hours: report of a clinical study. J Vasc Access. 2022;23(3):339–47.
32. BD™ intraosseous vascular access system [internet]. https://www.bd.com/en-us/products-and-solutions/products/product-families/bd-intraosseous-vascular-access-system. Accessed 9 June 2022.
33. Little A, Alsbrooks K, Jones D. Physician preferences associated with powered intraosseous access systems: safety features, reliability, and ease of use. J Am Coll Emerg Physicians Open. 2022;3(3):e12710.
34. Drozd A, Wolska M, Szarpak L. Intraosseous vascular access in emergency and trauma settings: a comparison of the most universally used intraosseous devices. Expert Rev Med Devices. 2021;18(9):855–64.
35. Lewis P, Wright C. Saving the critically injured trauma patient: a retrospective analysis of 1000 uses of intraosseous access. Emerg Med J. 2015;32(6):463.

Flow Rates with Intraosseous Catheterization

7

Nicholas Righi and James H. Paxton

Introduction

Intraosseous (IO) catheters can be used to provide medication for the treatment of a wide variety of medical conditions, including acute respiratory failure, uncontrolled pain, severe dehydration, cardiovascular collapse associated with shock states, and cardiac arrest. Patients experiencing severe hemodynamic instability associated with profound hypovolemia may require large infusions of crystalloid fluid or blood products to restore homeostasis. When large-volume infusion is needed, providers must consider whether available vascular access devices, including IO catheters, are capable of achieving adequate flow rates. Fluid flow rates are measured as volume (e.g., milliliters) infused per unit of time (e.g., minute) and are influenced by a wide variety of **extrinsic** (i.e., outside of the patient) and **intrinsic** (i.e., inside of the patient) factors. The dominant extrinsic factors affecting IO flow rates include the infusion pressure applied to the fluid infusate by the provider, resistance to flow imparted by the IV tubing and external portion (i.e., hub) of the IO catheter, and fluid viscosity. Key intrinsic factors include resistance to flow within the catheter itself (which is essentially a function of catheter length and diameter but can be influenced by the presence of debris and other physical impediments), ambient pressure within the medullary cavity, the capacitance of the venous system draining the intraosseous space, and realized pressure within the venous system (a function of intravascular fluid volume and venous capacity) [1, 2].

The venous channels draining the medullary space are of small caliber when compared to named peripheral or central veins. Consequently, this physiologic bottleneck limits the rate at which the medullary space can be drained and can rapidly lead to congestion within the local venous system. Intraosseous infusion should be

N. Righi (✉) · J. H. Paxton
Department of Emergency Medicine, Wayne State University School of Medicine, Detroit, MI, USA
e-mail: nicholas.righi@med.wayne.edu; james.paxton@wayne.edu

© The Author(s), under exclusive license to Springer Nature Switzerland AG 2024
J. H. Paxton (ed.), *Intraosseous Vascular Access*,
https://doi.org/10.1007/978-3-031-61201-5_7

considered **indirect** venous access, as substances deposited into the bone marrow must be picked up by medullary sinusoids and transported to perforating venules, which subsequently drain into the venous plexus and ultimately the efferent veins leading to the central circulation [3]. Although substances are deposited in the IO space, these substances cannot reach the central circulation without being picked up by the venous drainage system of the bone. By contrast, **direct** venous infusion (i.e., through a cannula inserted into a peripheral or central vein) benefits from the lower (often negative) intrinsic pressure of the venous system, which is associated with higher flow rates due to reduced resistance to flow and greater capacity to accept supraphysiologic volumes of fluid through venous distension [4–6].

To optimize flow rates associated with IO infusion, providers must be aware of the anatomic and physiologic factors that influence the **ingress** ("traveling into") and **egress** ("traveling out of") of fluids and medications deposited within the intramedullary space. Increased awareness of these factors can help providers to optimize the flow rates achievable with this technique, reduce the risk of certain complications associated with IO infusion, and guide future research leading to advancements in the efficacy of IO fluid infusion. This chapter will explore how and to what extent various factors affect IO flow rates, including a discussion on the differences between IO and IV infusion reflected in flow rate data provided in the available medical literature.

Fluid Dynamics

Poiseuille's law (Fig. 7.1) describes the laminar flow of fluids through a cylinder with a fixed diameter, and approximates the relationship between flow and pressure through a blood vessel or vascular catheter. In this equation, volumetric flow rate (Q) is shown to be directly proportional to the pressure gradient (ΔP) and inversely proportional to the resistance (R) encountered within the vascular system:

The resistance (R) associated with blood flow is further predicted by the viscosity (η) of the fluid flowing through a tube with a certain length (L) and radius (r) [7, 8]. As shown in Fig. 7.2, resistance increases with increasing tube length and fluid viscosity and decreases with increasing radius of the tubing (e.g., vein or catheter) through which the fluid is traveling:

Although Poiseuille's law offers only a simplified estimate of the factors influencing blood flow through a vascular bed or catheter, this law effectively predicts that veins with a small radius or longer length are associated with increased resistance. Therefore, reducing the resistance associated with IO infusion requires

Fig. 7.1 Poiseuille's law

$$Q = \frac{\Delta P}{R}$$

Fig. 7.2 Resistance to flow predicted by Poiseuille's law

$$R = \frac{8\eta L}{\pi r^4}$$

reduction in the viscosity of the infusate, decreased length of the vein, or increased radius/diameter of the vessel and/or IO infusion catheter. When resistance to flow is reduced, flow rates increase. Thus, this basic law of fluid dynamics predicts that IO flow rates should be greater when draining venules and veins are closer to the central circulation (e.g., shorter tubes) or are of larger caliber. When one considers the "tube" to be the medullary cavity, this law also suggests that larger medullary spaces should have reduced resistance to flow and increased flow rates when compared to smaller intramedullary spaces. Thus, **flow rates are generally higher when IO infusion sites are closer to the central circulation or provide larger intramedullary spaces within which the infusate can be deposited**. Smaller bones offer greater resistance to flow, and require higher infusion pressures to achieve forward flow when compared to larger bones. Similarly, small-caliber catheters likely require larger infusion pressures than large-caliber catheters.

One key difference between intravenous infusion and intraosseous infusion is the inability of the bone marrow cavity to expand or contract in response to changes in systemic blood pressure and whole-body fluid balance. This is an advantage in some ways, as venous collapse in hypovolemic states can make venous cannulation difficult but does not appreciably change the ability of providers to access the IO space. However, this **rigidity of the IO space may also serve as a limitation for IO fluid infusion rates**. While veins can expand appreciably to accommodate supraphysiologic increases in infusion pressure and fluid volume, the fixed diameter of the IO marrow space leads to increasing resistance with infusion rates above a certain physiologic threshold. Unfortunately, little is known about the true capacitance (i.e., ability to accept large volumes of fluid) of the IO drainage system at different IO infusion sites. The presence of bone marrow, various blood cells, and other materials in the IO space likely influences the maximal fluid infusion rate by increasing the resistance to flow and possibly even the viscosity of the infusate as it traverses the marrow space. After all, fluids infused into the intramedullary space will pick up and carry debris from the marrow cavity that are not present in venous channels. These additional materials undoubtedly contribute to increased fluid viscosity and resistance to flow with IO infusion that is not seen with IV infusion.

Patient-Related Factors

Many patient-related factors influence the flow rates achievable through IO catheters, including anatomic considerations, which may be somewhat static, as well as more dynamic factors introduced by the patient's presenting medical condition. As mentioned above, the capacitance of the IO space may be determined by the intramedullary diameter of the target bone as well as the degree to which draining veins can accept increased fluid volume within the bone. The capacitance of the bone drainage system is a function of both the number and size of the draining venules, as each intact venule adds to the total drainage capacity of the bone. Younger patients will have larger amounts of physiologically active **"red" marrow** within the IO space, as well as the more efficient drainage system required to transfer blood elements formed in the marrow into the general circulation. But as humans age, much of the "red" marrow is replaced with **"yellow" marrow** composed primarily of adipose tissue (i.e., fat), and the venous drainage system gradually atrophies with advancing age. This offers the advantage of increased physiologic "dead space" within the marrow cavity available to accept new infusates, but may also be associated with an impaired ability to remove the infusate from the IO space once it is infused. Thus, the ability of small draining veins within the bone to remove fluids from the intramedullary space may become a rate-limiting factor, especially in adult subjects.

Normal capillary venous pressure ranges from 10.5 to 22.5 mmHg [9], while peripheral venous pressure ranges from 8 to 12 mmHg [10], and central venous pressure is much lower at 0–6 mmHg [11]. In general, the ambient pressure within a vein increases with the effects of gravity and diminished vein caliber, so that **small veins in a dependent position have much higher intraluminal pressures than larger veins near the heart** [11]. This creates a system of decreasing intravenous pressure as deoxygenated blood travels from the peripheral tissues towards the heart, which serves to pull blood from the periphery and facilitates diastolic heart filling. This diminishing intraluminal pressure may also facilitate increased flow rates in larger veins due to both larger vein diameter and diminished resistance within the vein.

By comparison, baseline intraosseous pressure (IOP) in healthy subjects varies primarily according to arterial perfusion pressure and is generally 25–30% of systolic blood pressure [12, 13]. It has also been noted that IOP decreases with lowering of systemic arterial blood pressure and increases with elevated systemic venous pressure, suggesting that **IOP is highly dependent upon fluid status and arterial vasomotor tone** [12, 13]. Whatever the patient's resting systemic blood pressure, it is likely that the IOP is much higher than the intraluminal pressure associated with adjacent peripheral veins. However, IO infusion sites close to the heart enjoy some of this benefit of reduced resistance in the central venous circulation, contributing to better flow rates at "proximal" IO insertion sites (e.g., proximal humerus, sternum, clavicle) than is available at more "peripheral" IO sites (e.g., distal tibia, proximal tibia) due to lower resistance within the draining venules as it is transmitted from the larger central veins.

Considering Poiseuille's law, it may be assumed that the intrinsic pressure within smaller caliber veins draining the bone is much higher than the pressure within larger veins collecting the blood from these perforating vessels. Since the IO infusion pressure must overcome ambient IOP to yield a net positive driving pressure, the infusion pressures required for IO infusion are typically much higher than those required for peripheral or central venous infusion. Previous studies have shown that the sternum has the lowest resting IOP, followed (in order of increasing IOP) by the humerus, tibia, and femur [13]. This is largely reflective of the proximity of these infusion sites to the vena cava, including the shorter distance that blood must travel to reach the heart. **The further that an IO infusion site is from the heart, the greater its intrinsic resistance to fluid flow**. Thus, the anatomical factors that influence baseline IO pressures appear to include the size and shape of the marrow cavity, the total cross-sectional area of the associated sinusoidal outflow tract, and the proximity of the IO infusion site to the central veins. Of course, the size and shape of target bones may be different between patients, especially when comparing pediatric to adult subjects.

The physiologic mechanisms controlling blood flow through the bone are neural, hormonal, and metabolic [14], and each of these factors contributes to IO flow rates. It has been shown that stimulation of nerve fibers innervating a bone can produce decreased bone blood flow [15]. For example, lumbar sympathectomy has been shown to cause a 27% decrease in blood flow to the canine tibia [16]. Circulating sympathetic hormones, such as adrenaline, can also affect blood flow to and from the bone. Adrenaline (i.e., epinephrine) is a potent vasoconstrictor which, despite increasing mean arterial pressure, also decreases blood flow from bone due to venous constriction [17]. This leads to increased IO pressure due to congestion of blood within the bone [14]. **Of the three physiologic mechanisms of control, metabolic factors are likely the most influential** [18]. Metabolic factors include oxygen and carbon dioxide concentrations or the presence of acid metabolites and their effect on local pH. It has been shown that experimental administration of lactic acid increases bony blood flow [19], and prolonged femoral artery occlusion leads to reactive hyperemia due to vasodilatation of the nutrient vessels. This vasodilation of bone vessels after prolonged ischemia, and the resultant increase in bone blood flow, persists somewhat after reperfusion and cannot be overridden by nerve stimulation or by vasopressin administration [20]. The effect that this vasodilatation may have on IO infusion rates remains unknown, but deserves greater attention in future studies on the use of IO infusion to treat shock states.

Pathological states also affect bone blood flow and, in turn, influence IO flow rates. Intraosseous infusion into a fractured bone is contraindicated primarily for safety reasons due to the risk of extravasation of infusates into the surrounding soft tissues. However, experimental data have shown that fractures also dramatically reduce blood flow to the fractured bone, which may affect flow to nearby bones as well. In one study, subcapital fractures were associated with an 83% reduction in blood flow to the femoral head [21]. Although *osteogenesis imperfecta* is only a relative contraindication for IO use [22], it should be considered that misshapen bones could have impaired flow through the marrow cavity.

The effects of **hypovolemia** (i.e., low intravascular fluid volume) on IO blood flow are not yet fully understood. Some studies suggest that hypovolemia has no statistically significant effect on IO flow rates, while other studies have shown up to a 32% decrease in blood flow rates to bone under hypovolemic conditions with both IV and IO infusions [2, 23, 24]. Under normal circumstances, hypovolemia induces a number of physiological changes within the subject that serve to preferentially shunt blood flow towards vital organs and away from more peripheral tissues, including the bones. The systemic and local effects of hypovolemia on blood flow to the bone remain unclear, suggesting the need for further study.

Infusion Site Selection

As mentioned above, the IO site chosen for infusion is of paramount importance in predicting associated flow rates. In the earliest days of IO infusion, nearly a century ago, the **sternum** was the preferred site for volume infusion in adults due to its high degree of red marrow and proximity to the central venous circulation. However, increasing concerns about cardiac injury due to sternal perforation, especially among pediatric subjects, led to a gradual transition to use of the **proximal tibia** site among many providers. In recent years, increasing evidence has emerged suggesting the superiority of **proximal insertion sites** (e.g., sternum, proximal humerus) over more distal sites (e.g., distal tibia, proximal tibia) for large volume infusion, although the proximal tibia remains the IO insertion site most commonly used by modern providers [23, 25]. While the proximal tibia is clearly an easily accessible site, it may not be an optimal site for high-volume IO fluid infusion.

The **depth of the target bone** may have an effect on flow rates as well, especially if the targeted bone lies deep within a musculoskeletal compartment with relatively high intracompartmental pressure. Given that veins are highly susceptible to collapse from extraluminal pressure, it is intuitive that the venous outflow tract from a bone deep in a highly pressurized soft tissue compartment would have increased resistance to flow when compared to a more superficial target. Although most traditional IO insertion sites are quite superficial, the effect of overlying soft tissue on bone drainage may ultimately prove to be an important consideration.

Data on flow rates according to insertion site appear to differ depending upon the population studied, ranging across healthy human subjects, treated patients, and animal models. In general, the sternum appears to be associated with the highest reported infusion rates, although the **proximal humerus** is comparable to the sternum in most models [1, 26–33]. Reported flow rates at the proximal tibial site are highly variable, though usually reported to be lower than sternal or humeral flow rates when infusion is administered by gravity alone [1, 25, 26, 34, 35]. Recent studies by Ngo and Ong suggest that increased infusion pressure can augment flow rates at the proximal tibial site substantially, offering the potential for improved flow using pressure bags or syringe injection [35, 36].

Techniques for Pressurized Infusion

As mentioned previously, increased resistance within the flow tract can impede infusion through the IO space. While the use of gravity as the driving force for IO infusion is sufficient in some cases [5, 37], pressurized infusion may be required to achieve adequate flow rates. Manually pumped pressure bags are commonly used to provide pressurized infusion, as they are readily available and familiar to most clinicians. The use of a stopcock and the presence of a pressure-release valve allow the bag pressure to be maintained at a constant level, as long as the pressure bladder is frequently reinflated [38]. Other techniques for providing pressurized infusion include syringes and rate-controlled infusion pumps. The relative benefits and drawbacks for each method of producing pressurized flow are described in Table 7.1.

Table 7.1 Comparison of techniques for pressurized infusion

Technique	Benefits	Drawbacks	Flow rates (mL/min)
Syringe	Easy setup High pressures Rapid infusion	Increased pain with infusion [39]	96.5 (95% CI 81.9–111.1) at pH [31] 232.5 ± 131.2 at S [40]
Pressure bag	Relatively constant pressure	Limited infusion pressure options Requires periodic reinflation of bag	72.6 (95% CI 61.0–84.2)–115 at pH [31, 32] 81 at PT [32] 104.1 ± 46.5 in S [40]
Infusion pump	Precise infusion rate "Smart" pumps prevent infusion errors Can infuse multiple fluids simultaneously High-pressure alarms	Time required to set up Costly devices Limited availability Flow rates are limited (e.g., 1 L/h) [41] Requires electrical source	60.0 (95% CI 44.8–75.2)–79 in pH [31, 32] 47 in PT [32]

Notes: *pH* Proximal humerus, *PT* Proximal tibia, *S* Sternum

Infusion Pressures

Higher IO infusion pressures generally provide higher flow rates, within certain physiologic limits [25–27, 29, 31, 40]. The technique used to provide pressurized infusion greatly influences peak infusion pressures and the flow rates achievable with IO infusion. Syringe pressure can provide extremely high infusion pressures over a relatively short period of time. This can be useful for rapid infusion of fluids for resuscitation, but safety limitations must also be considered. Higher infusion pressures may exceed the capacitance of the intramedullary system, leading to rupture of the draining veins and concomitant fluid extravasation into the adjacent soft tissues [42].

Risks of Pressurized Infusion

Early investigators of IO infusion techniques were concerned about the risk of **fat embolism** with overaggressive infusion into the medullary space. However, this hypothetical risk has never been shown to be clinically significant [43]. Considering the small caliber of draining veins from the bone, the degree of adipose tissue displacement into the systemic circulation is likely to be minimal, although further research is needed to confirm this assumption.

A much more formidable and common complication of IO infusion is **extravasation** of infused materials into the adjacent soft tissues. Although the precise mechanism of extravasation with IO infusion remains unclear, it may occur as a result of the rupture of draining veins or via retrograde flow of infusate through the IO insertion site. Both of these events can be attributed to attempting an infusion pressure that exceeds the capacitance of the draining system. Since the medullary space has a fixed maximal rate of drainage and cannot expand to accommodate larger volumes of fluid, IO pressure in excess of the system's ability to evacuate fluid likely leads to a pressure gradient between the IO space and the surrounding soft tissue space that favors evacuation of fluid forcibly through whatever communicating channels are available. For this reason, providers are encouraged to avoid a second attempt at IO insertion on the same bone, since the previous attempt may have compromised the cortical integrity and created a convenient route for extravasation. One possible exception to this principle is the placement of a second functional IO catheter in the same bone, assuming that both IO catheters are well-seated in the cortex and maintain an infusion pressure greater than the IO pressure.

Infusate

Characteristics of the infusate itself must be considered when evaluating the ability of IO infusion to achieve a desired flow rate. While crystalloid solutions are the most common fluids infused via IO catheterization, the infusion of blood products, hetastarch, and other solutions with higher viscosity may require additional infusion pressure or other techniques to overcome the additional resistance to flow imparted by the fluid's viscosity. The temperature of a solution may also influence its flow through the IO space, as chilled solutions may have increased viscosity or induce a vasoconstrictive effect on local vascular tone.

Flow rates for crystalloid solutions are generally found to be higher than those for whole blood, without controlling for subject type [1, 4, 5, 28, 31]. Unfortunately, increased infusion pressure may also be associated with increased risk of hemolysis for blood products containing cellular components (e.g., whole blood, packed red blood cells) or have other undesired effects on acellular solutions such as plasma [30].

Infusion Tract

Resistance to flow is also introduced by the IO device and infusion tubing, with longer infusion tracts contributing to reduced flow, with all other factors being equal. Thus, the physical dimensions of the catheter, length of infusion tubing, presence of secondary Y-ports, and the presence of kinked or damaged tubing may reduce flow. One recent study of the effect of IV cannula length on flow rates showed that, for a given cannula gauge, flow rates increased between 5% and 18% with a 13 mm reduction in cannula length. This effect was most pronounced for 16-gauge cannulae [44]. While the effect of catheter design and length of infusion tubing has not yet been studied for IO catheters, it is possible that shorter and wider catheters and tubing could augment flow rates. This effect should be studied further as a means of improving IO flow rates.

Subject

Recent swine studies at the proximal humerus infusion site have shown a flow rate of 96.5 mL/min with the syringe push-pull method, versus 72.6–74.0 mL/min with pressure bag infusion and 60.0 mL/min with rapid infuser infusion ($p < 0.05$) [30, 31]. Infusion rates in the swine model are 55 mL/min at the sternum, 128 mL/min with simultaneous infusion at bilateral humeri, and 127 mL/min at the humerus and sternum simultaneously [30]. These findings suggest that the flow rate available at the swine humerus may be greater than that available at the sternum, and that bilateral humeral (or humeral plus sternal) flow may be substantially greater than flow rates achievable with cannulation of the humerus alone [30]. Flow rates with hetastarch are lower than with lactated Ringer's solution, likely due to increased viscosity [29].

A recent study by Lange reports a flow rate of 55.6 mL/min when saline was infused in the proximal humerus using the EZ-IO® catheter and a pressure bag. This rate is comparable to that reported in studies by Hammer (60 mL/min) and Pasley (57.1 mL/min), although the confidence intervals for the mean flow rates obtained in all three of these studies are quite large [1, 25, 26].

Reported IO flow rates vary widely in the medical literature, likely due to differences in patient intravascular fluid status, site selection, device selection, and other patient- or study-specific factors. This makes generalizations about IO flow rate by site or other individual factors very challenging. Table 7.2 shows rates of IO infusion flow as previously reported in the medical literature for a variety of IO insertion sites and devices.

Table 7.2 Studies reporting intraosseous flow rates

Study	Type (n)	CV state	Fluid	Site	Insertion device	Gauge, length	Pressure device (mmHg)	Mean flow rates (mL/min)
Auten (2019) [31]	SW (36)	HS	Blood	PH	EZ-IO	15G, 45 mm	PB (360)[a]	72.6 (95% CI 61.0–84.2)
							RI (301)[a]	60.0 (95% CI 44.8–75.2)
							SY (3058)[b]	96.5 (95% CI 81.9–111.1)
Bjerkvig (2018) [5]	HV (20)	E	Blood	S	FAST1	14G, 155 mm	Gr	Median 46.2 (range 39.3–51.2)
					TALON	15G, 38.5 mm	Gr	Median 32.4 (range 26.3–39.2)
Carness (2012) [29]	SW (8)	E	LR	S	Jamshidi	15G, variable	Gr	8 (SD ± 3)

(continued)

Table 7.2 (continued)

Study	Type (*n*)	CV state	Fluid	Site	Insertion device	Gauge, length	Pressure device (mmHg)	Mean flow rates (mL/min)
				TT	EZ-IO	15G, 25 mm	PB (300)	34 (SD ± 18)
							Gr	24 (SD ± 11)
			Hetastarch	S	Jamshidi	15G, variable	PB (300)	111 (SD ± 54)
							Gr	6 (SD ± 3)
				TT	EZ-IO	15G, 25 mm	PB (300)	26 (SD ± 14)
							Gr	10 (SD ± 4)
Douma (2015) [45]	SW (5)	n/a	NS	PH	EZ-IO	15G, 25 mm	PB (300)	44 (SD ± 24)
							IP[c]	32.87 (95% CI 32.61–33.15)
							PB (300)	42.28 (95% CI 37.81–47.96)
Hammer (2015) [26]	HC (65)	n/a	NS	S	FAST-R	14G, 155 mm	PB[d]	53 (SD ± 2)–112 (SD ± 47)
				PH	EZ-IO	15G, 45 mm		16 (SD ± 3)–60 (SD ± 44)
				PT	EZ-IO	15G, 25 mm		27 (SD ± 5)–69 (SD ± 54)
Hodge (1987) [2]	D (4)	Hypo	LR	PT	Monoject	20G, 63.5 mm	Gr	11 (range 7–14)
							BPU (300)	24 (range 14–30)
					Manual	13G, 88.9 mm	Gr	13 (range 9–17)
							BPU (300)	29 (range 24–34)
Johnson (2005) [4]	HC (106)	n/a	NS	S	FAST1	14G, 155 mm	Gr	102
Lairet (2010) [32]	SW (10)	E	Optirate 320	PH	EZ-IO	15G, 45 mm	RI (239)[a]	79 (range 77–114)
							PB (394)[a]	115 (range 77–144)
				PT	EZ-IO	15G, 25 mm	RI (270)[a]	47 (range 36–58)
							PB (471)[a]	81 (range 30–105)
Lange (2019) [25]	DC (11)	n/a	NS	PH	EZ-IO	15G, 15 mm	Gr	0.9405 mL/kg/min (SD ± 0.6045)
							PB (300)	2.068 mL/kg/min (SD ± 0.8707)

Table 7.2 (continued)

Study	Type (*n*)	CV state	Fluid	Site	Insertion device	Gauge, length	Pressure device (mmHg)	Mean flow rates (mL/min)
				IW	EZ-IO	15G, 15 mm	Gr	0.5295 mL/kg/min (SD ± 0.3176)
							PB (300)	1.515 mL/kg/min (SD ± 0.5951)
				PT	EZ-IO	15G, 15 mm	Gr	0.2948 mL/kg/min (SD ± 0.2927)
							PB (300)	0.6049 mL/kg/min (SD ± 0.4942)
				DF	EZ-IO	15G, 15 mm	Gr	1.029 mL/kg/min (SD ± 0.6646)
							PB (300)	2.102 mL/kg/min (SD ± 0.7135)
Larabee (2011) [6]	SW (5)	CA	CS	PT	Illinois	15G	PB (300)	1.153 mL/kg/min (SD ± 0.447)
Mader (2010) [46]	SW (8)	CA	CS	PT	EZ-IO	15G, 15 mm	IP (n/a)	1.8 cm³/kg/min (95% CI 1.3, 2.3)
Miller (2010) [34]	HV (16)	E	n/a	PH	EZ-IO	15G, 25 mm	PB (300)	84.9 (SD ± 43.9)
				Right PT	EZ-IO	15G, 25 mm	PB (300)	17.5 (SD ± 13.9)
				Left PT	EZ-IO	15G, 25 mm	PB (300)	13.8 (SD ± 3.9)
Ngo (2009) [35]	HV (18)	CA or Hypo	NS	PH	EZ-IO	15G, 25 or 45 mm	Gr	81.8 (SD ± 38.4)
							PB (300)	148.1 (SD ± 75.3)
				PT	EZ-IO	15G, 25 or 45 mm	Gr	68.2 (SD ± 42.1)
							PB (300)	204.6 (SD ± 156.0)
Ong (2009) [36]	HV (24)	CA or Hypo	NS	PH	EZ-IO	15G, 25 or 45 mm	Gr	84.4 (SD ± 37.5)
							PB (300)	153.2 (SD ± 65.0)
				PT	EZ-IO	15G, 25 or 45 mm	Gr	73.0 (SD ± 35.4)

(continued)

Table 7.2 (continued)

Study	Type (*n*)	CV state	Fluid	Site	Insertion device	Gauge, length	Pressure device (mmHg)	Mean flow rates (mL/min)
							PB (300)	165.3 (SD ± 112.5)
Pasley (2015) [1]	HC (16)	n/a	NS	S	FAST1	14G, 155 mm	PB (300)	93.7 (SD ± 37.9)
				PH	EZ-IO	15G, 25 or 45 mm	PB (300)	57.1 (SD ± 43.5)
				PT	EZ-IO	15G, 25 or 45 mm	PB (300)	30.7 (SD ± 18.7)
Puga (2016) [28]	HV (30)	E	NS	S	TALON	15G, 38.5 mm	PB (300)	159.8 (SD ± 45.1)
				PH	EZ-IO	n/a	PB (300)	104.9 (SD ± 54.6)
Sulava (2021) [30]	SW (24)	E	Blood	S	FAST1	14G, 155 mm	PB (360)	55
				PH	EZ-IO	15G, 45 mm	PB (360)	74
Tan (2012) [47]	HV (22)	CA or Hypo	NS	PT	EZ-IO	15G, 25 mm	Gr	3.96
							PB (300)	6.36
				DT	EZ-IO	15G, 25 mm	Gr	1.72
							PB (300)	3.28
Tiffany (1999) [40]	HV (5)	E	NS	S	FAST1	14G, 155 mm	Gr	17.9 (SD ± 9.1)
					FAST1	14G, 155 mm	PB (300)	104.1 (SD ± 46.5)
							SY (n/a)	232.5 SD ± 131.2)
Winkler (2017) [48]	HV (17)	E	Lohexol 350	Right PH	EZ-IO	15G, 45 mm	SY (n/a)	200
				Left PH	EZ-IO	15G, 45 mm	SY (n/a)	220
				Tibia	EZ-IO	15G, 25 mm	SY (n/a)	190

Notes: *BPU* Blood pump unit, *C* Calcaneus, *CA* Cardiac arrest, *CI* Confidence interval, *CS* Chilled saline, *D* Dog, *DC* Dog cadaver, *DF* Distal femur, *DT* Distal tibia, *E* Euvolemic, *HC* Human cadaver, *HV* Human volunteer (healthy subject), *Hypo* Hypovolemic, *IW* Iliac wing, *LR* Lactated Ringer's solution, *n/a* Data not available, *NS* 0.9% Normal saline solution, *PH* Proximal humerus, *PT* Proximal tibia, *S* Sternum, *SD* Standard deviation, *SY* Syringe.

[a]Mean infusion pressure
[b]Peak infusion pressure
[c]Infusion pump set at a flow rate of 999 mL/h
[d]Increased from 0 to 300 mmHg in 50 mmHg increments

Troubleshooting

Marrow Aspiration

The adequacy of flow through an IO catheter is ultimately a clinical determination, which should be evaluated on a case-by-case basis. The ability to aspirate bone marrow, which usually appears as a blood-tinged viscous fluid containing fat and particulate material, is commonly cited as evidence of appropriate penetration of the IO cavity with the potential for satisfactory IO infusion. While aspiration of bone marrow is certainly a reliable sign that the tip of the cannula is in the medullary space, **the inability to aspirate marrow is not definitive evidence that the catheter is malpositioned**. In some cases, the tip of the IO catheter may be within the medullary cavity even when marrow cannot be aspirated. This could be due to a variety of causes, including obstruction of retrograde flow due to partial or complete occlusion of the catheter tip from bony spicules or other material within the IO space. High resistance experienced with attempted syringe infusion immediately after IO catheter insertion should be considered to be evidence of suboptimal placement of the catheter, but the tip may still be within the medullary cavity. **The combination of absent marrow aspiration and substantial resistance to flow suggests that the tip of the IO catheter may not be appropriately seated**; in such cases, the provider should consider that the IO catheter may not be suitable for use. However, if the catheter can be easily flushed, and there is no evidence of local extravasation (i.e., swelling of the soft tissues in the area of insertion with subsequent infusion), it is reasonable to consider infusion through the IO catheter. In all cases, the insertion site should be monitored periodically for evidence of extravasation throughout the infusion process. If any signs of localized soft tissue swelling are identified, the infusion should be stopped.

Catheter Insertion

As a general rule, IO catheters are inserted at a right angle (90°, perpendicular) to the surface of the bone. This sounds simple, but it is often challenging to determine the plane in which the surface being cannulated is directed. The best rule of thumb is to **consider the direction of the limb (or sternal structure) being cannulated and base the angle of insertion on that plane**. Recommended IO insertion sites are relatively flat bony surfaces, but bones are not always flat surfaces. As mentioned above, the proximal humerus (for example) is not uniformly flat, so identification of the recommended insertion site is extremely important to ensure that a flat plane is cannulated. This is one of the reasons why it is important to cannulate the recommended site on a bone and not to cannulate a site on a bone that is different from the recommended anatomic site.

Providers should feel for the loss of resistance during insertion, indicating penetration of the cortex and entrance into the marrow space. It is not recommended to proceed past this point, as this could result in positioning the catheter tip against the inner surface of the opposing (*trans*) cortex and may prevent adequate forward flow. After insertion is complete, the provider should draw back on the syringe, aspirate, and look for blood and/or bone marrow in the connection tubing to confirm placement. A 10 mL flush with saline is recommended to confirm suitable flow, and providers should not proceed with the infusion if this saline flush is unsuccessful.

Obstacles to Flow

It is tempting to think of IO catheters in the same terms as peripheral intravenous (PIV) catheters, but they are not the same. One of the biggest differences between IO and PIV catheters is the angle of insertion. Peripheral IV catheters are inserted at a 15–30° angle from the plane of the target vessel, with optimal placement resulting in the tip of the catheter situated at the center of the lumen. Once the vein has been punctured, the provider usually drops their hand to advance the catheter, with the result that the catheter is more or less pointed in the same direction as the vein. This is absolutely different with IO catheters. In fact, the angle of insertion for an IO catheter is ideally 90° perpendicular to the bone surface. A perfectly placed IO catheter will penetrate the cortex of the target bone at a 90° angle and will be advanced through the bone cortex (which is usually 2–3 mm thick) until the tip of the cannula is situated at the center of the medullary space. But this bony space is not a vacant wide-open space. Rather, the medullary space is an epicenter of hematological activity, packed with mesenchymal stem cells and a host of more developed cells, including osteoblasts, osteoclasts, chondrocytes, myocytes, fibroblasts, macrophages, adipocytes, and endothelial cells. The intramedullary space also contains hematopoietic cells, such as red blood cells, white blood cells, and platelets, in various stages of development and is full of bony spicules and other calcified structures that readily obstruct free flow.

Because of this very important difference between PIV and IO catheters, a properly placed IO catheter may still function very poorly despite the best possible effort on the part of the clinician. It is true that peripheral veins have valves and some other anatomical causes for obstruction of flow. However, a well-placed PIV will usually function consistently well if proper insertion technique is followed. This is not always true for IO catheters. In many cases, perfect insertion technique still yields a poorly performing IO catheter. With the limitations of current imaging modalities, it is literally impossible to know what is impeding flow through the IO space. Syringe flush of at least 10 mL (preferably more) through the catheter immediately after insertion usually clears out some of the intramedullary space for the infusion of fluids and medications, but this only flushes out the mobile components of the IO space. It does not alter the bony architecture of the medullary cavity, which may be the cause for poor flow through an IO catheter.

If flow rates become inadequate during infusion, providers should check the catheter to confirm that it has not been dislodged. They should check the tubing as well to confirm that there are no kinks or punctures and that no connections have become loose. It is important to periodically check the device that is being used to create infusion pressure, whether it be a pressure bag or an infusion pump. Providers should ensure that the pressure bag is inflated or that the infusion pump is on, plugged in, and charged and that the infusion pump is set to the desired rate of infusion.

Future Directions

Additional research is needed to identify factors that contribute to optimal intraosseous flow rates for human subjects. The existing data on IO catheter flow are difficult to interpret, as investigators do not uniformly report the IO insertion site utilized, the associated infusion pressure, or the patient's comorbid medical conditions that could influence fluid flow. Certain medical conditions, such as hypovolemia, congestive heart failure, shock states, and other causes of vasoplegia must be reported along with relevant flow rate data. Common data elements that should be collected for all study subjects include:

- Subject type (e.g., healthy human subject, clinically treated patient, animal model)
- Cardiovascular state (e.g., cardiac arrest, hypotensive, fluid overloaded)
- Infusion site (e.g., sternum, proximal humerus, proximal tibia)
- Infusion pressure (e.g., gravity infusion, pressure bag, infusion pump, syringe)
- Device used (e.g., EZ-IO®, FAST1®) including length and gauge of catheter
- Volume and duration of infusion

Researchers should consider that animal subjects are not the same as human subjects and that various physiologic differences may complicate the extrapolation of animal data to the clinical management of human patients. Unfortunately, clinical data on IO flow rates among human subjects are currently inadequate to make any sound recommendations on device or site selection. However, better data may be available if researchers choose to focus upon clinically relevant outcomes and provide adequate detail on the manner in which IO infusion is performed. Even the most cursory review of the available literature confirms that all IO devices and all IO insertion sites do not perform the same.

In order to advance the science of IO infusion flow rates, we recommend that future studies include:

- Utilization of real-time measurement of intramedullary pressures to guide infusion pressures for efficient and safe IO infusion
- More robust comparative evaluation of IO flow rates in pathologic states, including hypovolemia, shock, and cardiac arrest
- Investigation on the effect of patient positioning on IO flow rates (e.g., elevating tibias in a supine patient during calcaneal IO infusion)
- Additional "double-barreled" IO infusion studies using two IO catheters at different sites simultaneously

Conclusion

In emergent situation requiring large-volume IO infusion of crystalloid fluids or blood products, clinicians should be aware of the various factors affecting IO catheter flow rates. These factors include the site and device selected, the patient's general intravascular fluid status, the applied infusion pressure, and the type of infusate that is being contemplated.

Existing data on IO flow rates are highly specific to the patient population being studied, and interpretation of these data is limited by inadequate data collection on many parameters that influence flow rate. It is very challenging for clinicians to extrapolate existing data on IO flow rates to their patient population due to significant variation in the variables reported by investigators and an inaccurate assumption that all IO flow rates are the same. Intrinsic factors such as the size and capacity of the target bone, the gauge and length of the catheter selected, the patient's current intravascular fluid volume, and the circulating concentration of hormonal modifiers to bony blood flow must be considered when estimating IO infusion rates.

Key Concepts

- The sternum generally provides the highest IO flow rates, followed by the humerus, the femur, and the proximal tibia. In general, more distal target bones provide lower effective fluid infusion rates
- Increasing infusion pressure can increase flow rates, but also requires greater surveillance for complications due to excessive pressure exerted on veins draining the medullary space
- Providers should use the shortest possible IO catheter and tubing setup to reduce resistance to forward flow
- Low serum O_2 concentration and acidic metabolites have been shown to increase intraosseous blood flow, while vasopressors and neural stimulation decrease it
- Future research on IO flow rates should include standardized data elements, including the infusion pressures used to achieve flow, systemic blood pressure, infusion site used, and other patient-specific factors that may significantly influence fluid flow rates

References

1. Pasley J, Miller CH, DuBose JJ, et al. Intraosseous infusion rates under high pressure: a cadaveric comparison of anatomic sites. J Trauma Acute Care Surg. 2015;78(2):295–9. https://doi.org/10.1097/TA.0000000000000516.
2. Hodge D 3rd, Delgado-Paredes C, Fleisher G. Intraosseous infusion flow rates in hypovolemic "pediatric" dogs. Ann Emerg Med. 1987;16(3):305–7. https://doi.org/10.1016/s0196-0644(87)80176-2.
3. Draenert K, Draenert Y. The vascular system of bone marrow. Scan Electron Microsc. 1980;4:113–22.
4. Johnson DL, Findlay J, Macnab AJ, Susak L. Cadaver testing to validate design criteria of an adult intraosseous infusion system. Mil Med. 2005;170(3):251–7. https://doi.org/10.7205/milmed.170.3.251.

5. Bjerkvig CK, Fosse TK, Apelseth TO, et al. Emergency sternal intraosseous access for warm fresh whole blood transfusion in damage control resuscitation. J Trauma Acute Care Surg. 2018;84(6S Suppl 1):S120–4. https://doi.org/10.1097/TA.0000000000001850.

6. Larabee TM, Campbell JA, Severyn FA, Little CM. Intraosseous infusion of ice cold saline is less efficacious than intravenous infusion for induction of mild therapeutic hypothermia in a swine model of cardiac arrest. Resuscitation. 2011;82(5):603–6. https://doi.org/10.1016/j.resuscitation.2011.01.007.

7. Sweeney MN. Vascular access in trauma: options, risks, benefits, and complications. Sem Anesth Periop Med Pain. 20(1):47–50. https://doi.org/10.1053/sa.2001.21100.

8. Laney JA, Friedman J, Fisher AD. Sternal intraosseous devices: review of the literature. West J Emerg Med. 2021;22(3):690–5. https://doi.org/10.5811/westjem.2020.12.48939.

9. Shore AC. Capillaroscopy and the measurement of capillary pressure. Br J Clin Pharmacol. 2000;50(6):501–13. https://doi.org/10.1046/j.1365-2125.2000.00278.x.

10. Shah P, Louis MA. Physiology, central venous pressure. StatPearls; 2022.

11. Tansey EA, Montgomery LEA, Quinn JG, Roe SM, Johnson CD. Understanding basic vein physiology and venous blood pressure through simple physical assessments. Adv Physiol Educ. 2019;43(3):423–9. https://doi.org/10.1152/advan.00182.2018.

12. Beverly M, Murray D. Factors affecting intraosseous pressure measurement. J Orthop Surg Res. 2018;13(1):187. https://doi.org/10.1186/s13018-018-0877-z.

13. De Lorenzo RA, Ward JA, Jordan BS, Hanson CE. Relationships of intraosseous and systemic pressure waveforms in a swine model. Acad Emerg Med. 2014;21(8):899–904. https://doi.org/10.1111/acem.12432.

14. Shim SS. Physiology of blood circulation of bone. J Bone Joint Surg. 1968;50(4):812–24.

15. Drinker CK, Drinker KR. A method for maintaining an artificial circulation thro ugh the tibia of the dog, with demonstration of a vasomotor control of the marrow vessels. Am J Phys. 1916;40(4):514–21.

16. Trotman NM, Kelly WD. The effect of sympathectomy on blood flow to bone. JAMA. 1963;183:121–2. https://doi.org/10.1001/jama.1963.63700020020013e.

17. Stein AH Jr, Morgan HC, Porras RF. The effect of pressor and depressor drugs on intramedullary bone-marrow pressure. J Bone Joint Surg Am. 1958;40-A(5):1103–10.

18. Shim SS, Patterson FP. A direct method of qualitative study of bone blood circulation. Surg Gynecol Obstet. 1967;125(2):261.

19. Woodhouse CF. Nutrient arterial circulation control problems in bone. Am J Orthop. 1963;5:290–5.

20. Cumming JD. A study of blood flow through bone marrow by a method of venous effluent collection. J Physiol. 1962;162(1):13–20. https://doi.org/10.1113/jphysiol.1962.sp006909.

21. Shim SS. Quantitative studies of factors affecting bone blood flow based on bone clearance of radiostrontium (Sr^{85}). Dissertation. University of British Columbia; 1965. p. 137.

22. Nutbeam T, Fergusson A. Intraosseous access in osteogenesis imperfecta (IO in OI). Resuscitation. 2009;80(12):1442–3.

23. Shoor PM, Berryhill RE, Benumof JL. Intraosseous infusion: pressure-flow relationship and pharmacokinetics. J Trauma. 1979;19(10):772–4.

24. Warren DW, Kissoon N, Sommerauer JF, Rieder MJ. Comparison of fluid infusion rates among peripheral intravenous and humerus, femur, malleolus, and tibial intraosseous sites in normovolemic and hypovolemic piglets. Ann Emerg Med. 1993;22(2):183–6. https://doi.org/10.1016/S0196-0644(05)80199-4.

25. Lange J, Boysen SR, Betley A, Atilla A. Intraosseous catheter flow rates and ease of placement at various sites in canine cadavers. Front Vet Med. 2019;6:312. https://doi.org/10.3389/fvets.2019.00312.

26. Hammer N, Möbius R, Gries A, Hossfeld B, Bechmann I, Bernhard M. Comparison of the fluid resuscitation rate with and without external pressure using two intraosseous infusion systems for adult emergencies, the CITRIN (Comparison of InTRaosseous infusion systems in emergency medicINe)-study. PLoS One. 2015;10(12):e0143726. Published 2015 Dec 2. https://doi.org/10.1371/journal.pone.0143726.

27. Sørgjerd R, Sunde GA, Heltne JK. Comparison of two different intraosseous access methods in a physician-staffed helicopter emergency medical service—a quality assurance study. Scand J Trauma Resusc Emerg Med. 2019;27(1):15. Published 2019 Feb 13. https://doi.org/10.1186/s13049-019-0594-6.

28. Puga T, Montez D, Philbeck T, Davlantes C. Adequacy of intraosseous vascular access insertion sites for high-volume fluid infusion. Crit Care Med. 2016;44(12):263.

29. Carness JM, Russell JL, Lima R, Navarro LH, Kramer GC. Fluid resuscitation using the intraosseous route: infusion with lactated Ringer's and hetastarch. Mil Med. 2012;177(2):222–8. https://doi.org/10.7205/milmed-d-11-00195.

30. Sulava E, Bianchi W, McEvoy CS, et al. Single versus double anatomic site intraosseous blood transfusion in a swine model of hemorrhagic shock. J Surg Res. 2021;267:172–81.

31. Auten JD, McEvoy CS, Roszko PJ, et al. Safety of pressurized intraosseous blood infusion strategies in a swine model of hemorrhagic shock. J Surg Res. 2020;246:190–9.

32. Lairet JR, Bebarta V, Lairet K, et al. Intraosseous pressure infusion comparison using a rapid infusion device and a pressure bag in a swine model. Ann Emerg Med. 2010;56(3):S26.

33. Krepela A, Auten JD, Mclean J, et al. A comparison of flow rates and hematologic safety between intraosseous blood transfusion strategies in a swine (Sus scrofa) model of hemorrhagic shock: a pilot study. Ann Emerg Med. 2017;70(4):S139.

34. Miller L, Philbeck T, Montez D, Puga T. A two-phase study of fluid administration measurement during intraosseous infusion. Ann Emerg Med. 2010;56(3):467.

35. Ngo AS, Oh JJ, Chen Y, Yong D, Ong ME. Intraosseous vascular access in adults using the EZ-IO in an emergency department. Int J Emerg Med. 2009;2(3):155–60. https://doi.org/10.1007/s12245-009-0116-9.

36. Ong ME, Chan YH, Oh JJ, Ngo AS. An observational, prospective study comparing tibial and humeral intraosseous access using the EZ-IO. Am J Emerg Med. 2009;27(1):8–15.

37. Nevin DG, Brohl K. Permissive hypotension for active hemorrhage in trauma. Anaes. 2017;72(12):1443–8.

38. Hug MI, Buettiker V, Cornelius A, Weiss M. Variability in infusion pressure and continuous flow rate delivered from pressurized bag pump flush systems. Anaesth Intensive Care. 2002;30(3):341–7.

39. Philbeck T, Miller L, Montez D. 407: pain management during intraosseous infusion through the proximal humerus. Ann Emerg Med. 2009;54(3):S128.

40. Tiffany BR, Horwood BT, Pollack CV, Kurbat J, Adams J, Kharrazi R, Diethrich EB. Sternal intraosseous infusion: flow rates and utility. Ann Emerg Med. 1999;4(34):S15.

41. Acme Revival. Abbott Plum A+ Operating Manual. https://acmerevival.com/wp-content/uploads/2020/10/Abbott-Plum-A-Op-Manual.pdf. Accessed 28 May 2022.

42. Hunsaker S, Hillis D. Intraosseous vascular access for alert patients. Am J Nurs. 2013;113(11):34–40.

43. Orlowski JP, Julius CJ, Petras RE, Porembka DT, Gallagher JM. The safety of intraosseous infusions: risks of fat and bone marrow emboli to the lungs. Ann Emerg Med. 1989;18(10):1062–7.

44. Jayanthi NV, Dabke HV. The effect of IV cannula length on the rate of infusion. Injury. 2006;37(1):41–5.

45. Douma MJ, Bara GS, O'Dochartaigh D, Brindley PG. Double-barreled resuscitation: a feasibility and simulation study of dual-intraosseous needles into a single humerus. Injury. 2015;46(11):2239–42.

46. Mader TJ, Walterscheid JK, Kellogg AR, Lodding CC. The feasibility of inducing mild therapeutic hypothermia after cardiac resuscitation using iced saline infusion via an intraosseous needle. Resuscitation. 2010;81(1):82–6.

47. Tan BK, Chong S, Koh ZX, Ong ME. EZ-IO in the ED: an observational, prospective study comparing flow rates with proximal and distal tibia intraosseous access in adults. Am J Emerg Med. 2012;30(8):1602–6.

48. Winkler M, Talley C, Woodward C, Kingsbury A, Appiah F, Elbelasi H, Landwher K, Li X, Fleischmann D. The use of intraosseous needles for injection of contrast media for computed tomographic angiography of the thoracic aorta. J Cardiovasc Comput Tomogr. 2017;11(3):203–7.

Intraosseous Medication Administration

8

Paul Dobry, Stephanie B. Edwin, Renée M. Paxton, Tsz Hin Ng, and Christopher A. Giuliano

Introduction

The earliest reported use of the intraosseous (IO) route for medication administration was in the treatment of pernicious anemia during the 1930s, evaluating the infusion of campolon (liver extract) into the sternum and manubrium of human patients as an alternative to peripheral intravenous (PIV) infusion [1]. Since that time, many other medications have been studied via the IO route, with variable degrees of demonstrated efficacy. While IO and PIV infusions have been suggested to be equivalent, evidence within the existing medical literature suggests that the effects realized by medication administration through direct and indirect (e.g., IO) venous infusion may not be uniformly equivalent. This chapter explores the existing evidence for the efficacy of IO infusion, including sometimes conflicting reports on the utility of the IO route for emergently delivering lifesaving fluids and medications.

Most medications studied with IO infusion are indicated for the emergent stabilization of critically ill patients, including those experiencing cardiac arrest, hemodynamic instability, respiratory failure, acute poisoning, and emergent neurological conditions. In the absence of human trials, animal models currently provide the bulk of the existing evidence for the efficacy of IO infusion. Unfortunately, translational studies confirming the utility of IO infusion suggested by preclinical animal data

P. Dobry (✉) · C. A. Giuliano
Department of Pharmacy, Eugene Applebaum College of Pharmacy and Health Sciences, Wayne State University, Detroit, MI, USA
e-mail: paul.dobry@wayne.edu; ek2397@wayne.edu

S. B. Edwin · R. M. Paxton · T. H. Ng
Department of Pharmacy, Ascension St John Hospital, Detroit, MI, USA
e-mail: stephanie.edwin@ascension.org; renee.paxton@ascension.org; tsz.hin.ng@ascension.org

© The Author(s), under exclusive license to Springer Nature Switzerland AG 2024   167
J. H. Paxton (ed.), *Intraosseous Vascular Access*,
https://doi.org/10.1007/978-3-031-61201-5_8

have not been forthcoming, leaving the evidence for IO infusion of medication in human subjects largely anecdotal and assumptive nearly a century after the introduction of therapeutic IO infusion techniques.

Medications that have been previously reported to have been safely administered to humans via the IO route are provided in Table 8.1. This chapter explores evidence for these different types of medications in the sections that follow.

Table 8.1 Medications reportedly infused via the intraosseous route among human subjects

Analgesic, anesthetic, sedative, and paralytic medications	
Acetaminophen [2]	Mivacurium [2]
Alfentanil [2]	Morphine [3–8]
Atracurium [2, 9, 10]	Nalbuphine [2]
Cisatracurium [11]	Pancuronium [5, 10, 12–14]
Diazepam [5, 15–17]	Phenobarbital [7, 14]
Etomidate [7, 18, 19]	Propofol [2, 6, 7, 20, 21]
Fentanyl [6–8, 18, 21, 22]	Remifentanil [2]
Haloperidol [11, 23]	Rocuronium [7, 18, 21, 24]
Hydromorphone [7]	Ropivacaine [25]
Ketamine [2, 6–8, 10, 24]	Sufentanil [19]
Lidocaine [7, 17, 18, 21, 26–33]	Succinylcholine [4, 6, 7, 9, 10, 15, 16, 18, 26]
Lorazepam [7, 11, 34]	Thiopental [4, 9]
Midazolam [5–7, 18, 22]	Vecuronium [4, 6, 7, 22]
Cardiac medications	
Adenosine [35–38]	Ephedrine [2]
Amiodarone [7, 18, 23, 33, 39]	Epinephrine [4, 6, 7, 13–19, 21, 22, 40–42]
Atropine [4, 6, 7, 10, 14–18, 20, 22, 23, 26, 28]	Isoproterenol [2, 14]
Bretylium [17]	Labetalol [11, 23]
Digoxin [43]	Furosemide [18]
Diltiazem [7]	Norepinephrine [7, 18]
Dobutamine [5, 7, 42, 44]	Phenylephrine [7, 23]
Dopamine [5, 7, 13, 16, 18, 42]	Vasopressin [7, 18]
Volume replacement medications	
Albumin [7, 13, 44, 45]	0.9% Normal saline [2, 5–7, 18, 22, 41, 46, 47]
Dextran-40 [28]	Plasma, human [6, 13, 21, 41, 47–49]
Dextran-60 [50]	Packed red blood cells [4, 6, 13, 21, 23, 41, 48, 51]
Dextran-70 [52]	Succinylated gelatin [53]
Dextrose 5, 10, 25, or 50% [7, 16–18, 40, 44, 45, 54, 55]	Whole blood, human [28, 46, 47, 49]
Hartmann's solution [6, 28, 47]	3% hypertonic saline [56, 57]
Hydroxyethyl starch [41]	7.5% hypertonic saline [50, 52]
Lactated Ringer's solution [2, 5, 12, 17, 18, 21, 28, 50, 54, 58]	23.4% hypertonic saline [59, 60]
Mannitol [4]	
Antimicrobial medications	
Acyclovir [61]	Fluconazole [7]
Ampicillin [7, 13, 15, 20, 54, 62]	Gentamicin [7, 13]
Aztreonam [7]	Linezolid [7]
Benzylpenicillin [6]	Penicillin [5, 43]

Table 8.1 (continued)

Cefazolin [5, 23]	Piperacillin-tazobactam [7]
Cefepime [7]	Sulfadiazine [46]
Cefotaxime [54, 62]	Sulfapyridine [63]
Ceftriaxone [7, 23]	Tobramycin [7]
Flucloxacillin [6]	Vancomycin [7, 20]
Antitoxin medications	
Antipneumococcal serum [46]	Influenza B serum [46]
Antitetanus serum [49]	Lipid emulsion [64, 65]
Centruroides immune F(ab')2 [66]	Naloxone [7, 16–18, 67]
Flumazenil [19, 23]	Meningococci antitoxin [46]
Hydroxocobalamin [19, 23, 68, 69]	Methylene blue [70]
Other medications	
Alteplase [71, 72]	Magnesium sulfate [7, 11]
Aminophylline [18, 73]	Methylprednisolone [7, 11, 23]
Calcium chloride [4, 7, 17, 40, 54]	Neostigmine [2, 10]
Calcium gluconate [27, 49]	Ondansetron [7]
Contrast media [28, 43, 49, 74–79]	Phentolamine [80]
Cryoprecipitate [48]	Phenytoin [4, 7, 14, 16, 81]
Dexamethasone [4, 11, 28]	Potassium chloride [11, 23]
Diazoxide [28]	Promethazine [7, 18]
Diphenhydramine [7]	Recombinant factor VIIa [6]
Enoxaparin [23]	Sodium bicarbonate [4, 7, 13–16, 18, 27, 40, 49, 54]
Fosphenytoin [7]	Sodium sulfate [49]
Glucose 5–50% in water [13, 46, 49, 58, 63]	Tenecteplase [22, 39]
Heparin [7, 23, 28, 39, 43]	Thiamine [7, 18]
Hydrocortisone [10]	Tranexamic acid [48, 82]
Insulin [7, 43, 83]	Vitamin K [13]
Levetiracetam [7]	3-factor prothrombin complex concentrate [84]

General Considerations

Efficient and timely administration of lifesaving medications can be crucial to the stabilization of critically ill patients. In such patients, oral or rectal administration of medications is often not considered to be appropriate, necessitating the emergent establishment of parenteral venous access for medication infusion. Patients who are hemodynamically unstable may have difficult venous access, suggesting the need for alternative **indirect** means of establishing access to the venous system when intravascular volume is low or patients do not have available venous targets for the establishment of **direct** venous access at the time of their presentation to the clinical team. Consequently, alternative routes for drug delivery can be required under specific clinical circumstances. Intraosseous (IO) infusion has emerged as a potentially invaluable route for indirect access to the venous system among critically ill patients, allowing providers to infuse substances directly into the medullary cavity of bones, harnessing the well-vascularized environment within the bone marrow to deliver fluids and other medications.

Although the equivalence of medication bioavailability via the IO and peripheral intravenous (PIV) routes has become broadly accepted over time, such assumptions are based largely upon historical and anecdotal evidence of moderate quality [85]. However, many medications considered to be safe for infusion via PIV catheter have also been administered through an IO catheter in clinical practice with little to no data to suggest inferiority. Historical data on the efficacy of IO infusion are mostly derived from preclinical animal studies. Of course, physiological differences between animals (e.g., swine, dogs, lambs) and human subjects in regard to bone perfusion, bone composition, and proximity of IO insertion site to the central venous system likely limit our ability to extrapolate the findings in these studies to the care of human patients.

Emerging literature evaluating IO infusion in out-of-hospital cardiac arrest (OHCA) patients may provide more relevant conclusions, but not without their own limitations. Many biases must be considered in the interpretation of the results of these studies, including what appears to be the use of IO cannulation in patients with poor prognosis (i.e., patients who have failed multiple PIV attempts or who have peripheral veins that are deemed to be inaccessible by providers). This is referred to as **resuscitation time bias**. Resuscitation time bias is inherent to many OHCA studies, as protocols often arbitrarily require PIV access attempts before resorting to IO access. This cultural bias, based upon familiarity with PIV access, limits the potential benefits of early IO access over delayed PIV or central venous catheter (CVC) access. As such, outcomes in most previously reported trials are likely biased against the use of IO infusion for resuscitative medications. The relative paucity of randomized control trials comparing early IO to early PIV access in OHCA provides a clear example of how traditional methods of human patient management likely minimize the potential benefits of early IO access for cardiac arrest victims.

Anecdotal evidence may support the widespread assumption that PIV and IO dosing should be the same for most indications, but this assumption is built largely upon the unproven premise that medications delivered via the IO route are absorbed immediately and transmitted entirely and without delay into the subject's venous system without sequestration in the marrow space. This premise is altogether unlikely, as different patients may have different concentrations of red and yellow marrow in the target bones commonly used for IO cannulation. **Red marrow** (as seen predominantly with pediatric subjects) is highly vascularized, while **yellow marrow** (with a high concentration of adipose tissue, as often seen in the long bones of adult subjects) is less well vascularized and may have inefficient transport of infused substances when compared to red marrow [86]. This distinction has potential implications for IO medication administration, as red and yellow marrow are not homogenous tissues and likely exert differing effects on medication binding within the marrow and soft tissues prior to entry in the venous circulation.

Red marrow consists of approximately 40% water, 40% fat, and 20% protein, while yellow marrow has a higher proportion of fatty tissue (80%), with a lower water (15%) and protein (5%) concentration [87]. The distribution phase of a medication's pharmacokinetics (PK) profile will depend largely upon its **octanol-water partition coefficient** (P). Hydrophobic drugs with high partition coefficients

($\log P > 0$) are preferentially distributed to hydrophobic compartments such as the yellow marrow, while hydrophilic drugs with low partition coefficients ($\log P < 0$) are found in more hydrophilic compartments such as those provided by the red marrow. Depending upon the composition of the medullary cavity and the octanol-water partition coefficient of the agent being infused, there may be delayed or incomplete entry into the venous system (i.e., the so-called **depot effect**). This may lead to reduced peak concentrations (C_{max}) and longer times to peak concentration (t_{max}) following infusion. Evidence of this phenomenon has already been shown with studies of IO infusion for many drugs including amikacin, epinephrine, ceftriaxone, chloramphenicol, phenytoin, tobramycin, and vancomycin [88–90]. This effect may be at least partially overcome by administration of a 3–10 mL 0.9% normal saline flush immediately following drug infusion [88–90]. While this phenomenon may suggest the need for larger doses with IO administration of these drugs than with IV infusion, further research is needed to determine optimal dosing.

In addition to differing constituents of the medullary cavity, other factors likely influence the PK profile of medications administered via the IO route. Shock states, such as hypovolemia and cardiac arrest, are generally associated with **reduced blood flow to bones and other nonessential organs** as blood is preferentially shunted towards the brain, heart, and other vital organs under such conditions. This likely affects the absorption of medications from extremity IO sites into the central vasculature. Even in the absence of shock, intramedullary bone pressures significantly surpass the intraluminal pressures typically encountered during PIV infusion [91]. Thus, **the infusion pressures required for IO infusion are likely much greater than those needed for PIV or CVC infusion**. Medications infused via the IO route must also be taken up by relatively small drainage veins, and the biochemical mediators regulating venous drainage of target long bones remain poorly understood. Although it has been hypothesized that IO infusion of certain substances may alter subsequent venous drainage from the medullary space, further research is needed to better characterize this effect.

Cannulation site is another variable that likely influences the PK of medications infused via the IO route. The vast majority of studies examining IO access have focused upon the proximal tibial IO insertion site, which is definitively a subdiaphragmatic infusion. **It has been well known for more than four decades that subdiaphragmatic PIV infusion sites are not capable of achieving optimal central venous concentrations of drug in low-flow states such as cardiac arrest and hypovolemia** [92]. Anatomically, IO infusion through the proximal or distal tibia is akin to PIV infusion through a leg vein. While most emergency care providers would not consider resuscitating a critically ill patient solely via a tibial or soleal leg vein, many clinicians seem comfortable resuscitating patients with a tibial IO catheter. This begs the question as to why so many resources are spent comparing antecubital PIV or CVC administration to tibial IO administration, rather than comparing upper extremity PIV infusion to infusion through an upper extremity (e.g., humeral) or centrally located (e.g., sternal or clavicular) IO infusion site. It is **unlikely that venous infusion of any drug (either directly via PIV or indirectly via IO infusion) from a subdiaphragmatic insertion site can provide bioavailability**

comparable to that achieved by a supradiaphragmatic insertion site in the setting of cardiac arrest or other conditions characterized by low systemic blood pressure.

Optimal IO insertion sites, such as the proximal humeral, sternum, and clavicle, are not well studied in the existing medical literature, but these sites may offer potential advantages over tibial IO infusion sites as they are closer to the heart and central venous circulation [93]. Evidence of these advantages exists, as in one swine PK study showing that the mean dose of epinephrine delivered via tibial IO route was 65% of the drug delivery provided via the sternal IO route [94]. In another swine PK study, 1 mg of epinephrine administered via humeral IO infusion was associated with a significantly higher C_{max} and a significantly shorter t_{max} when compared to tibial IO administration of the same drug dose [95]. In conditions characterized by low circulatory blood flow, when the primary target of action is the heart, such alternative sites may prove especially advantageous.

Despite all of the potential differences between IO and IV medication administration, limited PK data from human subjects in the existing medical literature suggest that the two routes may be bioequivalent under certain circumstances [3]. Many studies evaluating the resuscitation of cardiac arrest in various animal models have compared IO access with IV access and found no significant differences in rates of return of spontaneous circulation (ROSC) or the concentrations of common resuscitative medications as measured from the central vasculature [96–105]. These studies contribute to the prevailing opinion that IO and PIV administrations yield similar results. However, **controlled animal studies may not reflect real-world human subject use of the IO route in the setting of delayed clinical resuscitation**. Further research is needed to determine whether the PK and clinical outcomes of IO medication infusion in animal subjects are similar to those currently theorized for human subjects.

Conditions Treated with Intraosseous Medications

Cardiac Arrest/Dysrhythmias

The first modern guidelines for OHCA resuscitation were established in 1974 by the American Heart Association (AHA) [106], but these guidelines did not endorse or even describe the use of IO infusion for medication administration [106]. Although reports of fluid and medication infusion via the IO route were very common in the English-language medical literature of the 1940s and 1950s, it was not until a handful of clinicians including pediatrician James Orlowski publicly called for the resurgence of IO infusion in 1984 that modern resuscitative guidelines would suggest IO cannulation for the treatment of OHCA patients [107]. Even then, the trend began with pediatric patients—not adults. Orlowski's first-hand experience with IO infusion for crystalloid fluids during a cholera epidemic in India gave him unique insight into the lifesaving capabilities of IO cannulation under emergent conditions [107]. With input from Orlowski and others, the AHA guidelines were revised in 1986 to include a newly featured section on Pediatric Advanced Life Support (PALS). This section was the first to highlight tibial IO administration as an alternative to PIV infusion under emergent conditions [108]. The success of IO administration among pediatric patients and the advent of improved methods to cannulate the denser tibial bones of adult patients ultimately led to its inclusion into the 2005 AHA adult ACLS guidelines as the preferred route of drug administration (superior to endotracheal tube injection) when IV access was unobtainable [109]. In 2010, the AHA PALS guideline updated their endorsement for IO access to "the primary vascular entry point during cardiac arrest," classified as Class I, Level of Evidence C [110]. This revision appears to have effectively established parity between intravenous IV and IO access for resuscitative applications in the pediatric population. The IO route made its debut as an alternative to direct venous cannulation in the neonatal population in the 2020 update to the AHA guidelines while remaining the preferred route of infusion for both adult and pediatric patients in whom IV access was deemed difficult or impossible [85, 111, 112].

Epinephrine appears to be the medication most commonly used to treat cardiac arrest, so it is not surprising that IO epinephrine infusion has been relatively well studied when compared to other resuscitative medications. In his initial exploration of the IO route for administering epinephrine in various animal models (e.g., guinea pigs, cats, rabbits, dogs, rats), Macht observed that aqueous solutions of epinephrine were absorbed at a comparable rate whether administered via the IO or PIV route with similar duration of effect on subject heart rate and blood pressure [113]. However, **when epinephrine was suspended in oil, the medication exhibited a significantly prolonged duration of effect**. Macht theorized that these oil emulsions lingered within the marrow for an extended period, functioning as reservoirs for the drug, gradually releasing it through the oil medium [113]. These findings suggested that IO infusion of epinephrine may not always be bioequivalent to PIV infusion of epinephrine, with the difference in bioavailability predominantly a function of the solution in which the drug was dissolved.

Similar findings were noted in a comparison between an IO autoinjector prototype and PIV administration during cardiopulmonary resuscitation (CPR) in the swine model [89]. In this study, an IO autoinjector was used to administer a 2 mg (in 2 mL solution) IO epinephrine dose into the proximal tibia in studied subjects, compared with the standard 1 mg/mL PIV dose administered through a leg vein. Tracer radioisotopes were used to track epinephrine doses. Carotid arterial sampling and gamma camera imaging revealed comparable circulation times and arterial concentrations [89] between the PIV and IO groups. However, this study also identified a depot effect within the marrow, likely due to inadequate bone marrow perfusion in the porcine CPR model.

Spivey and colleagues noted that proximal tibial IO administration of epinephrine at conventional PIV doses (0.01 mg/kg) did not result in a notable change in diastolic or mean blood pressure in an anesthetized swine model. However, when administered at higher doses (i.e., 0.1 mg/kg), epinephrine induced a more distinct influence on blood pressure and circulating plasma epinephrine levels [114]. Other studies have also suggested that **higher doses of epinephrine may be necessary**

with IO infusion when compared to PIV infusion [115–117]. Wong et al. compared tibial IO to PIV administration of epinephrine during cardiac arrest in pigs and found that tibial IO administration was associated with significantly lower serum epinephrine concentrations at several time points and a significantly longer **time to maximal concentration** (t_{max}). Although the **maximal serum concentration** (C_{max}) was not significantly lower in the IO group ($p = 0.069$), the authors suggest that this difference would likely have been significant if more subjects were included in the study [116]. Similarly, Burgert et al. observed a significantly lower C_{max} of epinephrine following both tibial IO and sternal IO administration when compared to PIV infusion. The t_{max} for tibial IO administration was significantly faster than PIV infusion, but they found no significant difference in t_{max} between sternal IO and PIV infusion [115]. Given that epinephrine is a potent vasoconstrictor, it is likely that IO infusion of epinephrine exerts a considerable effect on blood flow to and from the target bone, although this potential vasoconstrictive effect of IO epinephrine on subsequent IO infusions remains poorly explored in the existing medical literature.

Despite evidence for a depot effect with IO epinephrine administration, many studies comparing IO to PIV administration of epinephrine during cardiac arrest in animal models have found no significant differences in either PK or clinical outcomes according to the route of infusion [94–96, 118–122]. This is surprising since the majority of these studies compared tibial IO to central venous epinephrine administration, which superficially appears to be an unfair comparison. Likely due in part to resuscitation time bias and the lack of PK data, these findings have only been reciprocated in one subgroup analysis of a large randomized controlled trial (RCT) in humans. Although this study randomized patients to epinephrine or saline (rather than IO or PIV), the placebo group was instrumental in minimizing the effects of resuscitation time bias. This study found no difference in the adjusted odds of **return of spontaneous circulation** (ROSC), long-term survival rates, or favorable neurological outcomes following IO or IV epinephrine infusion for the treatment of OHCA [123]. However, most human studies report a clinical benefit with PIV epinephrine administration during cardiac arrest [124, 125]. Regardless, patients enrolled into cardiac arrest studies are by definition not able to achieve ROSC until receiving the intervention (i.e., IO access). Since many EMS study protocols mandate previous PIV attempts prior to obtaining IO access, patients receiving IO tend to have longer duration of cardiac arrest when compared to patients receiving PIV access in such studies. This serves as a source of bias, as longer durations of cardiac arrest have previously been shown to be independently associated with worse outcomes. **This timing bias likely influences the results of such studies towards a harmful effect associated with IO access for OHCA** when compared to PIV infusion.

The timing of epinephrine administration may be more important than the route of infusion, especially for patients presenting with favorable prognostic factors (e.g., shockable rhythms, witnessed arrest, bystander CPR). It has been shown that early IO epinephrine administration produces superior neurological outcomes when compared to delayed PIV epinephrine in a swine model characterized by prolonged ventricular fibrillation [126]. Similarly, at least one study in humans experiencing OHCA demonstrated that for every 1-min delay between emergency medical service (EMS) call receipt and vasopressor administration, the odds of achieving ROSC declines by 4%. This same study also found that time to first drug (i.e., vasopressin or epinephrine) was significantly shorter with IO infusion when compared to PIV infusion [127]. Another retrospective cohort study in humans experiencing OHCA reported similar findings, concluding that IO administration is associated with significantly higher success rates in prehospital line placement, epinephrine administration, and shorter time to epinephrine administration when compared to PIV infusion of the drug [128].

Existing evidence also suggests that **intravascular volume status** plays a role in determining outcomes associated with IO versus PIV epinephrine administration. Long et al. studied a group of swine in cardiac arrest and found that proximal humeral IO epinephrine administration in normovolemic swine was associated with higher C_{max} levels, shorter T_{max} values, and faster ROSC times when compared to the humeral IO hypovolemic group ($p < 0.05$). All seven participants in the IO normovolemic group achieved ROSC, in contrast to three participants in the IO hypovolemic group. In hypovolemic swine, PIV epinephrine was associated with a higher C_{max} and shorter T_{max} ($p < 0.05$), but longer time to ROSC, although more patients were able to achieve ROSC when compared to those receiving IO drug administration [129]. Yauger and colleagues described a similar phenomenon in a pediatric swine model. In their normovolemic group treated with tibial IO epinephrine, all participants achieved ROSC. Conversely, in the hypovolemia-induced group, the likelihood of ROSC was significantly lower when epinephrine was administered via the tibial IO route compared to the PIV route ($P = 0.03$). The tibial IO hypovolemia group displayed significantly diminished plasma epinephrine concentrations compared to the PIV hypovolemia group at several time points, including the C_{max}. Furthermore, the tibial IO hypovolemia group experienced a significantly delayed t_{max} and a significantly lower AUC when compared to subjects with tibial IO normovolemia [130].

It has been hypothesized that potent vasoconstrictors such as epinephrine can compromise subsequent medication absorption into the central venous system from the medullary cavity. Eriksson et al. challenged this theory by randomizing pigs in hemorrhagic shock to receive a bolus of tibial IO gentamycin after either three IO boluses of epinephrine (0.01 mg/kg, each dose followed by a 10 mL normal saline bolus) or three IO boluses of normal saline (10 mL) through the same cannula. A third group received the same epinephrine regimen as described above and was also given CPR for an induced cardiac arrest. In the no-CPR groups, the mean gentamicin plasma concentrations at 5, 15, and 30 min as well as the AUC did not differ. Those subjects receiving CPR had significantly higher gentamycin concentrations at 15 and 30 min and a significantly higher mean AUC when compared to both other groups [118]. These authors suggest that IO administration of epinephrine may not impair the subsequent uptake of gentamicin administered through the same cannula. However, it is not clear whether IO infusion of epinephrine might reduce subsequent uptake of other drugs (besides gentamycin).

Voelckel et al. sought to elucidate the effects of epinephrine and vasopressin on bone marrow blood flow in pigs experiencing hemorrhagic shock and cardiac arrest. After ROSC was achieved, bone marrow blood flow remained at baseline after IO vasopressin infusion but was reduced significantly after IO epinephrine infusion. Bone vascular resistance was also significantly higher in the epinephrine group when compared to the vasopressin group. Although epinephrine was found to significantly decrease bone marrow blood flow and increase bone vascular resistance, these factors did not seem to affect drug absorption into the systemic circulation. Cerebral perfusion pressures at 30 s and 2 min after drug administration as well as **mean arterial pressure** (MAP) at 5 min post-resuscitation were higher in pigs that received epinephrine when compared to those receiving vasopressin [131]. These findings suggest that alterations in bone marrow blood flow may be a result of epinephrine's effect on the systemic circulation rather than its local effects on bone metabolism. Vasopressin and epinephrine are both potent vasopressors, but act by different mechanisms using different receptors. Studies comparing local IO infusion of vasopressin to epinephrine suggest that these two drugs may have differing effects on blood flow to and from the medullary space, suggesting that **vasopressin and epinephrine may have different effects on subsequent medication infusion when administered via the IO route**.

Similar to epinephrine, conflicting data exist regarding the equivalency of IO and PIV vasopressin administration during cardiac arrest. Four studies report no difference in both PK (C_{max}, t_{max}, and/or serum vasopressin concentrations) and clinical (i.e., rate of ROSC) outcomes. Two were conducted in a hypovolemic cardiac arrest swine model and evaluated at different IO sites (e.g., proximal tibia and proximal humerus) [102, 103], and two were conducted in a normovolemic cardiac arrest swine model and evaluated at different IO infusion sites [101, 132]. Vallier et al. did not assess clinical outcomes, but determined that there is no difference in C_{max}, t_{max}, or serum vasopressin concentrations when vasopressin was administered via sternal IO versus PIV in a normovolemic cardiac arrest swine model [100].

Adams et al. also conducted a study in a hypovolemic cardiac arrest swine model comparing three groups receiving vasopressin infusion: tibial IO, humeral IO, and PIV. They found no significant differences in the rate or timing of ROSC among these three groups. The C_{max} was significantly greater in the PIV group when compared to the tibial IO group, but no significant differences were observed between the other groups. The t_{max} was significantly shorter in the humeral IO group when compared to the tibial IO group, although no significant differences were seen between the other groups. Notably, higher odds of survival were recorded in the humeral IO group when compared to all other groups [133]. Johnson et al. came to a similar conclusion in their study of tibial IO versus PIV vasopressin administration in a normovolemic cardiac arrest swine model. They found that the C_{max} of vasopressin was significantly higher in the PIV group when compared to the IO groups. However, there were no significant distinctions observed between groups in terms of ROSC, time to ROSC, or t_{max} [134]. Several human studies have also reported the safe administration of IO vasopressin, although its efficacy in humans has not yet been established [7, 18].

Amiodarone is commonly given for pulseless ventricular tachycardia and ventricular fibrillation. O'Sullivan et al. sought to determine the differential effects of amiodarone on ROSC when given via the sternal IO, tibial IO, or PIV route in swine with ventricular fibrillation undergoing CPR. All swine received amiodarone, vasopressin, and at least one dose of parenteral epinephrine. The rate of ROSC was similar between all groups, but time to ROSC was significantly faster in the sternal IO group when compared to the tibial IO group, which was noted to be significantly slower than the PIV group. The time to ROSC was nearly five times faster when using the sternal IO site than with the proximal tibial IO site, suggesting the likelihood of PK differences between these two sites [135]. Burgert and colleagues evaluated potential PK differences by also comparing sternal IO, tibial IO, and PIV amiodarone in a cardiac arrest swine model. Although no significant differences in C_{max} were found, the t_{max} of amiodarone was significantly shorter in both the sternal IO and PIV groups than in the proximal tibial IO group [136]. Lipophilic amiodarone may have taken a longer time to distribute from the more adipose-dense proximal tibial site, reflecting the longer time to ROSC and maximum concentration; however, several competing factors for ROSC attainment in both studies likely hinder this assumption.

Three studies in a cardiac arrest swine model all detected no difference in both PK (C_{max}, t_{max}, and/or serum amiodarone concentrations) and clinically important (i.e., rate of ROSC) outcomes when IO and PIV amiodarone were compared [99, 104, 105]. Each study evaluated a different IO infusion site, allowing speculation into the potential depot effect of lipophilic amiodarone within the yellow marrow. Studies assessing the proximal tibial [105] and proximal humeral [104] IO infusion sites both used a 20 mL normal saline flush after amiodarone administration, rather than the traditional 10 mL flush used in the sternal IO study [99]. These findings suggest that **larger volume flushes into more lipophilic cortices may reduce the depot effect of IO infusion of lipophilic drugs**.

Although the Amiodarone, Lidocaine, or Placebo Study (ALPS) did not show a difference in survival or favorable neurologic outcome with amiodarone or lidocaine administration for OHCA due to initial shock-refractory ventricular fibrillation or pulseless ventricular tachycardia when compared to placebo, a secondary analysis of the study stratified by IO versus PIV dosing did identify significant findings. When compared to placebo, individuals who received PIV amiodarone or PIV lidocaine demonstrated a significantly higher discharge survival rate than those who received the drug via IO infusion. Conversely, discharge survival rates did not show significant differences for those administered IO amiodarone or IO lidocaine. No notable outcome variations were noted between PIV and IO placebo, indicating that patients with poorer prognosis were not more likely to receive IO drugs, as appears to be the case in many other human cardiac arrest trials [33].

Adenosine is often the drug of choice to terminate supraventricular tachycardia (SVT). Its efficacy and safety via IO administration were first demonstrated over three decades ago in the porcine model. However, researchers have concluded that the minimal effective IO dose of adenosine needed to induce atrioventricular blockade is less than the minimal effective dose via PIV administration and greater than the central venous dose, though these differences were not deemed to be significant [137]. Its efficacy via IO administration in humans was suggested in 1996, when an infant was administered IO adenosine resulting in successful termination of supraventricular tachycardia [35]. Fidanci et al. describe a similar case of an infant successfully treated with tibial IO adenosine for SVT [38]. Another neonatal patient receiving adenosine via tibial IO catheter achieved normal rhythm using a mixed method administration. In this case, adenosine (0.1 mg/kg) was diluted with normal saline to a 3 mL total volume and was rapidly pushed through the IO line without complications [36].

Goodman et al. documented conflicting findings when IO adenosine was administered to two pediatric patients. Both patients failed to achieve termination of SVT after multiple increasing doses of tibial IO adenosine followed by saline flushes. Ultimately, PIV adenosine was able to terminate the tachyarrhythmia in both cases [37]. Despite these controversial cases, it is still suggested that adenosine should be administered via IO infusion when PIV access cannot be obtained.

Four animal experiments have been conducted evaluating the PK parameters of **atropine** administered through various routes, including the IO, IV, and IM routes [98, 138–140]. Yost et al. investigated the kinetics of atropine administered via the IO, PIV, and IM routes among euvolemic and hypovolemic swine. Their data showed immediate T_{max} for IO and PIV routes in both euvolemic and hypovolemic swine (0 min), whereas the IM route required a longer time (6 min in normovolemic swine and 19.5 min in hypovolemic swine). The AUC values were comparable between all three routes with both volume statuses [140]. Cornell et al. also compared PK parameters among normovolemic and hypovolemic swine which received atropine via sternal IO infusion. This study demonstrated that hypovolemic swine had a significantly greater AUC, longer half-life, and slower clearance via IO infusion when compared to normovolemic swine. No significant differences were noted in V_d, C_{max}, or t_{max} [98]. In an anesthetized monkey model experiment by Prete et al., the authors observed a quicker average T_{max} with PIV (1.37 min) when compared to the IO route (3.87 min) and a slightly higher estimated AUC with IO administration when compared to PIV infusion [139].

Atropine has been safely and effectively administered to human subjects in many cases, although details of its use are rarely documented in the cardiac arrest/dysrhythmia literature. Iserson et al. described a case series involving two patients presenting to an emergency department in cardiac arrest. Both patients were cannulated via distal tibial IO and had a positive hemodynamic response within 1 min of IO atropine administration [141]. Other cases have been found to corroborate the safe and effective use of IO atropine in cardiac arrest [23, 142, 143]. Collectively, these findings suggest that the IO route is an effective means of administering atropine and that the sternal IO route may be comparable in efficacy to the tibial IO route even in cases of significant hypovolemia.

Calcium is another drug that is commonly infused for the treatment of cardiac arrest. Orlowski et al. conducted two animal experiments to explore the effects of IO calcium chloride administration [144, 145]. In this study, they assessed the safety of administering various emergency drugs and solutions (i.e., epinephrine, sodium bicarbonate, hydroxyethyl starch, dextrose 50%, lidocaine [1 mg/kg], and calcium chloride [10 mg/kg]) through the IO route in dogs. The dogs were subsequently sacrificed to measure the resulting bone marrow and fat emboli in the lungs. Autopsy examinations revealed a greater number of emboli in all treatment animals, except for those that received sodium bicarbonate, when compared to control subjects receiving saline, although none of the differences were statistically significant [144]. Fat embolization to the lungs has also been described in human cases, although the clinical significance of such emboli in the absence of an intracardiac shunt is questionable.

In a subsequent Orlowski study, researchers performed a comparison of IO, PIV, and CVC calcium chloride administration (10 mg/kg bolus) in the canine model [145]. No significant differences were observed in serum ionized calcium levels over time between the three routes of infusion [145]. Equal bioavailability between IO and PIV calcium administration has also been suggested in human studies. In one post hoc analysis, post-cardiac arrest patients had similar levels of ionized calcium after calcium chloride was infused via the IO or PIV route [146]. These findings are further supported by an RCT which reported no subgroup differences in the rate of ROSC, 30-day survival, or 30-day favorable neurological outcome according to IO versus PIV calcium chloride administration after out-of-hospital cardiac arrest. However, the utilization of calcium during cardiac arrest situations is under much scrutiny, and even this most recent RCT failed to show a clinical benefit of IO/PIV calcium chloride administration versus placebo [147]. In addition, calcium chloride is a known vesicant, and IO extravasation of this drug has deleterious consequences that have previously been reported in the literature [148].

Sodium bicarbonate is another drug that is commonly infused during cardiac arrest, although it is often reserved for prolonged cases of cardiac arrest or situations in which an accompanying metabolic acidosis is present. Three animal experiments have provided insights into the PK of IO sodium bicarbonate infusion using a 1 mEq/kg dose of sodium bicarbonate [145, 149, 150]. Spivey and colleagues conducted a randomized study involving 23 swine with induced cardiac arrest to investigate blood pH alterations following IO, CVC, and PIV administration of sodium bicarbonate. They found no significant disparity in femoral arterial blood pH between IO and CVC routes, though pH levels were markedly lower with PIV administration 4 min after infusion commencement and continued to remain lower for the duration of the experiment (30 min). The IO route demonstrated the slowest rate (4 min) towards achievement of peak pH when compared to the CVC and PIV routes (each approximately 2 min) [150].

Orlowski et al. performed a similar study on healthy dogs, analyzing the PK of sodium bicarbonate administered through the same three routes. This group assessed changes in end-tidal carbon dioxide percentage following sodium bicarbonate infusion. Mirroring Spivey's findings, subjects in the IO group exhibited the slowest time to achievement of peak effect, with a mean **end-tidal carbon dioxide** (ETCO$_2$) peak level falling between those of the CVC and PIV groups. In this study, the longest duration of ETCO$_2$ effect occurred in the IO group [145]. In a third study, Warren et al. conducted a prospective investigation on intubated, mechanically ventilated, and exsanguinated piglets to evaluate sodium bicarbonate response after administration through various IO sites (e.g., distal femur, proximal humerus, proximal tibia, malleolus) and PIV administration. Similarly, this study assessed end-tidal carbon dioxide change post-sodium bicarbonate infusion, allowing time for $ETCO_2$ to return to baseline values between injections. No significant differences emerged in the time to initial $ETCO_2$ elevation or maximal $ETCO_2$ elevation across sites [149].

Similar findings have been noted in humans. Iserson describes a case series involving seven patients who presented in cardiac arrest and were administered IO **sodium bicarbonate** without complication. Of these seven patients, four received arterial blood gas draws both pre- and post-bicarbonate administration, and all exhibited an increase in serum pH with IO infusion [141]. Reports of IO sodium bicarbonate administration are more abundant in pediatric subjects, with five case reports describing its use in cardiac arrest, none of which reported any complications of IO sodium bicarbonate administration [15, 44, 73, 151, 152]. Collectively, these data suggest that sodium bicarbonate can be safely and effectively administered via the IO route at the same doses commonly used for PIV infusion.

Shock States

Shock states, regardless of their etiology, are **characterized by low systemic blood pressure and poor perfusion to distal organs** including the bone marrow. Unlike the arterial vasculature, which is able to enhance blood pressure by contraction of smooth muscle within the vascular wall to enhance perfusion pressure, the venous vasculature is highly dependent upon systemic blood pressure to achieve adequate intravenous pressures. **Cannulation of the medullary cavity of long bones and other IO target bones allows providers to capitalize upon the presence of a non-collapsible pathway for the introduction of medications and fluids directly into the central venous circulation**. Current understanding suggests that even in states of shock, egress of fluids and medication from the marrow space might remain viable despite the collapse of the patient's venous system and reduced forward flow due to cardiac dysfunction or other causes of systemic hypotension. As a result, IO cannulation could provide benefits for individuals experiencing undifferentiated shock when compared to the employment of PIV or central venous cannulation.

Voelckel et al. sought to elucidate the effects of hemorrhagic shock on bone marrow blood flow in pigs with acute exsanguination of 35% of their estimated blood volume. In their model, bone marrow blood flow decreased up to 70–80% from baseline values [131]. Even in the presence of such severe hypovolemia, several agents such as dextran, normal saline, lactated Ringer's solution, and hydroxyethyl starch have been safely and effectively administered via the IO route in both animal and human subjects experiencing hemorrhagic shock [41, 50, 97, 153–155].

Neufeld et al. compared IO, PIV, and CVC administration of normal saline (50 mL/min over 20 min) in a hemorrhagic swine model. At the end of volume resuscitation, there was no significant difference seen between groups for any of the collected hemodynamic variables (i.e., blood pressure, MAP, central venous pressure, pulmonary capillary wedge pressure, and cardiac output). Additionally, they found no difference between groups in mixed venous oxygen saturation or arterial oxygen saturation at the end of resuscitation. Microscopic examination of the tibial bones targeted for IO saline delivery showed a 1 mm needle track in the cortex and a 2 × 4 mm cavity at the bottom of the track. Marrow proximal to the IO insertion site showed marked hypocellularity with areas of necrosis. Control tibial bones were subjected to the same microscopic evaluation and did not exhibit any of these abnormalities [156]. These findings suggest that IO infusion may reduce cellularity of the medullary cavities used for IO infusion, although the clinical impact of this alteration in IO constituency is on unclear clinical significance.

Crystalloid solutions such as 0.9% normal saline and lactated Ringer's solution exert their pharmacologic effects at a volume roughly tenfold higher than solutions such as hypertonic saline or dextran solution. Higher volumes of fluid infused over a short period of time likely lead to the morphologic changes in bone and other potentially adverse effects seen in subjects receiving IO infusion. Experiments involving rapid IO infusion of substantial quantities of isotonic crystalloid solutions to treat hemorrhagic shock in animal models have suggested that **IO infusions might provide adequate volume replacement to effectively resuscitate young children with a low body weight, but these benefits may not be universally extrapolated to larger adult subjects** [58, 156–159].

The limitations of infusing large volumes of crystalloid fluids via the IO route have prompted researchers to investigate IO resuscitation using **hypertonic saline** or **dextran-containing solutions** in a hemorrhagic animal model. Perron et al. first demonstrated that a 250 mL dose of hypertonic saline/dextran solution (i.e., the typical dose for an adult human) could be administered within a span of 4 min using a sternal IO access device [160]. By employing this sternal access device, Dubick et al. assessed the safety and efficacy of a 4 mL/kg bolus of 7.5% NaCl/6% dextran-70 via either the sternal IO or the PIV routes in euvolemic swine. During the initial 120 min following infusion, they observed nearly identical responses in terms of hemodynamic variables (e.g., MAP, cardiac output), expansion of plasma volume (20% above baseline in both groups), and shifts in plasma protein concentrations and plasma electrolytes [161]. Similarly, prompt reestablishment of hemodynamic stability was noted in hemorrhagic sheep following a 200 mL bolus of 7.5% NaCl/6% dextran-70 through a sternal IO catheter. No differences were noted when compared to administration through a CVC, and no local bone abnormalities or other adverse effects were noted on autopsy [162]. Other research has also highlighted the effectiveness of IO administration of hypertonic saline/dextran solutions in reviving animals from hemorrhagic shock [153, 163, 164]. These studies suggest that delivery of an effective dose of isotonic crystalloid solutions is hindered by the substantial volumes required and higher hydraulic resistance in the marrow than in the intraluminal venous space.

Chavez-Negrete et al. compared the efficacy of sternal IO and PIV infusion of 7.5% NaCl/6% dextran-60 (250 mL) to PIV infusion of lactated Ringer's in humans with hemorrhagic shock due to upper gastrointestinal bleeding. They found no difference in clinical response when comparing IO to PIV infusion of 7.5% NaCl/6% dextran-60 administration, so they were analyzed as the same group in the final analysis. Fifteen minutes after administration and thereafter, blood pressures of patients in the 7.5% NaCl/6% dextran-60 group rose significantly higher than blood pressures in the lactated Ringer's group. Patients in the 7.5% NaCl/6% dextran-60 group also had less supplemental fluid requirements, significantly higher urine output, and a significant improvement in neurological status at 24 h post-resuscitation compared to the group that received lactated Ringer's solution [50].

Hydroxyethyl starch is another colloid with the potential to provide adequate volume expansion using smaller volumes than required with crystalloid fluid infusion. Analysis of medium-molecular-weight hydroxyethyl starch concentrations over time in a hemorrhagic swine model revealed nearly identical peak plasma concentrations for tibial IO ($C_{max} = 5.82 \pm 0.44$ mg/mL) and PIV ($C_{max} = 5.73 \pm 0.88$ mg/mL) administration. Similar changes in MAP, cardiac output, central venous pressure, mean pulmonary capillary wedge pressure, and mean pulmonary artery pressure were seen between groups [155]. Several other animal model studies have also endorsed the safe and effective use of IO hydroxyethyl starch [97, 154, 165]. **Low (70–130 kDa) or medium (200 kDa) molecular weight hydroxyethyl starch should be used preferentially over higher molecular weight formulations with IO infusion**, as they are less likely to accumulate in the bone and surrounding tissues.

Tranexamic acid (TXA) is often used as an adjunctive agent during massive transfusions to reduce the risk of death in patients with hemorrhagic shock associated with hyperfibrinolysis. Timely administration is crucial, as evidence suggests that late administration beyond 3 h of the initial injury may be harmful [166]. Preclinical studies in swine models have concluded that IO infusion of TXA is equivalent to IV TXA in terms of efficacy (confirmed through viscoelastic testing) and that IO TXA is not associated with any major safety concerns [167, 168]. In terms of PK parameters, one study showed that the t_{max} occurred at the end of the infusion and the C_{max} was nonsignificantly lower than PIV TXA administration in a hemorrhagic swine model [167]. A second swine model study in nonhemorrhagic, normovolemic subjects demonstrated that the serum TXA concentration during the 5-min infusion was significantly larger in the PIV group as compared to the IO group, but no significant differences were seen between groups for t_{max}, C_{max}, V_d, AUC, plasma clearance, or half-life [168].

As previously mentioned, TXA is typically administered in conjunction with the massive transfusion of blood products. However, it remains unclear how TXA should be administered if a subject's IO line is already being used to transfuse blood products. Although IM administration is an option, Douma et al. conducted a feasibility study demonstrating the application of dual-IO insertion into the swine proximal humerus. Their simulation for trauma resuscitation involved the infusion of pRBCs at a pressure of 300 mmHg using a pneumatic pressure bag through one needle, while TXA (6 g over 1 h) was concurrently infused through a second needle. This trial demonstrated successful outcomes, with the blood product being infused on average for 771 s for a volume of 250 mL, equivalent to an average rate of 20 mL/min [169]. This technique has not yet been described in humans. Although IO delivery of TXA has been reported in humans, reports of its IO administration and downstream clinical effects are lacking. This justifies the need for further research into the IO infusion of TXA in humans, although its use in animal models seems to be both safe and effective.

Vasopressors/Inotropes

The IO administration of vasopressors has gained prominence in critical care settings as a rapid and effective alternative when direct IV access is challenging or delayed. While **norepinephrine** is the preferred vasopressor for most shock patients, limited data exist to support IO administration of the drug. Ward et al. conducted a swine study evaluating the effect of norepinephrine administration on MAP by both IO and IV routes. Various IO sites were used in this study (i.e., proximal tibia, distal femur, distal humerus, sternum, and proximal ulna). Baseline MAP was 66 ± 6 mmHg. Norepinephrine was infused to increase MAP (mean change 115%, range: 70–162%). Significant correlation ($p < 0.05$, $r = 0.5$) was noted throughout the range of MAP from 40% of the IO sites; however, the norepinephrine response showed **hysteresis** (i.e., a lag in timing between the intervention and its downstream effects) [170]. This delay between increases in IO pressure and MAP may be related to physiologic factors, mechanics of the vasculature, and interaction of norepinephrine within the IO system, among other causes.

Peshimam et al. conducted a retrospective, observational study evaluating the prevalence of vasopressor-associated adverse events according to the route of drug administration during prehospital transport. They found that IO access was utilized in 8.6% of cases ($n = 48$), with 21 patients receiving regimens containing norepinephrine. Overall, the adverse event rate was 10.4% in patients with IO access. Characterization of adverse events included four cases of leg swelling/discoloration and a single grade one extravasation in a patient receiving IO infusion of epinephrine [171]. Similarly, Charbel et al. specifically evaluated the risk of complications with PIV administration of norepinephrine to 37 pediatric patients in the prehospital setting. Norepinephrine concentrations ranged from 10 to 1270 µg/mL with maximum doses ranging from 0.03 to 2 µg/kg/min. Five patients in the study received norepinephrine via IO access (four via proximal tibial, one via distal femur). No IO infusion-related complications were noted in this subset [172].

Several case reports have also described the IO infusion of norepinephrine. The first case is of a 42-year-old morbidly obese female status post-cardiac arrest requiring norepinephrine through a distal tibial IO site while central venous access was being obtained. No evidence of IO-related complications was noted; the patient clinically improved and was subsequently discharged [173]. Suominen et al. reported a neonatal cardiac arrest necessitating insertion of three different IO needles. These include a catheter in the left tibia, which was removed following swelling with a bolus injection, an IO catheter in the left distal femur that was dislodged with movement of the patient's legs, and right proximal tibial IO cannula. Approximately 24 h following placement, the patient developed pallor and discoloration of the right lower extremity leading to a diagnosis of compartment syndrome eventually requiring a below-the-knee amputation. Both norepinephrine and epinephrine had previously been infused through this IO device [174]. Finally, Fetissov et al. reported a case of progressive skin necrosis following resuscitation of a 74-year-old with septic shock who received norepinephrine for approximately 45 min following insertion of a proximal tibial IO catheter. The authors hypothesized that the skin necrosis may have occurred due to norepinephrine extravasation, peri-osseous artery spasm, or ischemic lesions associated with multiorgan failure [175].

Dopamine and **dobutamine** are two other commonly used vasopressors with evidence to support their administration via the IO route. Two swine studies were conducted to evaluate the effects of dopamine (20 µg/kg/min) when administered through an 18-gauge spinal needle inserted into a variety of IO insertion sites (e.g., sternum, distal tibia, iliac crest). In the first study, average baseline systolic blood pressure was 105 ± 20 mmHg and heart rate was 82 ± 20 beats per minute in the nine pigs. The increase in systolic blood pressure was statistically significant 2 min into the dopamine infusion, with a rise in blood pressure noted at 5, 10, 15, and 20 min post-initiation of drug infusion. Significantly elevated heart rate was noted at 15 and 20 min [176]. Similarly, a second swine study separately evaluated the physiologic effects of dobutamine (20 µg/kg/min) and **isoproterenol** (20 µg/kg/min) when administered through a bone marrow biopsy needle inserted at the proximal tibia versus CVC infusion at the femoral vein. Heart rate, arterial pressure, and cardiac output were similar prior to drug infusion in all four groups. Following administration of either isoproterenol or dobutamine, heart rate and cardiac output roughly double by 20 min post-initiation of drug, regardless of the route of administration. The only significant difference between the physiologic effects of IO and CVC administration occurred in the dobutamine group, which demonstrated a higher mean heart rate (approximately 200 bpm vs. 160 bpm) at 5 min in the IO group when compared to the CVC group. This increased heart rate seen in the IO dobutamine group seemed to converge with the CVC group by 20 min post-initiation of infusion. No significant changes in arterial pressure were noted from baseline in either group [177].

In 1984, Berg reported the case of a 6-month-old infant experiencing hypoxic cardiac arrest attributed to an aspiration event [42]. Following infiltration of the child's PIV line and multiple failed attempts at direct venous access, an IO line was placed into the right proximal tibia. In response to hypotension (32/18 mmHg), IO dopamine (10 µg/kg/min) infusion was initiated. Blood pressure improved to 78/56 mmHg within seconds, but dropped to 55/40 mmHg over the next 15 min as a femoral vein cutdown was attempted. The IO access was inadvertently dislodged, leading the blood pressure to drop precipitously to 23/13 mmHg. A second IO catheter was placed in the left proximal tibia with subsequent initiation of dobutamine 10 µg/kg/min. This stabilized the patient's condition, allowing time for a new PIV catheter to be placed [42]. Goldstein et al. reported the case of a 3-year-old male with second- and third-degree burns covering 80% of his total body surface area. After multiple unsuccessful attempts at peripheral and central venous access, proximal tibial IO infusion was used for fluid resuscitation and subsequent dobutamine and dopamine infusion. The patient subsequently recovered [5].

Lidocaine/Analgesics

Pain is a common side effect of IO catheter insertion due to the highly innervated periosteum surrounding long bones and the presence of pressure receptors within the medullary cavity. Penetration of the cortex leads to the stimulation of periosteal pain fibers, inducing a sharp, localized perception of pain at the insertion site. Subsequent infusion of fluid or medication can further exacerbate this perception of pain by stimulating pressure sensors within the medullary space in response to increased intramedullary pressure [86]. Consequently, sensate patients should receive slow infusion (over 120 s, allowing a dwell time of at least 60 s) of 40 mg (2 mL) of **preservative-free 2% lidocaine** through the IO catheter immediately after placement to anesthetize the IO space prior to subsequent infusion of medications or fluids. Following lidocaine administration, the IO line should be flushed with 5–10 mL of normal saline, and an additional 20 mg of lidocaine may be infused over 60 s to provide additional anesthesia to the medullary space [11, 178]. For pediatric patients, the initial dose of IO lidocaine should be 0.5 mg/kg (not to exceed 40 mg), with subsequent doses of 0.25 mg/kg (not to exceed 20 mg). If pain or discomfort persists during prolonged IO infusions, repeat IO lidocaine dosing is permitted.

Although no consistent guidelines have been established for the frequency or maximum safe dose of IO lidocaine infusion, it is generally recommended that IO lidocaine boluses should not exceed 3 mg/kg in total per day or be given more frequently than every 45 min to avoid lidocaine toxicity (e.g., paresthesias, seizures, cardiovascular effects). The central nervous system effects (e.g., paresthesias, seizures) of lidocaine toxicity are generally seen at lower serum concentrations (i.e., >5 mcg/mL) than the drug's toxic cardiovascular effects (>12 mcg/mL). When provided as bolus or short infusions, the elimination half-life of lidocaine is 1.5–2.0 h, although the half-life may be even greater than 3 h when prolonged (e.g., >24 h) infusions are provided. Considering that lidocaine is 90% metabolized by the liver, patients with hepatic dysfunction should be monitored closely for signs of lidocaine toxicity after receiving boluses of IO lidocaine. It is important to remember that lidocaine infused via the IO route will be taken up rapidly into the venous circulation, which can limit the efficacy and duration of IO lidocaine analgesia and may also potentiate the risk of systemic lidocaine toxicity.

Contrary to other indications for local anesthesia (e.g., intradermal injection), lidocaine given via the IO route should not be mixed with epinephrine. It is also not necessary or recommended to routinely buffer IO lidocaine solution with sodium bicarbonate, although buffered lidocaine may improve drug efficacy for patients with profound intramedullary acidosis. Preservative- and epinephrine-free lidocaine is the preferred formulation for both IV and IO lidocaine delivery.

Alternative agents for local anesthesia following IO cannulation have also been explored. In the Safety and Efficacy of Intraosseous Ropivacaine in Lower Extremity (SORE) study, researchers randomized 15 patients undergoing anterior cruciate ligament reconstruction to receive either IO **ropivacaine** (1.5 or 2.0 mg/kg) or local infiltration of ropivacaine (300 mg in 150 mL) into the soft tissue as a control. When comparing the administration of ropivacaine through local infiltration and IO delivery, it is evident that the former results in a more gradual and sustained increase to its C_{max} over an extended duration of approximately 41 min following tourniquet deflation. In contrast, IO delivery leads to a quicker attainment of C_{max} shortly after tourniquet withdrawal (around 9 min) with a gradual decrease observed over the subsequent 2 h. These authors found no significant differences in pain scores or opioid requirements between the three groups [25].

If local analgesics cannot adequately control pain associated with IO infusion, it may be prudent to consider providing systemic analgesia. Fortunately, adequate systemic concentrations of opioid analgesics can likely be achieved through IO delivery. Von Hoff et al. described the only PK study of IO infusion in human subjects. Participants were randomly assigned to two groups: one group receiving an IO bolus of **morphine sulfate** (5 mg over 15 s) followed by an equivalent PIV bolus 24 h later, and a second group receiving the same regimen in opposite order. Serial blood samples were collected at prespecified time points for 8 h post-infusion, and PK parameters were calculated. For most of the PK parameters, including C_{max} (235 ± 107 vs. 289 ± 197 ng/mL, IO vs. PIV, respectively), T_{max} (1.3 ± 0.5 vs. 1.4 ± 0.5 min), and $AUC_{0-\infty}$ (4372 ± 1785 vs. 4410 ± 1930 ng min^{-1} mL^{-1}), no differences were observed between IO and PIV administration. However, a notable exception was detected in the **volume of distribution** (V_d), which was significantly greater for intraosseous infusion at 4.81 L ± 1.66 in the IO group and 3.62 liters ±1.41 in the PIV group ($p = 0.0247$). As V_d is a **proportionality constant** relating the amount of drug in the body to the plasma concentration of drug (i.e., amount of drug in body (mg) divided by plasma concentration of drug (mg/L)), drugs with a higher V_d appear to be more widely distributed outside of the bloodstream than drugs with a lower V_d. Thus, drugs with a higher V_d typically require higher doses to achieve the same serum concentrations as drugs with a lower V_d. The investigators speculate that this disparity in V_d was attributed to a minor deposition effect, likely occurring near the intraosseous port or within the bone marrow itself.

It is worth noting that the Von Hoff study [3] is the only study to date that has reported PK data for any drug in human subjects, all of whom were adult volunteers receiving IO infusion at the iliac crest. The iliac crest, which is not commonly cannulated in adults receiving IO infusion, has a higher proportion of red marrow than most long bones. Morphine sulfate is a very **hydrophilic** opioid, meaning that it is less avidly bound to adipose tissue than more **lipophilic** opioids such as **fentanyl citrate**. These facts suggest that opioid infusion at long bones (such as the proximal tibia and proximal humerus, which are commonly used in clinical practice) may be associated with a greater depot effect (i.e., higher V_d) than that seen with the Von Hoff study. Unfortunately, no subsequent PK studies have been done to investigate these potential differences according to the type of opioid administered or site of IO infusion.

At least one randomized controlled trial has been conducted to determine the clinical benefits of IO morphine sulfate administration during orthopedic surgery. Participants undergoing total knee arthroplasty surgery were randomized to receive either IO antibiotics alone or IO antibiotics plus IO morphine sulfate (10 mg). On average, patients who received IO morphine experienced superior pain relief and significantly lower postoperative opioid consumption (as measured by morphine milliequivalents) for up to 2 weeks after surgery [179]. These findings suggest that local IO infusion of analgesic medications near the operative site during orthopedic surgery may reduce postoperative analgesia requirements.

Hypoglycemia/Hyperglycemia

Dextrose is commonly utilized in the treatment of hypoglycemia, with typical concentrations including 5%, 10%, and 50% dextrose-containing solutions. In a canine study, the IO administration of 25 grams of 50% dextrose exhibited similar peak times and peak glucose concentrations to those achieved via CVC dextrose administration. In this study, glucose levels were found to be identical across various time intervals, up to 30 min post-administration. In this study as well as others, IO infusion of dextrose has been shown to achieve a superior peak glucose concentration when compared to PIV administration [145, 176]. There is a paucity of data evaluating 5 and 10% dextrose solutions infused via the IO route, likely due to the fact that such low dextrose concentrations are rarely utilized in emergent hypoglycemic conditions. Although 50% dextrose is the preferred agent for emergent treatment of severe hypoglycemia, lower concentrations of dextrose have also been shown to be safely administered via the IO route to both children and adults [7, 44, 45].

Insulin infusion is often required for hyperglycemic emergencies such as diabetic ketoacidosis (DKA) and hyperglycemic hyperosmolar state. Alawi et al. documented the successful management of a 5-year-old pediatric DKA patient with IO insulin infusion. Following multiple unsuccessful attempts at establishing PIV access, a 14-gauge, 3 cm disposable intraosseous infusion needle was inserted into the proximal tibia. Insulin infusion commenced at the standard rate of 0.1 units/kg/h and was continued for 14 h via the IO catheter, ultimately leading to the patient's recovery. No significant adverse events or electrolyte abnormalities were observed with IO insulin administration. The authors also reported that the glycemic correction pattern resembled that expected with PIV insulin therapy [180].

Poisoning/Antidote Infusion

In cases of emergent poisoning, timely and effective drug administration is needed to counteract toxic effects and improve patient outcomes. Hemodynamic instability associated with severe poisoning can make PIV access difficult to obtain. Although the IM route is feasible for some antidotes such as atropine and pralidoxime, the longer onset of action with IM delivery may preclude its use in some emergent situations. Because of this, IO antidote administration has emerged as a lifesaving intervention when the establishment of PIV access is not feasible. This section will discuss IO infusion of antidotes for emergent poisoning, including hydroxocobalamin, naloxone, lipid emulsion, methylene blue, scorpion antivenom, atropine, and pralidoxime.

Atropine/Pralidoxime

Atropine is the preferred antidote for the management of cholinergic toxicity resulting from exposure to agents such as organophosphates, carbamates, and muscarine-containing mushrooms. Pralidoxime, a cholinesterase reactivator, is often administered concomitantly with atropine to overcome these toxicities [181]. Despite frequent utility of these agents as antidotes, there are no human toxicity studies evaluating IO administration of pralidoxime, and only one human case report exists for atropine. Manley describes the case of a 2-year-old male presenting with organophosphate overdose successfully treated with IO atropine without any apparent complications [182].

Murray et al. compared PK parameters of atropine, **pralidoxime**, and **hydroxocobalamin** when administered to minipigs via the IO, CVC, and IM (except hydroxocobalamin) routes [138]. Peak plasma concentrations for atropine and pralidoxime occurred within 2 min (the earliest sampling point) for both CVC and IO groups, but not until 8 min in the IM group. For hydroxocobalamin, the t_{max} was shorter with IO administration (5 s) when compared to CVC infusion (6 s). The $AUC_{0-\infty}$ was comparable among all three routes for all three drugs; however, the C_{max} of atropine was higher when administered IO (117.1 ng/mL) compared to CVC (80.9 ng/mL) and IM (33.6 ng/mL) administration. Although no animals in the study were intoxicated prior to antidote administration and thus efficacy cannot be established, the data suggest that these antidotes exhibit rapid and adequate bioavailability without concerns for safety [138]. The potential for IO administration of hydroxocobalamin is of particular importance because it cannot be given via the IM route due to the large volume of diluent required.

Hydroxocobalamin

In addition to the hydroxocobalamin PK parameters discussed above, one case report documented the treatment of an infant with suspected cyanide poisoning due to smoke inhalation. This patient received 2.5 g of **hydroxocobalamin** via the IO route prior to hospital arrival. Following antidote administration, the patient's hemodynamic parameters stabilized, and she displayed significant overall improvement. She was discharged after 9 days of hospitalization with no sequelae [68]. Another case report of IO hydroxocobalamin administration in a 53-year-old female with suspected cyanide poisoning due to smoke inhalation offers similar conclusions. She was found unresponsive and pulseless in a burning building without spontaneous respiration. Cardiopulmonary resuscitation was initiated, and PIV access was attempted without success. Shortly after ROSC was achieved out of hospital, a left humeral IO line was placed and 5 grams of hydroxocobalamin was freely infused from the commercially available glass vial (Cyanokit®). Following administration of the antidote, she began to take spontaneous breaths, open her eyes, and bite the endotracheal tube, despite not following any commands. Upon hospital arrival, the patient was noted to have red-colored urine without the presence of red blood cells as confirmed by urinalysis. This suggests that IO hydroxocobalamin can adequately enter systemic circulation despite the non-compressible antidote vial. Although the patient improved initially, mental status declined by day 2 of hospitalization, and the family elected to pursue organ donation [69].

Bebarta et al. compared PIV versus IO hydroxocobalamin for the treatment of acute severe cyanide toxicity in 24 swine. Hydroxocobalamin (150 mg/kg) given over 2–3 min immediately after a continuous infusion of cyanide elicited a 50% drop in MAP. Following the 60-min study period, 10 out of 12 animals in the PIV group and 10 out of 12 in the IO group survived. No significant differences were detected between groups for cardiac output, oxygen saturation, systemic vascular resistance, bicarbonate, pH, and lactate levels. Whole-blood cyanide concentrations were undetectable after hydroxocobalamin administration in both groups [183]. Although the doses were larger and infused quicker than what is typically seen in practice, the results reinforce previous studies indicating that the PK profile achieved with IO hydroxocobalamin infusion closely resembles that of PIV administration and may be equally safe [138, 184].

Methylene Blue

Two studies investigated the IO administration of **methylene blue**, including an animal experiment and a pediatric case report. Herman et al. reported the case of a 6-week-old female infant with methemoglobinemia who received proximal tibial IO infusion of methylene blue (1 mg/kg over 3–5 min). The patient's severe cyanosis resolved after 8 min, oxygen saturation increased from 86% to 98–100%, and methemoglobin levels decreased from 29.8% to 8.2% within 3 h of IO drug administration. No apparent adverse effects resulted from the IO administration of methylene blue, and the infant ultimately recovered and was discharged after 3 days of hospitalization [70].

In an experimental study by Hosseinpour et al., 20 rabbits were randomized to receive either PIV or IO administration of 100 mg/10 mL of methylene blue over 20 s. Methylene blue was dosed at 38–71 mg/kg, much higher than the doses commonly seen in clinical management (1–2 mg/kg). The researchers assessed the drug's delivery into the systemic circulation by observing the time that it appeared in the aorta. There was no difference in the aorta entry time for methylene blue provided between the PIV and IO routes, and all the rabbits survived until the end of the experiment [185].

Lipid Emulsion

Several publications have described the use of IO infusion of **lipid emulsion** to treat various intoxicants. In one case report, tibial IO infusion of a lipid emulsion bolus

(12 mL of 20% solution) followed by a brief drip was used to successfully treat an infant experiencing tonic-clonic seizures due to lidocaine toxicity [64]. Another case report described the proximal tibial IO infusion of a lipid emulsion bolus (120 mL of 20% solution) at an undisclosed rate into an adult with verapamil overdose. In this case, the administration was initially painful for the patient, and the infusion was terminated only halfway through the bolus due to inadequate flow through the required filter and IO device. Despite these complications (and the patient's unfortunate demise 2 days later), the authors suggest that IO administration of lipid emulsion may be a viable alternative to IV infusion, especially when slower infusion rates can be tolerated [65].

Another animal experiment involving bupivacaine-intoxicated rats revealed comparable mortality and hemodynamic outcomes between IO and PIV administration of 30% lipid emulsion. In this study, 10 mL/kg of lipid emulsion was administered over 180 s with no reported complications [186]. These findings suggest that lipid emulsion doses much larger than what is typically seen in practice (1.5 mL/kg) can safely be administered by slow bolus infusion.

Scorpion Antivenom

Hiller et al. reported a case series including two children successfully treated with IO infusion of *Centruroides Immune F(ab')*2 (Anascorp®) following scorpion envenomation. In the first case, Anascorp® was infused via the IO catheter until infiltration was observed into the calf. One additional vial was given via the intramuscular (IM) route, leading to resolution of the patient's rotary nystagmus, jerking movements of the extremities, and apparent distress. In this case, the patient recovered with no identifiable complications. In the second case, three vials of Anascorp® were administered via IO infusion, and within minutes, respiratory failure was reversed and intubation was avoided. Within an hour, vital signs had returned to baseline, and the patient's nystagmus and other symptoms had resolved. This patient was discharged home the same day without any complications from the envenomation [66].

Naloxone

Although **naloxone** is supplied in several convenient and efficient dosage forms such as the IM autoinjector and an intranasal spray, it has also been safely administered to adults and pediatric patients via the IO route [7, 16–18, 67]. However, one case report noted ventricular tachycardia, a rare side effect of naloxone administration, after IO administration of naloxone (0.4 mg, ×2 doses) for an adult patient suspected of methadone overdose. The patient had several risk factors for dysrhythmia; thus, the authors could not conclude that the episode of ventricular tachycardia was related to the route of drug administration [187].

Seizures/Neurological Emergencies

Several animal experiments have investigated the IO administration of **diazepam**. One study was conducted using a pentylenetetrazol-induced seizure model in swine [188], while the second was executed in a healthy dog model [189]. In terms of PK outcomes, both studies demonstrated slightly elevated diazepam blood concentrations during the initial 5 min in the PIV group as compared to the IO group, albeit lacking statistical significance [188, 189]. Regarding the time taken to control seizure activity, Spivey et al. revealed no significant difference between the IO and IV routes (8 min versus 2 min, respectively) [188]. In this study, both the IO and IV groups received a 0.1 mg/kg bolus of diazepam, a dose comparable to that clinically used to treat status epilepticus in pediatric patients [188]. Similar findings have been reported when comparing IO to PIV **lorazepam** infusion in a swine model [190].

Only one case report details the IO administration of diazepam in a human subject. In this report, 1 mg of diazepam delivered via proximal tibial IO to a 6-month-old infant resulted in almost immediate cessation of seizure activity within 1 min. Prior to IO diazepam infusion, the patient had received approximately 120 mg (15 mg/kg) of IM phenobarbital without success [15]. This case underscores the utility of IO medication delivery under emergent conditions, suggesting that drugs administered via the IO route may be quickly and effectively absorbed into the systemic circulation, especially when compared to the IM route.

One PK study describing the IO infusion of **midazolam** has been reported using a swine model. In this study, pigs were administered midazolam via the IO, PIV, and IM routes, and serial blood samples were collected to determine PK parameters. The t_{max} for both the IO and PIV routes were identical (2 min), although the C_{max} for the PIV group was nonsignificantly larger. The C_{max} for both the IM and IO groups did not occur until approximately 10 min post-administration. Interestingly, the calculated bioavailability of IM midazolam (96%) was greater than that seen in the IO group (88%), although IO midazolam had an immediate anticonvulsive effect [191]. These results suggest that the clinical utility of midazolam infusion via all three routes may be similar, despite differing PK parameters.

Phenytoin is another drug commonly used to control seizure activity. In 1986, a case report was published describing the use of IO phenytoin infusion for seizure control in a 2-year-old boy presenting to the emergency department with status epilepticus. He had been previously prescribed phenytoin for a seizure disorder, but his initial phenytoin level on arrival was noted to be only 4 µg/mL, far less than the drug's therapeutic range of 10–20 µg/mL. Phenytoin (17 mg/kg) was subsequently infused into the patient's proximal tibial IO catheter at a rate of 25 mg/min, followed by a 17 mL/kg bolus of lactated Ringer's solution. After receiving IO phenytoin infusion, the patient returned to his baseline level of consciousness, and seizure activity resolved. After completion of the phenytoin infusion (140 min elapsed time), a repeat phenytoin level was drawn and found to be therapeutic at 28 µg/mL. Subsequent radiologic imaging revealed a cortical puncture wound at the IO infusion site, but no other complications were noted [81].

Preclinical studies of IO phenytoin infusion in animal models appear to provide conflicting results. Vinsel et al. administered a 15 mg/kg dose of phenytoin over 15 min to pigs using either the PIV or the tibial IO route. This group found no statistical difference in mean systemic concentrations of phenytoin levels between the two groups, although they found that 50% of the IO group never achieved a therapeutic drug level versus 100% in the PIV group. It has been suggested that alkaline substances such as phenytoin may damage the bone marrow. However, microscopic examination of the cortex and bone marrow at the IO infusion site in these pigs was noted to be normal as far as 5 weeks post-infusion [192].

In a similar experiment, Jaimovich et al. administered a 15 mg/kg dose of phenytoin (in addition to 20 mg/kg of **phenobarbital**) to pigs using both the PIV and tibial IO infusion routes. They found that the t_{max} was approximately 1 min for both anticonvulsants via either route; however, systemic concentrations of both anticonvulsants were significantly greater at all 11 time points within the PIV group compared to those pigs receiving IO infusion. Although IO infusion of phenobarbital yielded lower systemic concentrations than PIV infusion, the levels achieved with IO infusion were still within the therapeutic range throughout the study period. These authors found a more clinically significant difference with IO phenytoin infusion. Phenytoin levels within the IO group remained subtherapeutic for 30% of the study period, while phenytoin levels achieved in the PIV group were noted to be therapeutic throughout the study. For both anticonvulsants, the AUC was significantly higher when administered by the PIV route [193]. In a separate study with a very similar study design, the authors concluded that the bioavailability calculated from total phenytoin levels was 84% for IO phenytoin and 91% for IO fosphenytoin (a water-soluble prodrug of phenytoin) [194]. Although these preclinical data suggest suboptimal systemic absorption with IO phenytoin, future studies involving serum drug-level monitoring could inform dosage changes that would help alleviate this concern in clinical practice.

Brickman et al. conducted a series of experiments comparing IO to PIV phenobarbital infusion in the canine model. Their first study revealed that phenobarbital (10 mg/kg) infused over 1 min via the IO route resulted in nonsignificantly higher serum levels at all four time points when compared to the PIV group [189]. In their second study, the researchers used a 5 mg/kg bolus of phenobarbital to determine the PK/PD alterations that occur as a result of failed IO cannulation. In one group, three punctures were made in the tibia (one being used for infusion) to represent two failed IO attempts, and in the second group, only one tibial puncture was made where the drug was infused. The group with multiple IO punctures had significantly lower serum phenobarbital levels at all four of the assessed time points. In this study, the authors speculated that multiple IO attempts resulted in substantial extravasation into the adjacent soft tissues during infusion, leading to a considerably lower volume of medication escaping from the medullary cavity into the vascular system [195].

The efficacy of central venous infusion of **hypertonic (23.4%) saline** for the treatment of elevated intracranial pressure (ICP) has been well documented in the medical literature. However, placement of a CVC can be challenging in patients with intracranial hypertension (ICH) due to concerns about patient positioning during the procedure potentially worsening ICH. This suggests the potential value of alternative methods for infusing hypertonic saline. Not surprisingly, several cases have been reported on the IO delivery of 23.4% saline for patients with ICH. Farrokh et al. described a case series of six patients that were successfully treated with IO infusion of 23.4% saline for ICH [60]. In this report, three patients were being treated for intracranial bleed and herniation, one patient for subarachnoid hemorrhage (SAH) with herniation, one for cerebellar bleed with herniation, and one for a temporal lobe tumor with associated cerebral edema. Each patient received one 30 mL dose of IO 23.4% saline, except for the SAH patient who received three separate 30 mL doses. One of the patients with intracranial bleed had ICP measured before (43 mmHg) and after (28 mmHg) humeral IO hypertonic saline administration, which demonstrated efficacy of the IO infusion. No complications of IO administration were reported for any patient [60]. Similar findings were noted in a series of five patients administered IO 3% saline at 25–100 mL/h [57].

Wang et al. conducted a retrospective cohort study including patients who received 23.4% saline via IO or CVC infusion. In this study, most IO cannulae were placed in the proximal humerus (33/38, or 86.8%) or the proximal tibia (5/38). No local IO insertion site complications were reported. They found that the mean time to hypertonic saline administration was significantly shorter in the IO group. The increase in serum sodium after 23.4% saline administration was significantly larger in the CVC group as compared to the IO group, but there were no significant differences seen in Glasgow coma scale (GCS) score, herniation reversal, MAP change, hypotension, or survival to discharge. Although not statistically significant, this study showed a greater number of patients with successful herniation reversal in the IO group (36%) when compared to the CVC group (15.6%) [59]. These findings suggest that hypertonic saline can be effectively administered via IO infusion, although the small number of subjects reported is not adequate to provide definitive evidence of safety given the substantial risks associated with extravasation of hypertonic solutions into the soft tissues. The potential advantages of IO infusion when compared to CVC infusion in this clinical setting include a reduction in the time required to place the catheter and the ability to place an IO catheter without the need to place the patient in a recumbent or Trendelenburg position.

Utilization of IO hypertonic solutions is intriguing because of the reduced fluid volumes required to achieve physiological effects, but IO infusion of hypertonic saline may be associated with inherent risks. Saline concentrations >1% are direct vascular irritants and behave more like vesicants at higher concentrations such as 23.4%. Animals that have been administered IO hypertonic solutions have demonstrated leakage into adjacent soft tissues, skin necrosis, bone marrow necrosis, myonecrosis, deep vein thromboses, and superficial vein thromboses among other adverse effects [16, 196]. Consequently, the risk of hypertonic saline extravasation and subsequent soft tissue necrosis with IO catheter placement must be weighed against the potential advantages of IO infusion for these patients.

Hematologic Emergencies

Spencer et al. reported a case of tibial IO infusion of **alteplase** (100 mg over 2 h) administered for massive pulmonary embolism (PE). No repeat imaging was performed after thrombolytic administration, but the patient ultimately improved without any reported complications from IO administration of the drug [71]. Another case of IO thrombolytic administration involved a patient in cardiogenic shock resulting in out-of-hospital cardiac arrest. Empiric **tenecteplase** was administered before hospital transport, with subsequent imaging confirming the diagnosis of acute bilateral massive PE. Alongside IO delivery of resuscitation drugs, therapeutic hypothermia was applied. The treatment yielded favorable results, and the patient was discharged from the hospital 39 days later without significant complications [22].

Ruiz-Hornillos et al. described a case of a 64-year-old man with ST-segment elevation myocardial infarction and repeated episodes of ventricular fibrillation. Repeated attempts at PIV access failed, and the patient was subsequently cannulated via the tibial IO route. Tenecteplase (6000 IU) and unfractionated **heparin** (3000 IU) were delivered as a bolus, followed by a continuous IO heparin infusion. Thirty minutes after administration of these drugs, reperfusion dysrhythmias were noted, and the ST-segment elevation resolved. Within 25 min, the patient's chest pain had resolved. No complications of IO administration were identified [39].

More recently, the IO route has been used to administer alteplase for acute ischemic stroke. Bowry et al. described a series of three patients given standard doses of alteplase via a mobile stroke unit. Two patients were cannulated via tibial IO and one via humeral IO. In this report, IO access was left in place for 24 h post-administration in all patients, and no complications were reported [197].

Although IO administration of thrombolytics can be a lifesaving intervention in many instances, it does not come without risk. Landy et al. reported the case of an adult male in cardiac arrest with a suspected massive PE. Alteplase (0.6 mg/kg) was administered via a proximal tibia IO catheter, and sinus rhythm was restored 5 min later. Roughly 2 days later, the patient developed an extensive area of tissue necrosis on the anteromedial side of the leg surrounding the IO insertion site. Ultimately, surgical excision and subsequent skin grafting on the leg were required, as the soft tissue damage was not able to be managed adequately with conservative medical treatment [198]. Localized bleeding is an expected side effect of thrombolytic administration, and subcutaneous bleeding/hematoma may have induced pressure necrosis in this case.

One case report describes the humeral IO administration of **prothrombin complex concentrate** (human), Profilnine® SD (factors II, IX, X). Prothrombin complex concentrate (1490 U, 33 U/kg, a typical PIV dose) reconstituted in 10 mL of the manufacturer-provided diluent was administered at its maximum recommended rate (10 mL/min) to a 64-year-old man taking **rivaroxaban** (a factor Xa inhibitor) who presented with extensive bruising on all extremities and active melena. The patient was hypotensive on arrival and was noted to have an initial hemoglobin of 4.5 g/dL. The patient's hemodynamic status began to stabilize within 1 h of Profilnine®

SD administration, rectal bleeding resolved, and the patient's hemoglobin returned to an acceptable level within 2 days. Pain was the only described complication of IO administration, despite IO infusion of both 2% lidocaine and fentanyl citrate [84]. Although no lab values were available to confirm the efficacy of the drug in this case, this study suggests that IO administration of prothrombin complex concentrate is safe and can be used when clinically indicated.

Recombinant factor VIIa (rFVIIa) is a drug typically used in the treatment of hemophilia, as well as other bleeding disorders. Its use via IO administration has been described in one animal study, but evidence regarding IO use in humans is limited to one case without enough detail to determine safety and efficacy [6]. In the animal study, anesthetized pigs were subjected to hemorrhagic shock followed by resuscitation. Intraosseous infusion of rFVIIa (100 µg/kg) followed by a 20 mL saline bolus was delivered via tibial IO to six pigs. Subsequent PK analysis from serial blood draws revealed that rVIIa levels in the blood peaked within 2–5 min after IO infusion. Peak concentrations also quickly declined within 5 min, suggesting that no depot effect is associated with IO rFVIIa infusion. In this study, the calculated PK half-life was 60–80 min in the circulating blood. The results of this study suggest that rFVIIa can be safely and effectively delivered IO to pigs [199], although the effects of IO infusion in human subjects remain unknown.

Intraosseous Contrast Media

Computed tomography (CT) scans may require pre-infusion with contrast media in order for clinicians to be able to properly visualize potential pathology. Although there is a lack of extensive research on the use of IO infusion for CT contrast agents, numerous case reports have been published on the successful use of IO contrast-enhanced CT scans for both adults and pediatric subjects. These reports have suggested that safe image acquisition, with no documented adverse effects, can be achieved even when utilizing injection rates up to 5 mL/s with a maximum pressure of 300 PSI via power injector [74, 76–78, 200]. Collectively, these cases suggest that CT angiogram (CTA) of the thorax, abdomen, and pelvis after tibial, humeral, or sternal IO administration of iodinated contrast is both practical and adequate for diagnostic purposes.

Several cases have been reported describing the IO administration of contrast agents for both CTA and CT perfusion of the head and neck [201–203]. Krähling et al. described a case of suspected stroke where iodinated nonionic contrast medium was administered via tibial IO using their institutional IV stroke CT protocol. CT angiogram was conducted using 80 mL of contrast medium at a 4 mL/s flow rate, and a subsequent CT perfusion study was conducted using 30 mL of contrast at a 5 mL/s flow rate. The resulting images were reviewed by the performing radiologist and deemed to be of adequate quality and diagnostic value [201].

Schindler et al. conducted a case-control study comparing CT scans after IO or PIV contrast administration using both subjective and objective measures of image quality. Both groups were treated with the same CT protocol: cerebral CTA and CTA of the supra-aortic vasculature using 80 mL of contrast medium at a 4 mL/s flow rate and CTA of the chest/abdomen using 80 mL of contrast medium at a 3 mL/s flow rate. Assessment of objective image quality revealed no significant differences between groups in absolute CT attenuation, image noise, and contrast-to-noise ratio for head and neck, chest, and abdominal CT scans. Similarly, subjective image quality assessed by three different radiologists revealed no significant difference in image noise, delineation of vessels, or overall image quality between IO and PIV contrast administration. One patient also received IO contrast (40 mL at 5 mL/s and 80 mL at 3 mL/s) for a CTA of the lower limb vasculature, which was adequately visualized. No complications were reported in this study [202].

The preponderance of evidence suggests that **IO administration of contrast agents is both safe and effective**, leading to an endorsement of the IO route for contrast administration by the American College of Radiology in 2023 [204]. Additional study is needed on the IO delivery of non-iodinated contrast agents, such as gadolinium-based contrast media, although there is no pharmacologic distinction to suggest that these agents would be tolerated differently than iodinated agents.

Osteopathy

Ischemic osteonecrosis of the femoral head is a serious condition in which large, repeated doses of bisphosphonates (orally or subcutaneously) are typically given to inhibit osteoclast resorption. Because this is a localized disease affecting only one small portion of bone, researchers have hypothesized that localized IO injection of **bisphosphonates** may help to circumvent some of the common adverse effects with these drugs. To test this hypothesis, Aya-ay et al. surgically induced ischemic osteonecrosis in the right femoral head of 27 piglets and delivered various doses of IO **ibandronate** or saline at predetermined intervals. Ibandronate was dosed at 280 μg and 560 μg (2.5% and 5% of the typical subcutaneous dose, respectively). To determine distribution and retention of the drug, initial 560 μg and saline doses were labeled with a carbon 14 isotope. The authors determined that >99% of the radiolabeled ibandronate was retained in the femoral head at 48 h, 50% at 3 weeks, and 30% at 7 weeks. Both doses of ibandronate produced significant preservation of the femoral head structure, and the 560 μg dose produced significant preservation of the trabecular framework and bone volume when compared to saline control [205]. A similar study in pigs showed that combining IO ibandronate with bone morphogenetic protein-2 further decreased femoral head deformity while stimulating bone formation [206].

In 2021, this concept of localized ibandronate therapy was described in a human case series. Five patients with pre-collapse osteonecrosis of the femoral head received femoral head IO infusion of ibandronate (dose not reported) as adjuvant therapy to core decompression. At 1-year follow-up, all five patients showed no progression or collapse of the osteonecrosis of the femoral head on X-ray, and no complications were observed [207]. These results indicate that IO administration can promptly deliver and distribute ibandronate into an ischemic femoral head, which may help to decrease side effects and reduce the risk of repeated dosing associated with traditional methods of administration. Additional research is needed to determine optimal dosing.

Antibiotics

Localized IO administration of antibiotics to prevent postoperative infection has also been explored. Young et al. randomized adult patients undergoing total knee arthroplasty (TKA) to receive either 1 gram of **cefazolin** (in 200 mL normal saline) injected via tibial IO or 1 gram of cefazolin infusion via PIV. Tissue samples from fat and bone were analyzed at four separate time points. The IO group exhibited nearly 17 times higher mean fat cefazolin concentration and almost 12 times higher mean bone concentration without any reported complications [208]. The same team extended their research to assess tibial IO **vancomycin** delivery in the perioperative TKA setting. This study contrasted a standard 1 gram PIV vancomycin dose with IO vancomycin doses of 500 mg and 250 mg. Despite lower dosing, both IO groups yielded significantly higher subcutaneous fat and bone concentrations than the PIV group. The IO route was also able to avoid common side effects of systemic vancomycin such as vancomycin flushing syndrome, which was reported by one person in the PIV group [209]. Klasan et al. were also able to demonstrate better tolerability of IO administration compared to PIV in a review of 631 TKA cases. They found that tibial IO vancomycin (500 mg in 150 mL of saline) plus IV cefazolin prophylaxis did not elevate rates of acute kidney injury or neutropenia when compared to systemic cefazolin monotherapy [210].

Higher local antibiotic concentrations via IO administration may reasonably imply more effective infection prophylaxis. Young et al. validated this hypothesis in a mouse model. Mice received a knee prosthesis that was inoculated with standardized counts of *Staphylococcus aureus*. Antimicrobial prophylaxis occurred via PIV or IO vancomycin or cefazolin at various doses. Both IO vancomycin and IO cefazolin surpassed their PIV counterparts at the same dose, with fewer colony-forming units detected. Low-dose IO vancomycin (25 mg/kg) matched the efficacy of high-dose PIV vancomycin (110 mg/kg) [211]. Vancomycin concentration is important, as its PK/PD profile relies on its AUC divided by the bacteria's minimal inhibitory concentration (MIC) to maximize efficacy.

Rates of prosthetic joint infection have also been assessed in six human studies assessing IO vancomycin infusion [210, 212–216], although only two of them were adequately powered to detect a difference in treatment groups [214–215]. Both of the adequately powered studies detected a significantly lower rate of prosthetic joint infection in the IO group as compared to the PIV group [214–215]. It is important to note that all patients in the IO groups of the aforementioned human studies comparing IO to PIV antimicrobial prophylaxis had also received at least one dose of a first-generation cephalosporin via the PIV route.

Respiratory Failure

Common agents employed for the induction of rapid sequence intubation (RSI) include **etomidate**, **ketamine**, fentanyl, and midazolam. There are reports of the safe IO administration of etomidate in adult humans; however, details of its efficacy and PK parameters have not been described [7, 18, 19]. Ketamine, on the other hand, has been described more extensively. Aliman et al. evaluated IO versus PIV efficacy of ketamine, midazolam, and fentanyl in infants with congenital cardiac diseases undergoing hemodynamic studies requiring the use of general anesthesia. Ten infants in the PIV group received midazolam 0.20 mg/kg, fentanyl 2.24 µg/kg, and ketamine 2.24 mg/kg; 11 infants in the IO group received midazolam 0.28 mg/ kg, fentanyl 4.7 µg/kg, and ketamine 4.7 mg/kg. Additional boluses of all medications were provided to both groups as needed to maintain adequate anesthesia. Weight standardized mean doses of all three administered drugs were significantly larger in the IO group. Despite the higher initial and subsequent doses of IO-administered induction agents, the onset time of anesthesia was slower in the IO group (71.3 s) as compared to the IV group (56.3 s). All patients were reevaluated 1 year after the study, and no complications were reported [8].

Barnard et al. demonstrated that IO administration of ketamine, **succinylcholine**, and/or **rocuronium** were successfully used for RSI with a first-pass intubation success rate of 97% comparable to existing literature describing the use of these drugs via the PIV route. Median administered doses of ketamine, succinylcholine, and rocuronium were 100 mg, 200 mg, and 100 mg, respectively. Although patient weights were not reported, the authors speculated that succinylcholine doses were higher than what would typically be administered via PIV (1–1.5 mg/kg), likely due to hemodynamic compromise. One patient who received sternal IO ketamine experienced leakage in his traumatic chest wounds, highlighting the need to verify bone integrity prior to IO cannulation. No other complications were reported [24]. Another case report described successful RSI with 100 mg of IO ketamine, in addition to IO fentanyl (200 µg) and IO succinylcholine (100 mg) [217]. Based on these findings, a one-time dose of 100 mg of ketamine appears to be both safe and effective for the induction of RSI in adult patients.

The IO administration of succinylcholine has been documented in the literature more than any other neuromuscular blocking agent. Moore et al. compared the efficacy of IO, PIV, and IM administration of succinylcholine (1 mg/kg) in sheep. The average time to respiratory arrest was the longest in the IM group (230 ± 106 s), followed by the IO group (57.5 ± 10.3 s) and the PIV group (30.8 ± 7.3 s). Similarly, the loss of forefoot twitch took the longest in the IM group (291 ± 109 s), followed by the IO group (100.8 ± 24.2 s) and the PIV group (93.3 ± 34 s) [218]. Differences in both efficacy outcomes between the three groups were statistically significant, although the differences between IO and PIV administration are likely not clinically significant, as the values are comparable.

Katan et al. reported tibial IO administration of **thiopental** (20 mg, 2.7 mg/kg), succinylcholine (12 mg, 1.6 mg/kg), and **atracurium** at standard PIV doses to an infant with a presumed diagnosis of shaken child syndrome. A peripheral nerve stimulator confirmed that muscle relaxation was achieved within 60–70 s, and the patient was intubated without complications [9]. Similar findings were reported in a case series of two pediatric patients administered 1 mg/kg of succinylcholine via tibial IO route for intubation. Both patients experienced muscle relaxation within 45 s and were intubated without complications [26]. Likewise, muscle relaxation occurred within 45 s of IO succinylcholine and midazolam administration in another infant case. Shortly after succinylcholine administration, the patient experienced bradycardia, which was successfully controlled within 45 s of a 100 µg IO bolus of atropine. The patient was successfully intubated without any complications of IO delivery [219]. Hamed et al. reported on the IO administration of ketamine (1–2 mg/kg), succinylcholine (1–2 mg/kg), and pancuronium or atracurium for the induction of anesthesia in 26 pediatric patients prior to emergency surgery. Two patients were noted to have extravasation of fluids during surgery, and one patient developed postoperative cellulitis. The institution did not have access to specialized IO devices, so an 18-gauge PIV needle was used for IO cannulation, which may have influenced the rate of complications seen in this study [10].

Medina described a series of two pediatric cases in which lorazepam and vecuronium were administered via the IO route to achieve RSI. The first patient realized muscle relaxation at 90 s after lorazepam (0.05 mg/kg) and vecuronium (0.1 mg/kg) administration, and the second patient had muscle relaxation at 150 s after lorazepam (0.1 mg/kg) and vecuronium (0.15 mg/kg) administration. Both patients achieved successful RSI and did not have any complications of IO cannulation [220]. Adequate intubation conditions typically occur within 2–3 min following IV vecuronium administration, suggesting that the clinical effects realized with these two routes may be very similar.

Limited PK data exist surrounding the IO administration of medications commonly used to achieve RSI. Loughren et al. compared tibial IO to PIV administration of rocuronium (1.2 mg/kg) using electromyographic (EMG) data in a normovolemic swine model. The time from injection to the maximal reduction in EMG activity (a surrogate for the onset of paralysis) was not different between groups, and both groups began to recover within 20–30 min following rocuronium administration. However, the mean time to return to 50, 75, and 95% of baseline EMG activity was significantly longer in the IO group [221]. Nearly identical findings were reported in a follow-up study using the same methods in a hypovolemic swine model [222]. These results suggest that at least some portion of the relatively hydrophilic rocuronium had distributed within the tibial bone marrow and was slowly absorbed into systemic circulation over time. This is unlikely to be a clinically significant finding, as time to resolution of paralysis only differed by approximately 12 min between groups.

Conclusion

While direct venous access via PIV or CVC device insertion remains optimal for drug infusion, indirect venous access through intraosseous infusion may be adequate for the treatment of many emergent medical conditions. Over the last century, considerable evidence has accumulated suggesting that IO infusion may be comparable to direct peripheral venous infusion, although pharmacokinetic data in humans are lacking for nearly all drugs. Additional research is needed to support the claim that IO infusion is clinically equivalent to PIV or CVC infusion for most medications. Although many fluids and medications anecdotally appear to be safe and efficacious when delivered to human subjects via the IO route, limited data suggest that the bioavailability of drugs may differ according to the route of administration [90, 114, 197, 223]. Further study is needed to determine whether this potential reduction in bioavailability is also associated with diminished clinical efficacy of these drugs in human subjects.

Most medications administered via the IO route appear to exhibit an absorption phase. The degree to which medication absorption is influenced by the route of administration likely depends largely upon the lipophilicity of the infused drug. Drugs that bind avidly to adipose tissue are likely to have significant delay in regard to time of entry to the central circulation following IO delivery, and larger doses may be required to achieve the same clinical effects. Several factors such as intravascular volume status, medication flow rate, anatomical site of administration, and bone composition are likely to be implicated in this absorption process, although no clear trends have been identified based on the pharmacologic characteristics of the drug being infused. The absorption phase is important, as it will ultimately determine the fraction of the administered dose available to exert its pharmacologic action on the patient. Additional human PK studies are needed to elucidate the overall effects of this absorption phase on IO medication infusion.

Likely due to the limited data available on the safety and efficacy of IO medication administration, **the United States Food and Drug Administration (FDA) has not formally approved any drug to be given via the IO route**. As such, IO administration is considered off-label use, and it is ultimately left to the qualified clinical prescriber and their clinical discretion to ensure the safe and appropriate use of IO medication administration. Given the large number of studies reporting clinical use of IO infusion for various medications, providers appear to be generally comfortable assuming that the IO infusion of various medications will have their desired clinical effect. However, it is highly likely that future clinical research will continue to disrupt these assumptions, as has been shown with several high-profile studies in the realm of cardiac arrest. **Without additional research into the bioavailability and clinical efficacy of IO medication infusion at various infusion sites, drug doses, and medication formulations, conflicting clinical reports will likely further confuse the clinical picture of this method's utility**.

Nevertheless, IO infusion does offer many clinical advantages that should not be ignored despite questions about how to best administer drugs and fluids via this route. Perhaps the most beneficial aspect of IO delivery is the speed at which IO vascular access can be obtained. In many emergency conditions, faster time to medication delivery equates to better patient outcomes. Understanding the clinical utility of intraosseous infusion is of paramount importance to ensure its proper use.

Key Concepts
- Intraosseous drug administration offers several advantages over direct venous administration methods, including faster time to drug administration, and can be a lifesaving intervention in emergent situations where peripheral or central venous access cannot be rapidly established.
- Data comparing the pharmacokinetics of intraosseous and peripheral intravenous medication delivery are almost entirely limited to animal models and suggest that these two routes may be comparable, but not necessarily equivalent, for many drugs.
- Data to support the safety and efficacy of intraosseous drug administration in humans are largely anecdotal, and further research is warranted to determine optimal dosing strategies.
- Contrary to peripheral and central venous administration, most medications delivered via the IO route exhibit a prolonged absorption phase, or depot effect, that can be influenced by myriad factors including the composition of the intramedullary compartment and the octanol-water partition coefficient of the drug being administered.
- The most common complication of intraosseous drug administration is pain during infusion. Pain should be addressed in all sensate patients receiving medications via an intraosseous catheter.
- No medications have been formally approved by the United States Food and Drug Administration to be administered intraosseously. Clinicians must cautiously consider the risks and the benefits of intraosseous drug administration to ensure its safe and appropriate application.

References

1. Josefson A. A new method of treatment: intraosseous injection. Acta Med Scand. 1934;84(59 S):182–4.
2. Neuhaus D, Weiss M, Engelhardt T, Henze G, Giest J, Strauss J, et al. Semi-elective intraosseous infusion after failed intravenous access in pediatric anesthesia. Paediatr Anaesth. 2010;20(2):168–71. https://pubmed-ncbi-nlm-nih-gov.proxy.lib.wayne.edu/20078814/.
3. Von Hoff DD, Kuhn JG, Burris HA, Miller LJ. Does intraosseous equal intravenous? A pharmacokinetic study. Am J Emerg Med. 2008;26(1):31–8. https://pubmed-ncbi-nlm-nih-gov.proxy.lib.wayne.edu/18082778/.
4. Guy J, Haley K, Zuspan SJ. Use of intraosseous infusion in the pediatric trauma patient. J Pediatr Surg. 1993;28(2):158–61. https://pubmed-ncbi-nlm-nih-gov.proxy.lib.wayne.edu/8437069/.
5. Goldstein B, Doody D, Briggs S. Emergency intraosseous infusion in severely burned children. Pediatr Emerg Care. 1990;6(3):195–7. https://pubmed-ncbi-nlm-nih-gov.proxy.lib.wayne.edu/2216924/.
6. Cooper BR, Mahoney PF, Hodgetts TJ, Mellor A. Intra-osseous access (EZ-IO®) for resuscitation: UK military combat experience. BMJ Mil Health. 2007;153(4):314–6. https://militaryhealth-bmj-com.proxy.lib.wayne.edu/content/153/4/314.
7. Dolister M, Miller S, Borron S, Truemper E, Shah M, Lanford MR, et al. Intraosseous vascular access is safe, effective and costs less than central venous catheters for patients in the

hospital setting. J Vasc Access. 2013;14(3):216–24. https://pubmed-ncbi-nlm-nih-gov.proxy.lib.wayne.edu/23283646/.

8. Aliman AC, De Albuquerque PM, Piccioni JL, Oliva JL, Auler JOC. Intraosseous anesthesia in hemodynamic studies in children with cardiopathy. Rev Bras Anestesiol. 2011;61(1):41–9. https://pubmed-ncbi-nlm-nih-gov.proxy.lib.wayne.edu/21334506/.

9. Katan BS, Olshaker JS, Dickerson SE. Intraosseous infusion of muscle relaxants. Am J Emerg Med. 1988;6(4):353–4. https://pubmed-ncbi-nlm-nih-gov.proxy.lib.wayne.edu/3390254/.

10. Hamed RK, Hartmans S, Gausche-Hill M. Anesthesia through an intraosseous line using an 18-gauge intravenous needle for emergency pediatric surgery. J Clin Anesth. 2013;25(6):447–51. https://pubmed-ncbi-nlm-nih-gov.proxy.lib.wayne.edu/24008191/.

11. Paxton JH, Knuth TE, Klausner HA. Proximal humerus intraosseous infusion: a preferred emergency venous access. J Trauma. 2009;67(3):606–11. https://pubmed-ncbi-nlm-nih-gov.proxy.lib.wayne.edu/19741408/.

12. Stewart FC, Kain ZN. Intraosseous infusion: elective use in pediatric anesthesia. Anesth Analg. 1992;75(4):626–9. https://pubmed-ncbi-nlm-nih-gov.proxy.lib.wayne.edu/1306651/.

13. Martino Alba R, Ruiz Lopez MJ, Casado Flores J. Use of the intraosseous route in resuscitation in a neonate. Intensive Care Med. 1994;20(7):529. https://pubmed-ncbi-nlm-nih-gov.proxy.lib.wayne.edu/7995873/.

14. Smith RJ, Keseg DP, Manley LK, Standeford T. Intraosseous infusions by prehospital personnel in critically ill pediatric patients. Ann Emerg Med. 1988;17(5):491–5. https://pubmed-ncbi-nlm-nih-gov.proxy.lib.wayne.edu/3364831/.

15. McNamara RM, Spivey WH, Unger HD, Malone DR. Emergency applications of intraosseous infusion. J Emerg Med. 1987;5(2):97–101. https://pubmed-ncbi-nlm-nih-gov.proxy.lib.wayne.edu/3584924/.

16. Spivey WH. Intraosseous infusions. J Pediatr. 1987;111(5):639–43. https://pubmed-ncbi-nlm-nih-gov.proxy.lib.wayne.edu/3312550/.

17. Glaeser PW, Hellmich TR, Szewczuga D, Losek JD, Smith DS. Five-year experience in prehospital intraosseous infusions in children and adults. Ann Emerg Med. 1993;22(7):1119–24. https://pubmed-ncbi-nlm-nih-gov.proxy.lib.wayne.edu/8517560/.

18. Davidoff J, Fowler R, Gordon D, Klein G, Kovar J, Lozano M, et al. Clinical evaluation of a novel intraosseous device for adults: prospective, 250-patient, multi-center trial. JEMS. 2005;30(10):suppl 20–3. https://utsouthwestern.elsevierpure.com/en/publications/clinical-evaluation-of-a-novel-intraosseous-device-for-adults-pro.

19. Gazin N, Auger H, Jabre P, Jaulin C, Lecarpentier E, Bertrand C, et al. Efficacy and safety of the EZ-IO™ intraosseous device: out-of-hospital implementation of a management algorithm for difficult vascular access. Resuscitation. 2011;82(1):126–9. https://pubmed-ncbi-nlm-nih-gov.proxy.lib.wayne.edu/20947238/.

20. Joseph G, Tobias JD. The use of intraosseous infusions in the operating room. J Clin Anesth. 2008;20(6):469–73. https://pubmed-ncbi-nlm-nih-gov.proxy.lib.wayne.edu/18929292/.

21. Anson JA, Sinz EH, Swick JT. The versatility of intraosseous vascular access in perioperative medicine: a case series. J Clin Anesth. 2015;27(1):63–7. https://pubmed-ncbi-nlm-nih-gov.proxy.lib.wayne.edu/25547826/.

22. Valdés M, Araujo P, De Andrés C, Sastre E, Martin TE. Intraosseous administration of thrombolysis in out-of-hospital massive pulmonary thromboembolism. Emerg Med J. 2010;27(8):641–4. https://pubmed-ncbi-nlm-nih-gov.proxy.lib.wayne.edu/20522435/.

23. Santos D, Carron PN, Yersin B, Pasquier M. EZ-IO(®) intraosseous device implementation in a pre-hospital emergency service: a prospective study and review of the literature. Resuscitation. 2013;84(4):440–5. https://pubmed-ncbi-nlm-nih-gov.proxy.lib.wayne.edu/23160104/.

24. Barnard EBG, Moy RJ, Kehoe AD, Bebarta VS, Smith JE. Rapid sequence induction of anaesthesia via the intraosseous route: a prospective observational study. Emerg Med J. 2015;32(6):449–52. https://pubmed-ncbi-nlm-nih-gov.proxy.lib.wayne.edu/24963149/.

25. Stowers MDJ, Rahardja R, Nicholson L, Svirskis D, Hannam J, Young SW. Safety and efficacy of intraosseous ropivacaine in lower extremity (SORE) study. ANZ J Surg. 2023;93(1–2):328–33. https://pubmed-ncbi-nlm-nih-gov.proxy.lib.wayne.edu/36627759/.

26. Tobias JD, Nichols DG. Intraosseous succinylcholine for orotracheal intubation. Pediatr Emerg Care. 1990;6(2):108–9. https://pubmed-ncbi-nlm-nih-gov.proxy.lib.wayne.edu/2371145/.

27. Rosetti VA, Thompson BM, Miller J, Mateer JR, Aprahamian C. Intraosseous infusion: an alternative route of pediatric intravascular access. Ann Emerg Med. 1985;14(9):885–8. https://pubmed-ncbi-nlm-nih-gov.proxy.lib.wayne.edu/4025988/.

28. Valdes MM. Intraosseous fluid administration in emergencies. Lancet. 1977;1(8024):1235–6. https://pubmed-ncbi-nlm-nih-gov.proxy.lib.wayne.edu/68333/.

29. Ong MEH, Chan YH, Oh JJ, Ngo ASY. An observational, prospective study comparing tibial and humeral intraosseous access using the EZ-IO. Am J Emerg Med. 2009;27(1):8–15. https://pubmed-ncbi-nlm-nih-gov.proxy.lib.wayne.edu/19041528/.

30. Waisman M, Waisman D. Bone marrow infusion in adults. J Trauma. 1997;42(2):288–93. https://pubmed-ncbi-nlm-nih-gov.proxy.lib.wayne.edu/9042884/.

31. Frascone RJ, Jensen JP, Kaye K, Salzman JG. Consecutive field trials using two different intraosseous devices. Prehosp Emerg Care. 2007;11(2):164–71. https://pubmed-ncbi-nlm-nih-gov.proxy.lib.wayne.edu/17454802/.

32. Gillum L, Kovar J. Powered intraosseous access in the prehospital setting: MCHD EMS puts the EZ-IO® to the test. JEMS. 2005:30, 24–6.

33. Daya MR, Leroux BG, Dorian P, Rea TD, Newgard CD, Morrison LJ, et al. Survival after intravenous versus intraosseous amiodarone, lidocaine, or placebo in out-of-hospital shock-refractory cardiac arrest. Circulation. 2020;141(3):188–98. https://pubmed-ncbi-nlm-nih-gov.proxy.lib.wayne.edu/31941354/.

34. McMahon K, Paster J, Baker KA. Local anesthetic systemic toxicity in the pediatric patient. Am J Emerg Med. 2022;54:325.e3–6. https://pubmed-ncbi-nlm-nih-gov.proxy.lib.wayne.edu/34742600/.

35. Friedman FD. Intraosseous adenosine for the termination of supraventricular tachycardia in an infant. Ann Emerg Med. 1996;28(3):356–8. https://europepmc.org/article/med/8780485.

36. Helleman K, Kirpalani A, Lim R. A novel method of intraosseous infusion of adenosine for the treatment of supraventricular tachycardia in an infant. Pediatr Emerg Care. 2017;33(1):47–8. https://pubmed-ncbi-nlm-nih-gov.proxy.lib.wayne.edu/28045841/.

37. Goodman IS, Lu CJ. Intraosseous infusion is unreliable for adenosine delivery in the treatment of supraventricular tachycardia. Pediatr Emerg Care. 2012;28(1):47–8. https://pubmed-ncbi-nlm-nih-gov.proxy.lib.wayne.edu/22217885/.

38. Fidancı İ, Güleryüz OD, Yenice ÖD. Successful intraosseous adenosine administration in a newborn infant with supraventricular tachycardia. Turk J Pediatr. 2020;62(6):1064–8. https://pubmed-ncbi-nlm-nih-gov.proxy.lib.wayne.edu/33372446/.

39. Ruiz-Hornillos PJ, Martínez-Cámara F, Elizondo M, Jiménez-Fraile JA, Del Mar Alonso-Sánchez M, Galán D, et al. Systemic fibrinolysis through intraosseous vascular access in ST-segment elevation myocardial infarction. Ann Emerg Med. 2011;57(6):572–4. https://pubmed-ncbi-nlm-nih-gov.proxy.lib.wayne.edu/20947209/.

40. Brunette DD, Fischer R. Intravascular access in pediatric cardiac arrest. Am J Emerg Med. 1988;6(6):577–9. https://pubmed-ncbi-nlm-nih-gov.proxy.lib.wayne.edu/3178949/.

41. Burgert JM. Intraosseous infusion of blood products and epinephrine in an adult patient in hemorrhagic shock. AANA J. 2009;77. www.aana.com/aanajournal.aspx.

42. Berg RA. Emergency infusion of catecholamines into bone marrow. Am J Dis Child. 1984;138(9):810–1. https://pubmed-ncbi-nlm-nih-gov.proxy.lib.wayne.edu/6475867/.

43. Tarrow AB, Turkel H, Thompson MS. Infusions via the bone marrow and biopsy of the bone and bone marrow. Anesthesiology. 1952;13(5):501–9. https://pubmed-ncbi-nlm-nih-gov.proxy.lib.wayne.edu/12976731/.

44. Ramet J, Clybouw C, Benatar A, Hachimi-Idrissi S, Corne L. Successful use of an intraosseous infusion in an 800 grams preterm infant. Eur J Emerg Med. 1998;5(3):327–8.

45. Kelsall AWR. Resuscitation with intraosseous lines in neonatal units. Arch Dis Child. 1993;68(3 Spec No):324–5. https://pubmed-ncbi-nlm-nih-gov.proxy.lib.wayne.edu/8466272/.

46. Meola F. Bone marrow infusions as a routine procedure in children. J Pediatr. 1944;25:13–6.

47. Gunz FW, Dean RFA. Tibial bone-marrow transfusions in infants. Br Med J. 1945;1(4389):220. https://pubmed-ncbi-nlm-nih-gov.proxy.lib.wayne.edu/20785909/.

48. Lewis P, Wright C. Saving the critically injured trauma patient: a retrospective analysis of 1000 uses of intraosseous access. Emerg Med J. 2015;32(6):463–7. https://pubmed-ncbi-nlm-nih-gov.proxy.lib.wayne.edu/24981009/.

49. Heinild S, Søndergaard T, Tudvad F. Bone marrow infusion in childhood; experiences from a thousand infusions. J Pediatr. 1947;30(4):400–12. https://pubmed-ncbi-nlm-nih-gov.proxy.lib.wayne.edu/20290362/.

50. Chavez-Negrete A, Majluf Cruz S, Frati Munari A, Perches A, Arguero R. Treatment of hemorrhagic shock with intraosseous or intravenous infusion of hypertonic saline dextran solution. Eur Surg Res. 1991;23(2):123–9. https://pubmed-ncbi-nlm-nih-gov.proxy.lib.wayne.edu/1718756/.

51. Sherren P, Burns B. Prehospital blood transfusion: 5-year experience of an Australian helicopter emergency medical service. Crit Care. 2013;17(S2).

52. Dubick MA, Kramer GC. Hypertonic saline dextran (HSD) and intraosseous vascular access for the treatment of haemorrhagic hypotension in the far-forward combat arena. Ann Acad Med Singap. 1997;26(1):64–9. https://europepmc.org/article/med/9140581.

53. Chatterjee DJ, Bukunola B, Samuels TL, Induruwage L, Uncles DR. Resuscitation in massive obstetric haemorrhage using an intraosseous needle. Anaesthesia. 2011;66(4):306–10. https://pubmed-ncbi-nlm-nih-gov.proxy.lib.wayne.edu/21401545/.

54. Moscati R, Moore GP. Compartment syndrome with resultant amputation following intraosseous infusion. Am J Emerg Med. 1990;8(5):470–1. https://pubmed-ncbi-nlm-nih-gov.proxy.lib.wayne.edu/2206153/.

55. Singh Tomar R, Gupta A. Resuscitation by Intraosseous infusion in newborn. Med J Armed Forces India. 2006;62(2):202–3. https://pubmed-ncbi-nlm-nih-gov.proxy.lib.wayne.edu/27407899/.

56. Luu JL, Wendtland CL, Gross MF, Mirza F, Zouros A, Zimmerman GJ, et al. Three-percent saline administration during pediatric critical care transport. Pediatr Emerg Care. 2011;27(12):1113–7. https://pubmed-ncbi-nlm-nih-gov.proxy.lib.wayne.edu/22134236/.

57. Lawson T, Hussein O, Nasir M, Hinduja A, Torbey MT. Intraosseous administration of hypertonic saline in acute brain-injured patients: a prospective case series and literature review. Neurologist. 2019;24(6):176–9. https://pubmed-ncbi-nlm-nih-gov.proxy.lib.wayne.edu/31688708/.

58. Glaeser PW, Losek JD. Emergency intraosseous infusions in children. Am J Emerg Med. 1986;4(1):34–6. https://pubmed-ncbi-nlm-nih-gov.proxy.lib.wayne.edu/3004527/.

59. Wang J, Fang Y, Ramesh S, Zakaria A, Putman MT, Dinescu D, et al. Intraosseous administration of 23.4% NaCl for treatment of intracranial hypertension. Neurocrit Care. 2019;30(2):364–71. https://pubmed-ncbi-nlm-nih-gov.proxy.lib.wayne.edu/30397844/

60. Farrokh S, Cho SM, Lefebvre AT, Zink EK, Schiavi A, Puttgen HA. Use of intraosseous hypertonic saline in critically ill patients. J Vasc Access. 2019;20(4):427–32. https://pubmed-ncbi-nlm-nih-gov.proxy.lib.wayne.edu/30328363/.

61. De Marca S, Calafatti M, Romaniello L, Pesce S, Lapolla R, Gizzi C. Intraosseous infusion of acyclovir in a neonate. Ital J Pediatr. 2022;48(1). https://pubmed-ncbi-nlm-nih-gov.proxy.lib.wayne.edu/36068631/.

62. Vidal R, Kissoon N, Gayle M. Compartment syndrome following intraosseous infusion. Pediatrics. 1993;91(6):1201–2.

63. Papper EM. The bone marrow route for injecting fluids and drugs into the general circulation. Anesthesiology. 1942;3(3):307–13. https://doi.org/10.1097/00000542-194205000-00008.

64. French L, Kusin S, Hendrickson R. Pediatric lidocaine toxicity following intraosseous injection: a case series. Clin Toxicol. 2012;50(4):329–30.
65. Sampson CS, Bedy SME. Lipid emulsion therapy given intraosseously in massive verapamil overdose. Am J Emerg Med. 2015;33(12):1844.e1.
66. Hiller K, Jarrod MM, Franke HA, Degan J, Boyer LV, Fox FM. Scorpion antivenom administered by alternative infusions. Ann Emerg Med. 2010;56(3):309–10.
67. Stephens RJ, Filip AB, Baumgartner KT, Schwarz ES, Liss DB. Benzonatate overdose presenting as cardiac arrest with rapidly narrowing QRS interval. J Med Toxicol. 2022;18(4):344–9. https://pubmed-ncbi-nlm-nih-gov.proxy.lib.wayne.edu/35790679/.
68. Fortin J, Capellier G, Manzon C, Giocanti J, Gall O. Intraosseous administration in the acute treatment of cyanide poisoning. Burns. 2009;35:S15–6.
69. Mastenbrook J, Zamihovsky R, Brunken N, Olsen T. Intraosseous administration of hydroxocobalamin after enclosed structure fire cardiac arrest. BMJ Case Rep. 2021;14(3):239523.
70. Herman MI, Chyka PA, Butler AY, Rieger SE. Methylene blue by intraosseous infusion for methemoglobinemia. Ann Emerg Med. 1999;33(1):111–3. https://pubmed-ncbi-nlm-nih-gov.proxy.lib.wayne.edu/9867898/.
71. Spencer TR. Intraosseous administration of thrombolytics for pulmonary embolism. J Emerg Med. 2013;45(6). https://pubmed-ncbi-nlm-nih-gov.proxy.lib.wayne.edu/24054882/.
72. Northey LC, Shiraev T, Omari A. Salvage intraosseous thrombolysis and extracorporeal membrane oxygenation for massive pulmonary embolism. J Emerg Trauma Shock. 2015;8(1):55–7. https://pubmed-ncbi-nlm-nih-gov.proxy.lib.wayne.edu/25709256/.
73. Nafiu OO, Olumese PE, Gbadegesin RA, Osinusi K. Intraosseous infusion in an emergency situation: a case report. Ann Trop Paediatr. 1997;17(2):175–7. https://pubmed-ncbi-nlm-nih-gov.proxy.lib.wayne.edu/9230983/.
74. Knuth TE, Paxton JH, Myers D. Intraosseous injection of iodinated computed tomography contrast agent in an adult blunt trauma patient. Ann Emerg Med. 2011;57(4):382–6. https://pubmed-ncbi-nlm-nih-gov.proxy.lib.wayne.edu/21111513/.
75. Iwama H, Katsumi A, Shinohara K, Kawamae K, Ohtomo Y, Akama Y, et al. Clavicular approach to intraosseous infusion in adults. Fukushima J Med Sci. 1994;40(1):1–8. https://europepmc.org/article/med/7988980.
76. Ahrens KL, Reeder SB, Keevil JG, Tupesis JP. Successful computed tomography angiogram through tibial intraosseous access: a case report. J Emerg Med. 2013;45(2):182–5. https://pubmed-ncbi-nlm-nih-gov.proxy.lib.wayne.edu/23726677/.
77. Cambray EJ, Donaldson JS, Shore RM. Intraosseous contrast infusion: efficacy and associated findings. Pediatr Radiol. 1997;27(11):892–3. https://pubmed-ncbi-nlm-nih-gov.proxy.lib.wayne.edu/9361053/.
78. Geller E, Crisci KL. Intraosseous infusion of iodinated contrast in an abused child. Pediatr Emerg Care. 1999;15(5):328–9. https://pubmed-ncbi-nlm-nih-gov.proxy.lib.wayne.edu/10532661/.
79. Winkler M, Talley C, Woodward C, Kingsbury A, Appiah F, Elbelasi H, et al. The use of intraosseous needles for injection of contrast media for computed tomographic angiography of the thoracic aorta. J Cardiovasc Comput Tomogr. 2017;11(3):203–7. https://pubmed-ncbi-nlm-nih-gov.proxy.lib.wayne.edu/28341196/.
80. Greenstein YY, Koenig SJ, Mayo PH, Narasimhan M. A serious adult intraosseous catheter complication and review of the literature. Crit Care Med. 2016;44(9):e904–9. https://pubmed-ncbi-nlm-nih-gov.proxy.lib.wayne.edu/27058467/.
81. Walsh-Kelly CM, Berens RJ, Glaeser PW, Losek JD. Intraosseous infusion of phenytoin. Am J Emerg Med. 1986;4(6):523–4. https://pubmed-ncbi-nlm-nih-gov.proxy.lib.wayne.edu/3778598/.
82. Strong D, Powell E, Tilney PVR. A 20-year-old-male with hemorrhagic shock. Air Med J. 2016;35(1):8–11. https://pubmed-ncbi-nlm-nih-gov.proxy.lib.wayne.edu/26856652/.
83. Fiorito BA, Mirza F, Doran TM, Oberle AN, Vince Cruz EC, Wendtland CL, et al. Intraosseous access in the setting of pediatric critical care transport. Pediatr Crit Care Med. 2005;6(1):50–3. https://pubmed-ncbi-nlm-nih-gov.proxy.lib.wayne.edu/15636659/.

84. Means L, Gimbar RP. Prothrombin complex concentrate administration through intraosseous access for reversal of rivaroxaban. Am J Emerg Med. 2016;34(3):685.e1–2. https://pubmed-ncbi-nlm-nih-gov.proxy.lib.wayne.edu/26403851/.

85. Panchal AR, Bartos JA, Cabañas JG, Donnino MW, Drennan IR, Hirsch KG, et al. Part 3: Adult basic and advanced life support: 2020 American Heart Association guidelines for cardiopulmonary resuscitation and emergency cardiovascular care. Circulation. 2020;142(16_suppl_2):S366–468.

86. Standring S, editor. Gray's anatomy: the anatomical basis of clinical practice. 42nd ed. Elsevier; 2020.

87. Vogler JB, Murphy WA. Bone marrow imaging. Radiology. 1988;168(3):679–93. https://pubmed-ncbi-nlm-nih-gov.proxy.lib.wayne.edu/3043546/.

88. Buck ML, Wiggins BS, Sesler JM. Intraosseous drug administration in children and adults during cardiopulmonary resuscitation. Ann Pharmacother. 2007;41(10):1679–86. https://pubmed-ncbi-nlm-nih-gov.proxy.lib.wayne.edu/17698894/.

89. Brown C, Wiklund L, Bar-Joseph G, Miller B, Bircher N, Paradis N, et al. Future directions for resuscitation research. IV. Innovative advanced life support pharmacology. Resuscitation. 1996;33(2):163–77. https://pubmed-ncbi-nlm-nih-gov.proxy.lib.wayne.edu/9025133/

90. Butt TD, Bailey JV, Dowling PM, Fretz PB. Comparison of 2 techniques for regional antibiotic delivery to the equine forelimb: intraosseous perfusion vs. intravenous perfusion. Can Vet J. 2001;42(8):617.

91. De Lorenzo RA, Ward JA, Jordan BS, Hanson CE. Relationships of intraosseous and systemic pressure waveforms in a swine model. Acad Emerg Med. 2014;21(8):899–904. https://doi.org/10.1111/acem.12432.

92. Kuhn GJ, White BC, Swetnam RE, Mumey JF, Rydesky MF, Tintinalli JE, et al. Peripheral vs central circulation times during CPR: a pilot study. Ann Emerg Med. 1981;10(8):417–9. https://pubmed-ncbi-nlm-nih-gov.proxy.lib.wayne.edu/7020494/.

93. Dev SP, Stefan RA, Saun T, Lee S. Videos in clinical medicine. Insertion of an intraosseous needle in adults. N Engl J Med. 2014;370(24):e35. https://pubmed-ncbi-nlm-nih-gov.proxy.lib.wayne.edu/24918394/.

94. Hoskins SL, do Nascimento P, Lima RM, Espana-Tenorio JM, Kramer GC. Pharmacokinetics of intraosseous and central venous drug delivery during cardiopulmonary resuscitation. Resuscitation. 2012;83(1):107–12. https://pubmed-ncbi-nlm-nih-gov.proxy.lib.wayne.edu/21871857/.

95. Beaumont LD, Baragchizadeh A, Johnson C, Johnson D. Effects of tibial and humerus intraosseous administration of epinephrine in a cardiac arrest swine model. Am J Disaster Med. 2016;11(4):243–51. https://pubmed-ncbi-nlm-nih-gov.proxy.lib.wayne.edu/28140439/.

96. Andropoulos DB, Solfer SJ, Schreiber MD. Plasma epinephrine concentrations after intraosseous and central venous injection during cardiopulmonary resuscitation in the lamb. J Pediatr. 1990;116(2):312–5. https://pubmed-ncbi-nlm-nih-gov.proxy.lib.wayne.edu/2299508/.

97. Blouin D, Gegel BT, Johnson D, Garcia-Blanco JC. Effects of intravenous, sternal, and humerus intraosseous administration of Hextend on time of administration and hemodynamics in a hypovolemic swine model. Am J Disaster Med. 2016;11(3):183–92. https://pubmed-ncbi-nlm-nih-gov.proxy.lib.wayne.edu/28134417/.

98. Cornell M, Kelbaugh J, Todd B, Christianson K, Grayson K, O'Sullivan J, et al. Pharmacokinetics of sternal intraosseous atropine administration in normovolemic and hypovolemic swine. Am J Disaster Med. 2016;11(4):233–6. https://pubmed-ncbi-nlm-nih-gov.proxy.lib.wayne.edu/28140437/.

99. Smith S, Borgkvist B, Kist T, Annelin J, Johnson D, Long R. The effects of sternal intraosseous and intravenous administration of amiodarone in a hypovolemic swine cardiac arrest model. Am J Disaster Med. 2016;11(4):271–7. https://pubmed-ncbi-nlm-nih-gov.proxy.lib.wayne.edu/28140442/.

100. Vallier DJ, Torrence AD, Stevens R, Arcinue PN, Johnson D. The effects of sternal and intravenous vasopressin administration on pharmacokinetics. Am J Disaster Med. 2016;11(3):203–9. https://pubmed-ncbi-nlm-nih-gov.proxy.lib.wayne.edu/28134419/.

101. Wenzel V, Lindner KH, Augenstein S, Voelckel W, Strohmenger HU, Prengel AW, et al. Intraosseous vasopressin improves coronary perfusion pressure rapidly during cardiopulmonary resuscitation in pigs. Crit Care Med. 1999;27(8):1565–9. https://pubmed-ncbi-nlm-nih-gov.proxy.lib.wayne.edu/10470765/.

102. Fulkerson J, Lowe R, Anderson T, Moore H, Craig W, Johnson D. Effects of intraosseous tibial vs. intravenous vasopressin in a hypovolemic cardiac arrest model. West J Emerg Med. 2016;17(2):222–8. https://pubmed-ncbi-nlm-nih-gov.proxy.lib.wayne.edu/26973756/.

103. Wimmer MH, Heffner K, Smithers M, Culley R, Coyner J, Loughren M, et al. The comparison of humeral intraosseous and intravenous administration of vasopressin on return of spontaneous circulation and pharmacokinetics in a hypovolemic cardiac arrest swine model. Am J Disaster Med. 2016;11(4):237–42. https://pubmed-ncbi-nlm-nih-gov.proxy.lib.wayne.edu/28140438/.

104. Holloway CMM, Jurina CSL, Orszag CJD, Bragdon LGR, Green LRD, Garcia-Blanco JC, et al. Effects of humerus intraosseous versus intravenous amiodarone administration in a hypovolemic porcine model. Am J Disaster Med. 2016;11(4):261–9. https://pubmed-ncbi-nlm-nih-gov.proxy.lib.wayne.edu/28140441/.

105. Hampton K, Wang E, Argame JI, Bateman T, Craig W, Johnson D. The effects of tibial intraosseous versus intravenous amiodarone administration in a hypovolemic cardiac arrest procine model. Am J Disaster Med. 2016;11(4):253–60. https://pubmed-ncbi-nlm-nih-gov.proxy.lib.wayne.edu/28140440/.

106. Standards for cardiopulmonary resuscitation (CPR) and emergency cardiac care (ECC). JAMA. 1974;227(7):833. https://pubmed-ncbi-nlm-nih-gov.proxy.lib.wayne.edu/28834958/.

107. Orlowski JP. My kingdom for an intravenous line. Am J Dis Child. 1984;138(9):803. https://pubmed-ncbi-nlm-nih-gov.proxy.lib.wayne.edu/6475866/.

108. Standards and guidelines for cardiopulmonary resuscitation (CPR) and emergency cardiac care (ECC). JAMA. 1986;255(21):2905–84. https://jamanetwork-com.proxy.lib.wayne.edu/journals/jama/fullarticle/404537.

109. Nolan JP, Deakin CD, Soar J, Böttiger BW, Smith G. European resuscitation council guidelines for resuscitation 2005: section 4. Adult advanced life support. Resuscitation. 2005;67(SUPPL. 1):S39–86.

110. Kleinman ME, Chameides L, Schexnayder SM, Samson RA, Hazinski MF, Atkins DL, et al. Part 14: Pediatric advanced life support: 2010 American Heart Association guidelines for cardiopulmonary resuscitation and emergency cardiovascular care. Circulation. 2010;122(SUPPL. 3):S876–908. https://doi.org/10.1161/CIRCULATIONAHA.110.971101.

111. Topjian AA, Raymond TT, Atkins D, Chan M, Duff JP, Joyner BL, et al. Part 4: Pediatric basic and advanced life support: 2020 American Heart Association guidelines for cardiopulmonary resuscitation and emergency cardiovascular care. Circulation. 2020;142(16_suppl_2):S469–523.

112. Aziz K, Lee HC, Escobedo MB, Hoover AV, Kamath-Rayne BD, Kapadia VS, et al. Part 5: Neonatal resuscitation: 2020 American Heart Association guidelines for cardiopulmonary resuscitation and emergency cardiovascular care. Circulation. 2020;142(16_suppl_2):S524–50. https://doi.org/10.1161/CIR.0000000000000902.

113. Macht DI. Studies on intraosseous injections of epinephrine. Am J Physiol. 1943;138:269–72.

114. Spivey WH, Crespo SG, Fuhs LR, Schoffstall JM. Plasma catecholamine levels after intraosseous epinephrine administration in a cardiac arrest model. Ann Emerg Med. 1992;21(2):127–31. https://pubmed-ncbi-nlm-nih-gov.proxy.lib.wayne.edu/1739196/.

115. Burgert J, Gegel B, Loughren M, Ceremuga T, Desai M, Schlicher M, et al. Comparison of tibial intraosseous, sternal intraosseous, and intravenous routes of administration on pharmacokinetics of epinephrine during cardiac arrest: a pilot study. AANA J. 2012;80(4 Suppl):S6–S10.

116. Wong MR, Reggio MJ, Morocho FR, Holloway MM, Garcia-Blanco JC, Jenkins C, et al. Effects of intraosseous epinephrine in a cardiac arrest swine model. J Surg Res. 2016;201(2):327–33.

117. Neill MJ, Burgert JM, Blouin D, Tigges B, Rodden K, Roberts R, et al. Effects of humeral intraosseous epinephrine in a pediatric hypovolemic cardiac arrest porcine model. Trauma Surg Acute Care Open. 2020;5(1). https://pubmed-ncbi-nlm-nih-gov.proxy.lib.wayne.edu/32154374/.

118. Eriksson M, Larsson A, Lipcsey M, Strandberg G. The effect of hemorrhagic shock and intraosseous adrenaline injection on the delivery of a subsequently administered drug—an experimental study. Scand J Trauma Resusc Emerg Med. 2019;27(1). https://pubmed-ncbi-nlm-nih-gov.proxy.lib.wayne.edu/30850019/.

119. Burgert JM, Johnson AD, Garcia-Blanco J, Froehle J, Morris T, Althuisius B, et al. The effects of proximal and distal routes of intraosseous epinephrine administration on short-term resuscitative outcome measures in an adult swine model of ventricular fibrillation: a randomized controlled study. Am J Emerg Med. 2016;34(1):49–53.

120. Johnson D, Garcia-Blanco J, Burgert J, Fulton L, Kadilak P, Perry K, et al. Effects of humeral intraosseous versus intravenous epinephrine on pharmacokinetics and return of spontaneous circulation in a porcine cardiac arrest model: a randomized control trial. Ann Med Surg (Lond). 2015;4(3):306–10. https://pubmed-ncbi-nlm-nih-gov.proxy.lib.wayne.edu/26468375/.

121. Roberts CT, Klink S, Schmölzer GM, Blank DA, Badurdeen S, Crossley KJ, et al. Comparison of intraosseous and intravenous epinephrine administration during resuscitation of asphyxiated newborn lambs. Arch Dis Child Fetal Neonatal Ed. 2022;107(3):311–6. https://pubmed-ncbi-nlm-nih-gov.proxy.lib.wayne.edu/34462318/.

122. Sapien R, Stein H, Padbury JF, Thio S, Hodge D. Intraosseous versus intravenous epinephrine infusions in lambs: pharmacokinetics and pharmacodynamics. Pediatr Emerg Care. 1992;8(4):179–83. https://pubmed-ncbi-nlm-nih-gov.proxy.lib.wayne.edu/1513725/.

123. Nolan JP, Deakin CD, Ji C, Gates S, Rosser A, Lall R, et al. Intraosseous versus intravenous administration of adrenaline in patients with out-of-hospital cardiac arrest: a secondary analysis of the PARAMEDIC2 placebo-controlled trial. Intensive Care Med. 2020;46(5):954–62. https://pubmed-ncbi-nlm-nih-gov.proxy.lib.wayne.edu/32002593/.

124. Mody P, Brown SP, Kudenchuk PJ, Chan PS, Khera R, Ayers C, et al. Intraosseous versus intravenous access in patients with out-of-hospital cardiac arrest: insights from the resuscitation outcomes consortium continuous chest compression trial. Resuscitation. 2019;134:69–75. https://pubmed-ncbi-nlm-nih-gov.proxy.lib.wayne.edu/30391366/.

125. Zhang Y, Zhu J, Liu Z, Gu L, Zhang W, Zhan H, et al. Intravenous versus intraosseous adrenaline administration in out-of-hospital cardiac arrest: a retrospective cohort study. Resuscitation. 2020;149:209–16. https://pubmed-ncbi-nlm-nih-gov.proxy.lib.wayne.edu/31982506/.

126. Zuercher M, Kern KB, Indik JH, Loedl M, Hilwig RW, Ummenhofer W, et al. Epinephrine improves 24-hour survival in a swine model of prolonged ventricular fibrillation demonstrating that early intraosseous is superior to delayed intravenous administration. Anesth Analg. 2011;112(4):884–90. https://pubmed-ncbi-nlm-nih-gov.proxy.lib.wayne.edu/21385987/.

127. Hubble MW, Johnson C, Blackwelder J, Collopy K, Houston S, Martin M, et al. Probability of return of spontaneous circulation as a function of timing of vasopressor administration in out-of-hospital cardiac arrest. Prehosp Emerg Care. 2015;19(4):457–63. https://pubmed-ncbi-nlm-nih-gov.proxy.lib.wayne.edu/25909945/.

128. Yang SC, Hsu YH, Chang YH, Chien LT, Chen IC, Chiang WC. Epinephrine administration in adults with out-of-hospital cardiac arrest: a comparison between intraosseous and intravenous route. Am J Emerg Med. 2023;67:63–9. https://pubmed-ncbi-nlm-nih-gov.proxy.lib.wayne.edu/36806977/.

129. Long LRP, Gardner LSM, Burgert J, Koeller LCA, O'Sullivan LJ, Blouin D, et al. Humerus intraosseous administration of epinephrine in normovolemic and hypovolemic porcine model. Am J Disaster Med. 2018;13(2):97–106. https://pubmed-ncbi-nlm-nih-gov.proxy.lib.wayne.edu/30234916/.

130. Yauger YJ, Johnson MD, Mark J, Le T, Woodruff T, Silvey S, et al. Tibial intraosseous administration of epinephrine is effective in restoring return of spontaneous circulation in

a pediatric normovolemic but not hypovolemic cardiac arrest model. Pediatr Emerg Care. 2022;38(4):E1166–72. https://pubmed-ncbi-nlm-nih-gov.proxy.lib.wayne.edu/32453255/.

131. Voelckel WG, Lurie KG, McKnite S, Zielinski T, Lindstrom P, Peterson C, et al. Comparison of epinephrine with vasopressin on bone marrow blood flow in an animal model of hypovolemic shock and subsequent cardiac arrest. Crit Care Med. 2001;29(8):1587–92. https://pubmed-ncbi-nlm-nih-gov.proxy.lib.wayne.edu/11505132/.

132. Burgert JM, Johnson AD, Garcia-Blanco J, Fulton LV, Loughren MJ. The resuscitative and pharmacokinetic effects of humeral intraosseous vasopressin in a swine model of ventricular fibrillation. Prehosp Disaster Med. 2017;32(3):305–10. https://pubmed-ncbi-nlm-nih-gov.proxy.lib.wayne.edu/28270248/.

133. Adams TS, Blouin D, Johnson D. Effects of tibial and humerus intraosseous and intravenous vasopressin in porcine cardiac arrest model. Am J Disaster Med. 2016;11(3):211–8. https://pubmed-ncbi-nlm-nih-gov.proxy.lib.wayne.edu/28134420/.

134. Johnson D, Giles K, Acuna A, Saenz C, Bentley M, Budinich C. Effects of tibial intraosseous and IV administration of vasopressin on kinetics and survivability in cardiac arrest. Am J Emerg Med. 2016;34(3):429–32. https://pubmed-ncbi-nlm-nih-gov.proxy.lib.wayne.edu/26778642/.

135. O'Sullivan M, Martinez A, Long A, Johnson M, Blouin D, Johnson AD, et al. Comparison of the effects of sternal and tibial intraosseous administered resuscitative drugs on return of spontaneous circulation in a swine model of cardiac arrest. Am J Disaster Med. 2016;11(3):175–82. https://pubmed-ncbi-nlm-nih-gov.proxy.lib.wayne.edu/28134416/.

136. Burgert JM, Martinez A, O'Sullivan M, Blouin D, Long A, Johnson AD. Sternal route more effective than tibial route for intraosseous amiodarone administration in a swine model of ventricular fibrillation. Prehosp Emerg Care. 2018;22(2):266–75. https://pubmed-ncbi-nlm--nih-gov.proxy.lib.wayne.edu/28910187/.

137. Dietrich A, Franklin W, Getschman S, Allen H. Can adenosine be given by intraosseous infusion as effectively as peripherally or centrally? Pediatr Emerg Care. 1992;8(5):308. https://journals.lww.com/pec-online/Citation/1992/10000/CAN_ADENOSINE_BE_GIVEN_BY_INTRAOSSEOUS_INFUSION_AS.38.aspx.

138. Murray DB, Eddleston M, Thomas S, Jefferson RD, Thompson A, Dunn M, et al. Rapid and complete bioavailability of antidotes for organophosphorus nerve agent and cyanide poisoning in minipigs after Intraosseous administration. Ann Emerg Med. 2012;60(4):424–30.

139. Prete MR, Hannan CJ, Burkle FM. Plasma atropine concentrations via intravenous, endotracheal, and intraosseous administration. Am J Emerg Med. 1987;5(2):101–4. https://pubmed--ncbi-nlm-nih-gov.proxy.lib.wayne.edu/3828010/.

140. Yost J, Baldwin P, Bellenger S, Bradshaw F, Causapin E, Demotica R, et al. The pharmacokinetics of intraosseous atropine in hypovolemic swine. Am J Disaster Med. 2015;10(3):217–22. https://pubmed-ncbi-nlm-nih-gov.proxy.lib.wayne.edu/26663305/.

141. Iserson KV. Intraosseous infusions in adults. J Emerg Med. 1989;7(6):587–91. https://pubmed-ncbi-nlm-nih-gov.proxy.lib.wayne.edu/2625519/.

142. Frascone R, Kaye K, Dries D, Solem L. Successful placement of an adult sternal intraosseous line through burned skin. J Burn Care Rehabil. 2003;24(5):306–8. https://pubmed-ncbi-nlm--nih-gov.proxy.lib.wayne.edu/14501399/.

143. Sacchetti AD, Linkenheimer R, Lieberman M, Haviland P, Kryszczak LB. Intraosseous drug administration: successful resuscitation from asystole. Pediatr Emerg Care. 1989;5(2):97–8. https://pubmed-ncbi-nlm-nih-gov.proxy.lib.wayne.edu/2664724/.

144. Orlowski JP, Julius CJ, Petras RE, Porembka DT, Gallagher JM. The safety of intraosseous infusions: risks of fat and bone marrow emboli to the lungs. Ann Emerg Med. 1989;18(10):1062–7. https://pubmed-ncbi-nlm-nih-gov.proxy.lib.wayne.edu/2802282/.

145. Orlowski JP, Porembka DT, Gallagher JM, Lockrem JD, Vanlente F. Comparison study of intraosseous, central intravenous, and peripheral intravenous infusions of emergency drugs. Am J Disease Child. 1990;144(1):112–7. https://jamanetwork-com.proxy.lib.wayne.edu/journals/jamapediatrics/fullarticle/514962.

146. Andersen LW, Holmberg MJ, Granfeldt A, Vallentin MF. Calcium administration and post-cardiac arrest ionized calcium values according to intraosseous or intravenous administration—a post hoc analysis of a randomized trial. Resuscitation. 2022;170:211–2. https://pubmed-ncbi-nlm-nih-gov.proxy.lib.wayne.edu/34929298/.

147. Vallentin MF, Granfeldt A, Meilandt C, Povlsen AL, Sindberg B, Holmberg MJ, et al. Effect of intravenous or intraosseous calcium vs saline on return of spontaneous circulation in adults with out-of-hospital cardiac arrest: a randomized clinical trial. JAMA. 2021;326(22):1.

148. Oesterlie GE, Petersen KK, Knudsen L, Henriksen TB. Crural amputation of a newborn as a consequence of intraosseous needle insertion and calcium infusion. Pediatr Emerg Care. 2014;30(6):413–4. https://pubmed-ncbi-nlm-nih-gov.proxy.lib.wayne.edu/24892680/.

149. Warren DW, Kissoon N, Mattar A, Morrissey G, Gravelle D, Rieder MJ. Pharmacokinetics from multiple intraosseous and peripheral intravenous site injections in normovolemic and hypovolemic pigs. Crit Care Med. 1994;22(5):838–43. https://pubmed-ncbi-nlm-nih-gov.proxy.lib.wayne.edu/8181294/.

150. Spivey WH, Lathers CM, Malone DR, Unger HD, Bhat S, McNamara RN, et al. Comparison of intraosseous, central, and peripheral routes of sodium bicarbonate administration during CPR in pigs. Ann Emerg Med. 1985;14(12):1135–40. https://pubmed-ncbi-nlm-nih-gov.proxy.lib.wayne.edu/2998236/.

151. Mortensen ME, Bolon CE, Kelley MT, Walson PD, Cassidy S. Encainide overdose in an infant. Ann Emerg Med. 1992;21(8):998–1001. https://pubmed-ncbi-nlm-nih-gov.proxy.lib.wayne.edu/1497172/.

152. McNamara RM, Spivey WH, Sussman C. Pediatric resuscitation without an intravenous line. Am J Emerg Med. 1986;4(1):31–3. https://pubmed-ncbi-nlm-nih-gov.proxy.lib.wayne.edu/3004526/.

153. Runyon DE, Bruttig SP, Dubick MA, Clifford CB, Kramer GC. Resuscitation from hypovolemia in swine with intraosseous infusion of a saturated salt-dextran solution. J Trauma. 1994;36(1):11–9. https://pubmed-ncbi-nlm-nih-gov.proxy.lib.wayne.edu/7507529/.

154. Wilson J, Passmore A, Leger S, Lannan J, Bentley M, Johnson D. Effects of tibial intraosseous and intravenous administration of Hextend on time of administration and hemodynamics in a hypovolemic swine model. Am J Disaster Med. 2016;11(3):193–201. https://pubmed-ncbi-nlm-nih-gov.proxy.lib.wayne.edu/28134418/.

155. Kentner R, Haas T, Gervais H, Hiller B, Dick W. Pharmacokinetics and pharmacodynamics of hydroxyethyl starch in hypovolemic pigs; a comparison of peripheral and intraosseous infusion. Resuscitation. 1999;40(1):37–44. https://pubmed-ncbi-nlm-nih-gov.proxy.lib.wayne.edu/10321846/.

156. Neufeld JD, Marx JA, Moore EE, Light AI. Comparison of intraosseous, central, and peripheral routes of crystalloid infusion for resuscitation of hemorrhagic shock in a swine model. J Trauma. 1993;34(3):422–8. https://pubmed-ncbi-nlm-nih-gov.proxy.lib.wayne.edu/8483186/.

157. Morris RE, Schonfeld N, Haftel AJ. Treatment of hemorrhagic shock with intraosseous administration of crystalloid fluid in the rabbit model. Ann Emerg Med. 1987;16(12):1321–4. https://pubmed-ncbi-nlm-nih-gov.proxy.lib.wayne.edu/3688591/.

158. Hodge D, Delgado-Paredes C, Fleisher G. Intraosseous infusion flow rates in hypovolemic "pediatric" dogs. Ann Emerg Med. 1987;16(3):305–7. https://pubmed-ncbi-nlm-nih-gov.proxy.lib.wayne.edu/3813165/.

159. Schoffstall JM, Spivey WH, Davidheiser S, Lathers CM. Intraosseous crystalloid and blood infusion in a swine model. J Trauma. 1989;29(3):384–7. https://pubmed-ncbi-nlm-nih-gov.proxy.lib.wayne.edu/2926854/.

160. Perron P, Gunther R, Kramer G. Pressure-flow relationships of intraosseous infusions. Circ Shock. 1988;24:282.

161. Dubick MA, Pteiffer JW, Clifford CB, Runyon DE, Kramer GC. Comparison of intraosseous and intravenous delivery of hypertonic saline/dextran in anesthetized, euvolemic pigs. Ann Emerg Med. 1992;21(5):498–503. https://pubmed-ncbi-nlm-nih-gov.proxy.lib.wayne.edu/1373937/.

162. Halvorsen L, Bay BK, Perron PR, Gunther RA, Holcroft JW, Blaisdell FW, et al. Evaluation of an intraosseous infusion device for the resuscitation of hypovolemic shock. J Trauma. 1990;30(6):652–9. https://pubmed-ncbi-nlm-nih-gov.proxy.lib.wayne.edu/1693696/.
163. Okrasinski EB, Krahwinkel DJ, Sanders WL. Treatment of dogs in hemorrhagic shock by intraosseous infusion of hypertonic saline and dextran. Vet Surg. 1992;21(1):20–4. https://pubmed-ncbi-nlm-nih-gov.proxy.lib.wayne.edu/1374577/.
164. Watson J, Pascual J, Runyon D, Kramer G, Wisner S. Intraosseous resuscitation from hemorrhage: restoration of cardiac output using normal saline (NS) and 7.5% hypertonic saline 6% dextran (HSD). Circ Shock. 1990;31:69.
165. Johnson D, Penaranda C, Phillips K, Rice D, Vanderhoek L, Gegel B, et al. Effects of sternal intraosseous and intravenous administration of Hextend on time of administration and hemodynamics in a swine model of hemorrhagic shock. Am J Disaster Med. 2015;10(1):61–7. https://pubmed-ncbi-nlm-nih-gov.proxy.lib.wayne.edu/26102046/.
166. Olldashi F, Kerçi M, Zhurda T, Ruçi K, Banushi A, Traverso MS, et al. Effects of tranexamic acid on death, vascular occlusive events, and blood transfusion in trauma patients with significant haemorrhage (CRASH-2): a randomised, placebo-controlled trial. Lancet. 2010;376(9734):23–32. https://pubmed-ncbi-nlm-nih-gov.proxy.lib.wayne.edu/20554319/.
167. Lallemand MS, Moe DM, McClellan JM, Loughren M, Marko S, Eckert MJ, et al. No intravenous access, no problem: intraosseous administration of tranexamic acid is as effective as intravenous in a porcine hemorrhage model. J Trauma Acute Care Surg. 2018;84(2):379–85. https://pubmed-ncbi-nlm-nih-gov.proxy.lib.wayne.edu/29194320/.
168. Boysen SR, Pang JM, Mikler JR, Knight CG, Semple HA, Caulkett NA. Comparison of tranexamic acid plasma concentrations when administered via intraosseous and intravenous routes. Am J Emerg Med. 2017;35(2):227–33. https://pubmed-ncbi-nlm-nih-gov.proxy.lib.wayne.edu/27816438/.
169. Douma MJ, Bara GS, O'Dochartaigh D, Brindley PG. Double-barrelled resuscitation: a feasibility and simulation study of dual-intraosseous needles into a single humerus. Injury. 2015;46(11):2239–42. https://pubmed-ncbi-nlm-nih-gov.proxy.lib.wayne.edu/26372229/.
170. Ward JA, DeLorenzo RA, Rubal BJ, Jordan BS, Medina JS, Holbrook-Emmons VL, et al. Phase relationships between mean arterial pressure and intraosseous (IO) pressure. FASEB J. 2011:25. https://www.embase.com/search/results?subaction=viewrecord&id=L70759296&from=export.
171. Peshimam N, Bruce-Hickman K, Crawford K, Upadhyay G, Randle E, Ramnarayan P, et al. Peripheral and central/intraosseous vasoactive infusions during and after pediatric critical care transport: retrospective cohort study of extravasation injury. Pediatr Crit Care Med. 2022;23(8):626–34. https://pubmed-ncbi-nlm-nih-gov.proxy.lib.wayne.edu/35481954/.
172. Charbel RC, Ollier V, Julliand S, Jourdain G, Lode N, Tissieres P, et al. Safety of early norepinephrine infusion through peripheral vascular access during transport of critically ill children. J Am Coll Emerg Physicians Open. 2021;2(2). https://pubmed-ncbi-nlm-nih-gov.proxy.lib.wayne.edu/33718927/.
173. Zuckerman O, Ferrara S, Guevarra KP. Considerations for intraosseous access in obese patients. In: American Thoracic Society International Conference Meetings Abstracts American Thoracic Society International Conference Meetings Abstracts. 2019. p. A3490. www.atsjournals.org.
174. Suominen PK, Nurmi E, Lauerma K. Intraosseous access in neonates and infants: risk of severe complications—a case report. Acta Anaesthesiol Scand. 2015;59(10):1389–93. https://pubmed-ncbi-nlm-nih-gov.proxy.lib.wayne.edu/26300243/.
175. Fetissof H, Nadaud J, Landy C, Millot I, Paris R, Plancade D. Amines on intraosseous vascular access: a case of skin necrosis. Ann Fr Anesth Reanim. 2013;32(5). https://pubmed-ncbi-nlm-nih-gov.proxy.lib.wayne.edu/23623399/.
176. Neish SR, Macon MG, Moore JWM, Graeber GM. Intraosseous infusion of hypertonic glucose and dopamine. Am J Dis Child. 1988;142(8):878–80. https://pubmed-ncbi-nlm-nih-gov.proxy.lib.wayne.edu/3394678/.

177. Bilello JF, O'Hair KC, Kirby WC, Moore JW. Intraosseous infusion of dobutamine and iso-proterenol. Am J Dis Child. 1991;145(2):165–7. https://pubmed-ncbi-nlm-nih-gov.proxy.lib.wayne.edu/1994681/.

178. Philbeck TE, Miller LJ, Montez D, Puga T. Hurts so good. Easing IO pain and pressure. JEMS. 2010;35(9). https://pubmed-ncbi-nlm-nih-gov.proxy.lib.wayne.edu/20868946/.

179. Brozovich AA, Incavo SJ, Lambert BS, Sullivan TC, Wininger AE, Clyburn TA, et al. Intraosseous morphine decreases postoperative pain and pain medication use in Total knee Arthroplasty: a double-blind, randomized controlled trial. J Arthroplasty. 2022;37(6S):S139–46. https://pubmed-ncbi-nlm-nih-gov.proxy.lib.wayne.edu/35272897/.

180. Alawi KA, Morrison GC, Fraser DD, Al-Farsi S, Collier C, Kornecki A. Insulin infusion via an intraosseous needle in diabetic ketoacidosis. Anaesth Intensive Care. 2008;36(1):110–2. https://pubmed-ncbi-nlm-nih-gov.proxy.lib.wayne.edu/18326143/.

181. Howland M. Antidotes in depth. In: Howland MA, Hoffman RS, Howland MA, Lewin NA, Nelson LS, Goldfrank LR, editors. Goldfrank's Toxicologic emergencies, 10e. New York, NY: McGraw-Hill Education; 2015.

182. Manley L. Intraosseous infusion—a lifesaving technique that should be used more widely. J Intraven Nurs. 1989;12(6):367–8.

183. Bebarta VS, Pitotti RL, Boudreau S, Tanen DA. Intraosseous versus intravenous infusion of hydroxocobalamin for the treatment of acute severe cyanide toxicity in a swine model. Acad Emerg Med. 2014;21(11):1203–11. https://doi.org/10.1111/acem.12518.

184. Borron SW, Arias JC, Bauer CR, Sanchez M, Fernández M, Jung I. Hemodynamics after intraosseous administration of hydroxocobalamin or normal saline in a goat model. Am J Emerg Med. 2009;27(9):1065–71. https://pubmed-ncbi-nlm-nih-gov.proxy.lib.wayne.edu/19931752/.

185. Hosseinpour M, Khodaiari M. Appearance time of methylene blue in the aorta: intra-osseous vs peripheral intravenous route. Trauma Mon. 2012;17(1):239–41. https://pubmed-ncbi-nlm--nih-gov.proxy.lib.wayne.edu/24829890/.

186. Fettiplace MR, Ripper R, Lis K, Feinstein DL, Rubinstein I, Weinberg G. Intraosseous lipid emulsion: an effective alternative to IV delivery in emergency situations. Crit Care Med. 2014;42(2). https://pubmed-ncbi-nlm-nih-gov.proxy.lib.wayne.edu/24145832/.

187. Lameijer H, Azizi N, Ligtenberg JJM, Ter Maaten JC. Ventricular tachycardia after naloxone administration: a drug related complication? Case report and literature review Drug Saf Case Rep. 2014;1(1). https://pubmed-ncbi-nlm-nih-gov.proxy.lib.wayne.edu/27747471/.

188. Spivey WH, Unger HD, Lathers CM, McNamara RM. Intraosseous diazepam suppression of pentylenetetrazol-induced epileptogenic activity in pigs. Ann Emerg Med. 1987;16(2):156–9. https://pubmed-ncbi-nlm-nih-gov.proxy.lib.wayne.edu/3800088/.

189. Brickman KR, Rega P, Guinness M. A comparative study of intraosseous versus peripheral intravenous infusion of diazepam and phenobarbital in dogs. Ann Emerg Med. 1987;16(10):1141–4. https://pubmed-ncbi-nlm-nih-gov.proxy.lib.wayne.edu/3662161/.

190. Jim KF, Lathers CM, Farris VL, Pratt LF, Spivey WH. Suppression of pentylenetetrazol-elicited seizure activity by intraosseous lorazepam in pigs. Epilepsia. 1989;30(4):480–6. https://pubmed-ncbi-nlm-nih-gov.proxy.lib.wayne.edu/2752999/.

191. Eisenkraft A, Gilat E, Chapman S, Baranes S, Egoz I, Levy A. Efficacy of the bone injection gun in the treatment of organophosphate poisoning. Biopharm Drug Dispos. 2007;28(3):145–50. https://pubmed-ncbi-nlm-nih-gov.proxy.lib.wayne.edu/17315239/.

192. Vinsel PJ, Moore GP, O'Hair KC. Comparison of intraosseous versus intravenous loading of phenytoin in pigs and effect on bone marrow. Am J Emerg Med. 1990;8(3):181–3. https://pubmed-ncbi-nlm-nih-gov.proxy.lib.wayne.edu/2331255/.

193. Jaimovich DG, Shabino CL, Ringer TV, Peters GR. Comparison of intraosseous and intravenous routes of anticonvulsant administration in a porcine model. Ann Emerg Med. 1989;18(8):842–6. https://pubmed-ncbi-nlm-nih-gov.proxy.lib.wayne.edu/2757281/.

194. Khan TM, Kissoon N, Hasan MY, Saldajeno V, Murphy S, Lima J. Comparison of plasma levels and pharmacodynamics after intraosseous and intravenous administration of fosphenytoin

and phenytoin in piglets. Pediatr Crit Care Med. 2000;1(1):60–4. https://pubmed-ncbi-nlm-nih-gov.proxy.lib.wayne.edu/12813289/.

195. Brickman K, Rega P, Choo M, Guinness M. Comparison of serum phenobarbital levels after single versus multiple attempts at intraosseous infusion. Ann Emerg Med. 1990;19(1):31–3. https://pubmed-ncbi-nlm-nih-gov.proxy.lib.wayne.edu/2297152/.

196. Alam HB, Punzalan CM, Koustova E, Bowyer MW, Rhee P. Hypertonic saline: intraosseous infusion causes myonecrosis in a dehydrated swine model of uncontrolled hemorrhagic shock. J Trauma. 2002;52(1):18–25. https://pubmed-ncbi-nlm-nih-gov.proxy.lib.wayne.edu/11791047/.

197. Bowry R, Nour M, Kus T, Parker S, Stephenson J, Saver J, et al. Intraosseous administration of tissue plasminogen activator on a mobile stroke unit. Prehosp Emerg Care. 2019;23(4):447–52. https://pubmed-ncbi-nlm-nih-gov.proxy.lib.wayne.edu/30235055/.

198. Landy C, Plancade D, Gagnon N, Schaeffer E, Nadaud J, Favier JC. Complication of intraosseous administration of systemic fibrinolysis for a massive pulmonary embolism with cardiac arrest. Resuscitation. 2012;83(6). https://pubmed-ncbi-nlm-nih-gov.proxy.lib.wayne.edu/22394696/.

199. Wright JK, Christy RJ, Tharp RV, Kalns JE. Evaluation of intraosseous delivery of factor VIIa during hemorraghic shock in the pig. Mil Med. 2009;174(2):119–23. https://pubmed-ncbi-nlm-nih-gov.proxy.lib.wayne.edu/19317190/.

200. Plancade D, Nadaud J, Lapierre M, Fétissof H, Schaeffer E, Mellati N, et al. Feasibility of a thoraco-abdominal CT with injection of iodinated contrast agent on sternal intraosseous catheter in an emergency department. Ann Fr Anesth Reanim. 2012;31(12):e283–4. https://pubmed-ncbi-nlm-nih-gov.proxy.lib.wayne.edu/23159517/.

201. Krähling H, Masthoff M, Schwindt W, Stracke CP, Schindler P. Intraosseous contrast administration for emergency stroke CT. Neuroradiology. 2021;63(6):967.

202. Schindler P, Helfen A, Wildgruber M, Heindel W, Schülke C, Masthoff M. Intraosseous contrast administration for emergency computed tomography: a case-control study. PLoS One. 2019;14(5):e0217629. https://pubmed-ncbi-nlm-nih-gov.proxy.lib.wayne.edu/31150466/.

203. Winter J, Haas N, Olivieri M, Trumm C, Hermann M, Hopfner C, et al. Successful cerebral CT angiography via intraosseous contrast administration in an 18-month-old child with acute stroke. Klin Padiatr. 2023;235(1):50–1. https://pubmed-ncbi-nlm-nih-gov.proxy.lib.wayne.edu/35785804/.

204. ACR manual on contrast media 2023 ACR committee on drugs and contrast media. 2023.

205. Aya-Ay J, Athavale S, Morgan-Bagley S, Bian H, Bauss F, Kim HKW. Retention, distribution, and effects of intraosseously administered ibandronate in the infarcted femoral head. J Bone Miner Res. 2007;22(1):93–100. https://pubmed-ncbi-nlm-nih-gov.proxy.lib.wayne.edu/17166092/.

206. Vandermeer JS, Kamiya N, Aya-ay J, Garces A, Browne R, Kim HKW. Local administration of ibandronate and bone morphogenetic protein-2 after ischemic osteonecrosis of the immature femoral head: a combined therapy that stimulates bone formation and decreases femoral head deformity. J Bone Joint Surg Am. 2011;93(10):905–13. https://pubmed-ncbi-nlm-nih-gov.proxy.lib.wayne.edu/21593365/.

207. Kumar P, Aggarwal S, Jindal K, Patel S, Sharma S, Mahan M. Core decompression combined with intraosseous Ibandronate for pre-collapse osteonecrosis of the femoral head: report of a novel technique, its safety and early outcomes in five cases. J Orthop Case Rep. 2021;11(12):96–100. https://pubmed-ncbi-nlm-nih-gov.proxy.lib.wayne.edu/35415142/.

208. Young SW, Zhang M, Freeman JT, Vince KG, Coleman B. Higher cefazolin concentrations with intraosseous regional prophylaxis in TKA. Clin Orthop Relat Res. 2013;471(1):244–9. https://pubmed-ncbi-nlm-nih-gov.proxy.lib.wayne.edu/22773397/.

209. Young SW, Zhang M, Freeman JT, Mutu-Grigg J, Pavlou P, Moore GA. The Mark Coventry award: higher tissue concentrations of vancomycin with low-dose intraosseous regional versus systemic prophylaxis in TKA: a randomized trial. Clin Orthop Relat Res. 2014;472(1):57–65. https://pubmed-ncbi-nlm-nih-gov.proxy.lib.wayne.edu/23666589/.

210. Klasan A, Patel CK, Young SW. Intraosseous regional administration of vancomycin in primary total knee arthroplasty does not increase the risk of vancomycin-associated complications. J Arthroplast. 2021;36(5):1633–7. https://pubmed-ncbi-nlm-nih-gov.proxy.lib.wayne.edu/33468344/.

211. Young SW, Roberts T, Johnson S, Dalton JP, Coleman B, Wiles S. Regional intraosseous administration of prophylactic antibiotics is more effective than systemic administration in a mouse model of TKA. Clin Orthop Relat Res. 2015;473(11):3573–84. https://pubmed-ncbi-nlm-nih-gov.proxy.lib.wayne.edu/26224291/.

212. Young SW, Zhang M, Moore GA, Pitto RP, Clarke HD, Spangehl MJ. The John N. Insall award: higher tissue concentrations of vancomycin achieved with intraosseous regional prophylaxis in revision TKA: a randomized controlled trial. Clin Orthop Relat Res. 2018;476(1):66–74. https://pubmed-ncbi-nlm-nih-gov.proxy.lib.wayne.edu/29529618/.

213. Harper KD, Lambert BS, O'Dowd J, Sullivan T, Incavo SJ. Clinical outcome evaluation of intraosseous vancomycin in total knee arthroplasty. Arthroplast Today. 2020;6(2):220–3. https://pubmed-ncbi-nlm-nih-gov.proxy.lib.wayne.edu/32577466/.

214. Park KJ, Chapleau J, Sullivan TC, Clyburn TA, Incavo SJ. Intraosseous vancomycin reduces periprosthetic joint infection in primary total knee arthroplasty at 90-day follow-up. Bone Joint J. 2021;103-B(6 Supple A):13–7. https://pubmed-ncbi-nlm-nih-gov.proxy.lib.wayne.edu/34053300/.

215. Parkinson B, McEwen P, Wilkinson M, Hazratwala K, Hellman J, Kan H, et al. Intraosseous regional prophylactic antibiotics decrease the risk of prosthetic joint infection in primary TKA: a multicenter study. Clin Orthop Relat Res. 2021;479(11):2504–12. https://pubmed-ncbi-nlm-nih-gov.proxy.lib.wayne.edu/34397615/.

216. Chin SJ, Moore GA, Zhang M, Clarke HD, Spangehl MJ, Young SW. The AAHKS clinical research award: intraosseous regional prophylaxis provides higher tissue concentrations in high BMI patients in total knee arthroplasty: a randomized trial. J Arthroplast. 2018;33(7S):S13–8. https://pubmed-ncbi-nlm-nih-gov.proxy.lib.wayne.edu/29655497/.

217. Davis J, Bates L. Rapid sequence induction via an intraosseous needle. J Intensive Care Soc. 2016;17(2):178.

218. Moore GP, Pace SA, Busby W. Comparison of intraosseous, intramuscular, and intravenous administration of succinylcholine. Pediatr Emerg Care. 1989;5(4):209–10. https://pubmed-ncbi-nlm-nih-gov.proxy.lib.wayne.edu/2602189/.

219. Selby IR, James MR. The intraosseous route for induction of anaesthesia. Anaesthesia. 1993;48(11):982–4. https://pubmed-ncbi-nlm-nih-gov.proxy.lib.wayne.edu/8250197/.

220. Medina FA. Rapid sequence induction/intubation using intraosseous infusion of vecuronium bromide in children. Am J Emerg Med. 1992;10(4):359–60. https://pubmed-ncbi-nlm-nih-gov.proxy.lib.wayne.edu/1352102/.

221. Loughren MJ, Banks S, Naluan C, Portenlanger P, Wendorf A, Johnson D. Onset and duration of intravenous and intraosseous rocuronium in swine. West J Emerg Med. 2014;15(2):241.

222. Nemeth M, Williams GN, Prichard D, McConnico A, Johnson D, Loughren M. Onset and duration of intravenous and intraosseous rocuronium in hypovolemic swine. Am J Disaster Med. 2016;11(4):279–82. https://pubmed-ncbi-nlm-nih-gov.proxy.lib.wayne.edu/28140443/.

223. Pollack CV, Pender ES, Woodall BN, Parks BR. Intraosseous administration of antibiotics: same-dose comparison with intravenous administration in the weanling pig. Ann Emerg Med. 1991;20(7):772–6. https://pubmed-ncbi-nlm-nih-gov.proxy.lib.wayne.edu/2064098/.

Complications of Intraosseous Access

Stephanie Cox, Aleksandria Bartosiewicz, Erin Rieck,
Jacob Fanning, Amanda Pierce, Jonathon Verde,
Sameer Jagani, and James H. Paxton

Introduction

Intraosseous (IO) infusion has been used to deliver fluids and medications to critically ill patients for most of a century and can be absolutely lifesaving for patients with difficult or impossible vascular access. Despite the great utility of this technique, emergency care providers must be aware of certain complications known to be associated with IO infusion. Some complications, such as pain, may be unavoidable even with meticulous attention and care taken by the provider. Broadly speaking, avoidable complications can be attributed to one or more of the following factors: **improper insertion technique**, **device malfunction**, **patient-specific factors**, **inappropriate infusion pressures**, **technological limitations**, or **inadequate monitoring**. This chapter discusses each of these factors, including unique complications associated with each factor and how to prevent or reduce the risk of their occurrence. It is important to note that complications can occur at any time during the insertion, use, or removal of IO catheters, underscoring the need for proper insertion and management techniques. Complications may be further categorized as **major** (i.e., life- or limb-threatening), **moderate** (i.e., requiring specific medical intervention to treat), or **minor** (i.e., transient, or with no specific intervention required) in severity, although a patient's clinical condition must also influence determinations of complication severity. A list of potential complications associated with the use of IO catheters is provided in Table 9.1.

S. Cox (✉) · A. Bartosiewicz · E. Rieck · J. Fanning · A. Pierce · J. Verde · S. Jagani
Michigan State University College of Osteopathic Medicine, East Lansing, MI, USA
e-mail: coxstep3@msu.edu; bartosi9@msu.edu; rieckeri@msu.edu; fanning8@msu.edu; pierc118@msu.edu; verdejo1@msu.edu; jaganisa@msu.edu

J. H. Paxton
Department of Emergency Medicine, Wayne State University School of Medicine, Detroit, MI, USA
e-mail: james.paxton@wayne.edu

© The Author(s), under exclusive license to Springer Nature Switzerland AG 2024
J. H. Paxton (ed.), *Intraosseous Vascular Access*,
https://doi.org/10.1007/978-3-031-61201-5_9

Table 9.1 Complications of intraosseous catheter use, according to relative severity

Minor	Moderate	Major
Bleeding	Bony injury (e.g., fracture)	Compartment syndrome
Catheter bending/fracture	Cellulitis	Mediastinitis
Dermal abrasion/friction burn	Intra-articular placement	Necrotizing fasciitis
Device malfunction	Osteomyelitis	Pulmonary embolism (air/fat)[a]
Dislodgement	Retained catheter tip	Sternal perforation
Extravasation	Skin laceration	
Pain	Soft tissue ischemia/necrosis	
Slow (or no) infusion		

[a] Demonstrated in an animal model, but not yet reported clinically in human subjects

Each of these complications can be associated with adverse health effects for the patient, depending upon the patient's clinical condition and disease severity. For example, device malfunction may have little effect on a stable patient, but could be catastrophic for a patient in cardiac arrest with no other vascular access readily available. Similarly, extravasation may be inconsequential if noted immediately, but can lead to compartment syndrome or other more serious complications if identification is delayed. There are also many factors that can mitigate or worsen the downstream effects of these complications. Consequently, **determination of the severity of a complication ultimately depends upon the patient's unique clinical condition and subsequent management of the complication**.

Historically, IO cannulation has been considered to be a safe and effective technique for the delivery of fluids and medications when other routes of venous infusion are unavailable, unreliable, or unsafe. Several reviews and meta-analyses have been published on the topic of IO complications, with estimates on the overall rate of complications ranging from 0.3 to 9.7%, depending upon the types/definitions of complications included and the age range of subjects [1–8]. Reporting of complications in the existing medical literature remains inconsistent, poorly standardized, and subject to interpretation by study authors [8].

Pediatric vs. Adult Complications

Differences in complication rates between pediatric and adult patients receiving IO cannulation may relate to differing bone anatomy and physiology. Target bones in pediatric patients are generally smaller than those of adults, with smaller intramedullary cavities, increased bony elasticity, and active epiphyseal growth plates. Proper placement of the IO catheter tip within the marrow cavity can be quite difficult in pediatric subjects as the target intramedullary space is much smaller. Decreased volume capacity of the intramedullary space in smaller bones such as those of children can also generate increased resistance to forward flow of infusate and may increase the risk of extravasation. **Although bone fracture is a theoretical risk for any patient receiving an IO catheter, this complication is almost exclusively seen among pediatric subjects** following an insertion attempt employing excessive force. Unfortunately, IO infusion into a fractured bone can lead to extravasation, which may place the patient at risk of compartment syndrome if the extravasation is not identified in a timely manner. If there is any question about the cortical integrity of a target bone, a plain film (or dynamic ultrasound) of the bone should be done to confirm the absence of a fracture before IO infusion is permitted at that site. When clinically indicated, dynamic ultrasound monitoring may also be used to detect early extravasation before significant soft tissue injury can occur.

The **epiphyseal growth plate** is an area of hyaline cartilage located between the epiphysis and the metaphysis of the long bones where active bone growth occurs in children [9]. This area is 1–2 cm proximal to the recommended proximal tibial IO insertion site in children, which led to concern among early IO investigators about growth plate injuries as a result of proximal tibial IO cannulation. These fears have never been realized, and multiple studies have confirmed the absence of growth plate injuries following proper IO device insertion [10]. Cadaveric studies have shown that the growth plate in newborns is usually at or just proximal (within 5 mm) to the tibial tuberosity, suggesting that IO insertion should be 1 cm distal to the tibial tuberosity to avoid potential growth plate injury [11]. Some older references to manual IO catheter insertion recommend that the catheter be inserted at an angle of 10–45° away from the growth plate (i.e., pointing slightly distal, or away from the knee) [12], but there is no scientific basis for this suggestion. In fact, modern recommendations no longer include this directive; proper insertion of an IO catheter is generally perpendicular to the bone surface, regardless of the insertion site.

One major complication reported for both the adult and pediatric population is **compartment syndrome**, which is often more severe in pediatric cases due to the infusion of higher volumes relative to the compartment space and increased risk of iatrogenic bone fracture during the IO catheter insertion attempt [13]. Early diagnosis and treatment are the best prognostic predictors in compartment syndrome, but identification is often delayed among pediatric patients due to difficulties in communicating symptoms. Compartment syndrome is characterized by the "Five Ps" (i.e., pain, pulselessness, paresthesia, paralysis, and pallor), but paresthesias are usually the earliest symptom to present in the clinical course of the condition [14]. The other symptoms of compartment syndrome may present much later, after soft tissue ischemia has already begun to occur.

Early (Placement) Complications

Inability to Cannulate

Careful site and device selection can greatly enhance a provider's ability to place an IO catheter. **Excessive soft tissue depth** overlying the targeted site can lead to inability to adequately penetrate the cortex, preventing use of the catheter or promoting inadvertent infusion into the soft tissues surrounding the bone. Commercially available IO catheters generally range from 15 to 45 mm in length, although overlying soft tissue depths may fall outside of this range [15]. One recent study reported that difficulty in identifying anatomic landmarks due to obesity contributed to humeral or proximal tibial IO catheter placement failure in 2% (4/247) of cardiac arrest patients [16]. Kehrl et al. studied intraosseous placement in obese patients and concluded that a 25 mm IO catheter is usually adequate to cannulate the proximal tibia in adult patients with a body mass index (BMI) ≤43 and the distal tibia with a BMI ≤60, as the predicted soft tissue depths at these locations are generally <20 mm [15]. Although BMI ranges can be used as general guidelines in such cases, it is important to note that subcutaneous adipose and muscle may be distributed differently in individuals according to many patient-specific factors including genetic predisposition, sex, medication use, and level of physical activity. Additional study is needed to determine typical soft tissue depths associated with the most common IO insertion sites. To date, no clinical studies have been done in emergency care patients to aid providers in predicting the depth of soft tissue anticipated with different IO insertion sites. Consequently, providers are left to estimate the soft tissue depth required for IO cannulation on a case-by-case basis.

Bone fragility due to *osteogenesis imperfecta*, osteoporosis, or other medical conditions can contribute to IO catheter failure due to immediate dislodgement after placement. Nutbeam and Fergusson described a patient with type III *osteogenesis imperfecta* for whom three IO attempts were made, each becoming loose and unable to be secured or flushed [17]. The patient ultimately required PIV access after multiple failed IO cannulation attempts [17]. Patients with severe osteopenia or genetic disorders of bony metabolism should be monitored very closely for extravasation and subsequent compartment syndrome after IO catheter placement, especially when large-volume infusions are required.

Device Malfunction

In this context, **device malfunction** should be defined as **failure of a device to perform as expected**. This can be very difficult to distinguish from operator error, especially when using complicated semiautomatic devices that may require careful guidance by the operator to achieve proper insertion. Generally speaking, device malfunctions are characterized by manufacturing defects or inadequacies of the device that lead to unsuccessful placement or immediate failure of the infusion attempt. Common examples of device failure include battery failure (e.g., in placement drills), failure to deploy (e.g., with spring-loaded semiautomatic devices), catheter fracture or bending during routine placement (without exceptional force applied either during or following the placement attempt), or fracture/separation of the plastic hub during insertion or use. While certain categories of IO devices may share common failure-prone characteristics, these devices often have unique characteristics that can lead to specific types of device failure depending upon the device selected for use. For this reason, it is important that providers understand the types of device failures that they can expect to encounter with the specific device that they are using, in order to properly monitor for and identify complications due to device failures that can negatively affect patient outcomes.

Hafner and colleagues published their study comparing manual IO catheters to drill-assisted IO catheters in 2013 [18]. They found a 100% insertion success rate for the EZ-IO® drill-assisted catheter system and a 76.2% success rate with the Cook™ manual IO catheter. The most common cause of insertion failure was catheter bending with 33.3% of all manual IO insertion attempts, felt to be due to either device malfunction (i.e., structural weakness of the catheter needle) or improper technique with excessive force of insertion [18]. Brenner et al. reported similar results, with 15.4% of Cook™ manual catheters breaking or bending during insertion attempts [19]. Only one EZ-IO® patient required three attempts to achieve successful placement, although this was attributed to user error and lack of experience with the device [19]. Early reports on the EZ-IO® system suggested that "binding" of the drill motor and battery failure were occasionally seen [20], which led to device improvements that appear to have effectively eliminated those issues. Although they can be used for hundreds (or even thousands) of IO insertion attempts, many commercially available battery-operated drill insertion devices employ lithium ion batteries that are not rechargeable and do eventually become depleted.

Sørgjerd and colleagues published their comparison of the EZ-IO® at the proximal tibia or humerus to the sternal FAST-Responder® (FAST-R®) device in 2019 [20]. Both devices performed very well, with insertion times rarely greater than 30 s (4.8% and 12.5%, respectively). They reported on so-called **aspiration failure** (i.e., inability to aspirate bone marrow after insertion), with a reported rate of 11.9% for this complication among studied EZ-IO® patients. This also occurred with the FAST-R® device, but the rate was not reported. The significance of this "complication" is unclear, as it is widely known that **successful aspiration of bone marrow following IO catheter insertion is not required to confirm proper placement**. Although the ability to aspirate marrow certainly confirms successful cannulation of the target bone (and suggests optimal placement of the catheter tip within the intramedullary space), the absence of marrow on aspiration of the catheter does not uniformly indicate unsuccessful placement. When marrow is not aspirated, other methods can be used to confirm correct tip placement, such as dynamic ultrasound (to detect flow with a small flush through the catheter) or plain-film imaging to confirm that the catheter tip is within the marrow space. Sørgjerd also detected soft tissue extravasation of infusates in 2.3% of EZ-IO® cases and found much higher flow rates associated with sternal IO catheters than with proximal humerus or tibial IO infusion [20]. Hammer and colleagues found that flow rates are inconsistent between sites but may be augmented with pressure bag infusion [21]. While aspiration failure may be a sign of misplacement, this is not generally considered to be a complication of IO catheter insertion per se.

Considering the diversity of modern IO access devices, the specific complication rates reported in these studies are of less importance than provider recognition of the wide range of device-related failures that can be encountered in clinical practice. Adequate awareness of these complications, user training, and vigilant monitoring can help to reduce the impact of complications due to device failure on patient outcomes.

In some cases of IO catheter fracture, the proximal (i.e., deep) end of the catheter can be retained in the bone after the distal (i.e., more superficial) portion of the device has been removed. This is a rare complication, but has been reported with both sternal IO devices (e.g., FAST-1®, FAST-R®) [22–24] and humeral and tibial EZ-IO® devices [3, 23]. Among the FAST-1® series of devices, the steel catheter tip is attached to a clear polyvinylchloride (PVC) infusion tubing, which can become separated from the steel tip, leaving the tip in the sternum when the tubing is pulled out forcefully. It can be unclear whether this complication is due to inappropriate placement technique (e.g., insertion at a non-perpendicular angle, excessive force of insertion), inappropriate removal technique (i.e., excessive force with removal, removal force in the wrong direction), or device malfunction (i.e., poor design or manufacturing). Early versions of the FAST-1® device included an "extraducer" tool, intended to facilitate intact removal of the catheter [24], but more modern versions of the device does not require this tool. Catheter fractures involving EZ-IO® devices tend to occur between the plastic hub and the surface of the bone, sometimes leaving more than half (e.g., 15 mm) of the steel needle in situ. In one case, care providers attempted to remove a tibial EZ-IO® catheter with pliers, leading to catheter fracture and retained catheter tip requiring surgical intervention to remove it [3]. Although surgical intervention may be required, long-term follow-up of these patients after catheter tip removal suggests a low likelihood of long-term complications from retained catheter tip once it is removed [22]. The potential infectious or algetic complications of a retained catheter tip that is not promptly removed remain poorly described. Consequently, it is recommended that retained catheter tips be removed as soon as feasible and that catheters be examined after attempted removal to ensure that the entire device has been extracted.

As mentioned above, device malfunction can be difficult to distinguish from user error associated with improper insertion technique. Providers should be adequately trained on the insertion of IO devices before being asked to place them under clinical circumstances. Clinical studies suggest that "first-attempt" success with IO insertion is generally possible in >90% of all attempts [25], although this rate may be much lower in neonates or very young children. In one study, proper placement of a tibial IO catheter among pediatric patients (3 weeks to 16 years of age) was achieved in only 60% of cases (25/42 cases) [26]. Most of these patients were ≤6 months old. The causes of 17 failed placement attempts reported in this study included "needle missed the bone" (five cases), "tip of the needle embedded in the tibial cortex" (six cases), and **transcortical** (i.e., through both the *cis* (i.e., superficial) and *trans* (i.e., deep) cortices, resulting in through-and-through penetration with catheter tip in the nearby soft tissues) in six cases. The authors concluded that many of these placement failures may have been avoided with more appropriate selection of shorter IO catheters for very small patients, although factors such as provider experience and training are also very important [26]. **Many complications attributed to device failure in reported studies may be due to inappropriate device selection, improper insertion site selection, or poor insertion technique.** When studies report a placement failure rate significantly greater than 10%, improper catheter selection, incorrect insertion site, or lack of adequate provider training on insertion technique should be suspected. In one cadaveric study of children treated with IO catheters, providers who were trained in Pediatric Advanced Life Support (PALS) realized IO catheter insertion success rates almost twice as high as those experienced by non-PALS-trained EMS providers [27]. This study also found that placement of a 15 mm EZ-IO® catheter at the proximal tibia in children <6 months old was generally successful, while use of a 25 mm EZ-IO® catheter at the same site was almost always unsuccessful due to excessive catheter length

[27]. Selection of an inappropriately short IO catheter can also lead to high rates of immediate or delayed line failure, such as the use of a 25 mm catheter at the adult proximal humerus where a 45 mm or longer catheter is often required [28]. If improper catheter placement is not detected immediately, this user error can lead to other complications such as extravasation when subsequent infusion of fluids or medications is attempted.

Immediate Dislodgement/Extravasation

When properly placed, IO catheters should have their shaft securely lodged in the cortical bone with the catheter tip positioned as close as possible to the center of the medullary cavity and their hub stabilized at the skin surface. **If the catheter is not long enough to achieve cortical penetration, providers may try to over-advance the catheter in an attempt to reach the bone, leading to the catheter hub indenting the skin surface.** If the catheter is securely lodged in an over-advanced position, this can lead to significant pressure on the skin and subcutaneous tissues by the catheter hub and will promote soft tissue necrosis and dermal injury. Once compressed in this manner, the skin and subcutaneous will attempt to return to their normal anatomical position by exerting a retrograde force on the catheter hub that gradually pushes the catheter back out. Thus, a catheter that appears to be well positioned after initial insertion can be gradually backed out and eventually be retracted to such a degree that the tip is no longer within the medullary space. If this is not detected prior to infusion attempts, the infusate will be injected into the soft tissue adjacent to the bone and can accumulate there with resultant poor absorption and the potential for complications due to the effects of the accumulated fluid.

Although some automatic IO catheters have a preset depth of insertion, semiautomatic and manual IO catheters generally have some form of marking on the catheter to help the provider gauge whether the catheter is long enough to provide satisfactory cannulation of the target bone. For example, the EZ-IO® catheter system features black markings every 10 mm along the steel cannula that can be used to gauge the depth of the bone surface from the skin surface. The manufacturer recommends that at least one black line (the most proximal line, which is 5 mm from the catheter hub flange) should be visible above the skin surface after the catheter has been advanced through the soft tissues following contact with the bone surface. If no black lines are visible, a longer catheter should be selected instead to avoid placement of an inappropriately short catheter. This concept is illustrated in Fig. 9.1. In this figure, the top two examples are appropriate, and IO insertion can be performed; the bottom example demonstrates an inappropriate attempt to use an IO catheter of inadequate length, which is demonstrated by the lack of a visible black line above the skin surface. In this case, the bone should not be penetrated, and a longer catheter should be selected. Ideally, the hub flange should be at or above the skin surface; when an inadequately long catheter is selected, the hub flange will likely indent the skin, causing excessive pressure on the soft tissues and increasing the risk of catheter dislodgement or soft tissue injury. Figure 9.2 shows a

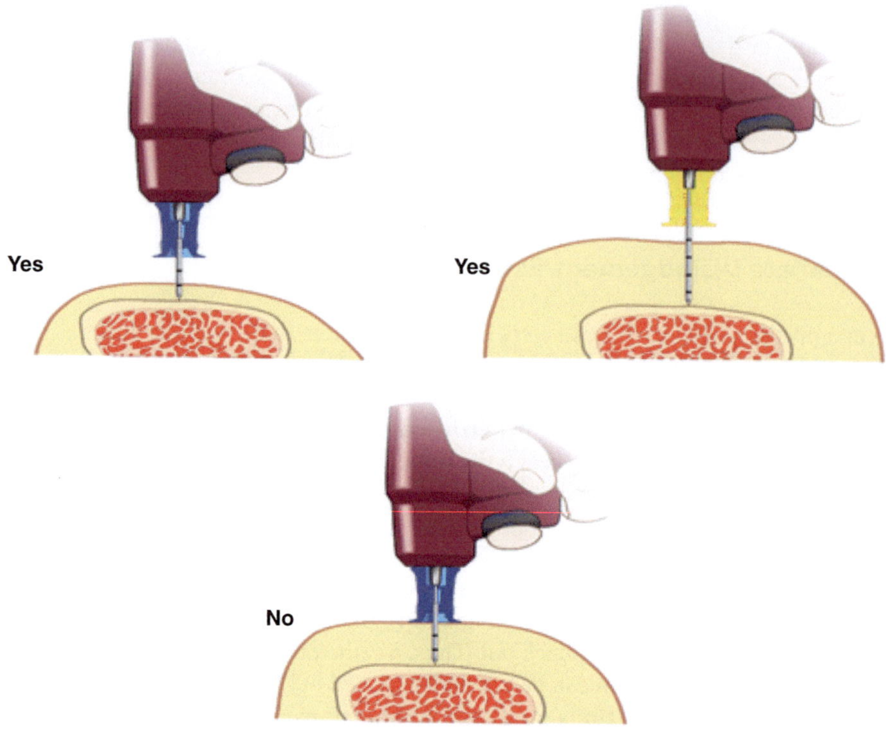

Fig. 9.1 Proper and improper intraosseous catheter length. (Image courtesy of Scotty Bolleter)

Fig. 9.2 Skin indentation due to excessive advancement of a 25 mm IO catheter at the proximal humerus. (*Image courtesy of the authors*)

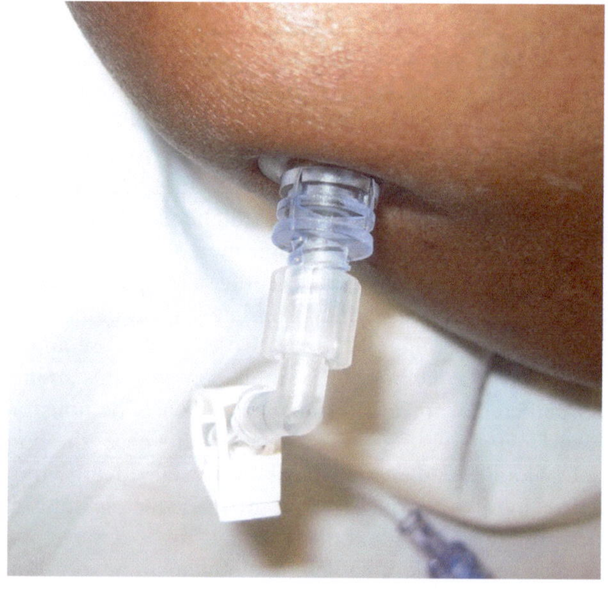

25 mm IO catheter inserted at the proximal humerus with skin indentation suggesting excessive insertion depth.

In addition to this risk of soft tissue injury, an over-advanced catheter will experience backward force from the soft tissues attempting to return to their previous as a result of skin and soft tissue elasticity. This can ultimately lead to catheter dislodgement. **Dislodgement** refers to the inadvertent extraction of a previously lodged catheter out of the bone and into the superficial soft tissues. This can (but does not universally) lead to extravasation of fluids and medications infused through the catheter into the soft tissue space. **Extravasation** refers to unintentional leakage of infused substances from the IO catheter tip or medullary space during attempted catheter infusion. This can be due to catheter dislodgement, but is also seen with IO infusion into a bone with discontinuity of the bony cortex (e.g., target bone fracture, multiple IO insertion holes). One common cause of proximal humeral IO catheter dislodgement is lifting the subject's arm above the head, which causes the IO catheter to be levered out of the humeral bone due to lateral pressure applied by the acromion process. A properly placed proximal humerus IO catheter is very close to the acromion process, as depicted in Fig. 9.3. As Fig. 9.4 illustrates, humeral IO catheters can become bent due to raising of the subject's arm above the head during clinical treatment, as with preparation for CT imaging of the thorax.

Extravasation can also potentially occur when the **osteotomy** (i.e., hole made in the bony cortex by the IO catheter during insertion) is oversized and does not snugly approximate the sides of the catheter shaft. In this context, extravasation can occur when the volume of fluid being infused into the medullary space exceeds the capacity of the bone venous drainage system to remove the infused substance, leading to high intramedullary pressure. Fluids in a rigid space such as the medullary cavity will seek the path of least resistance under high pressure; if a potential space exists between the catheter and the surrounding cortical bone, this space can provide a

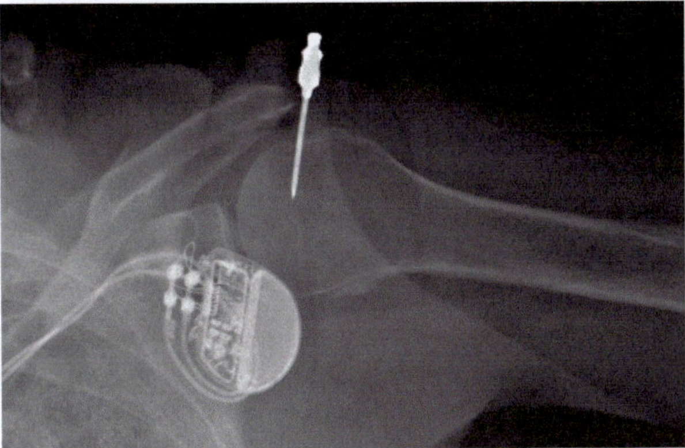

Fig. 9.3 Position of a proximal humerus IO catheter relative to the acromion process of the shoulder, as visible on plain film. Note that the catheter has been inserted much higher on the humerus than the usual insertion site, and that the patient's arm has also been abducted substantially. Both of these management choices make damage to the catheter and patient likely. (*Image courtesy of the authors*)

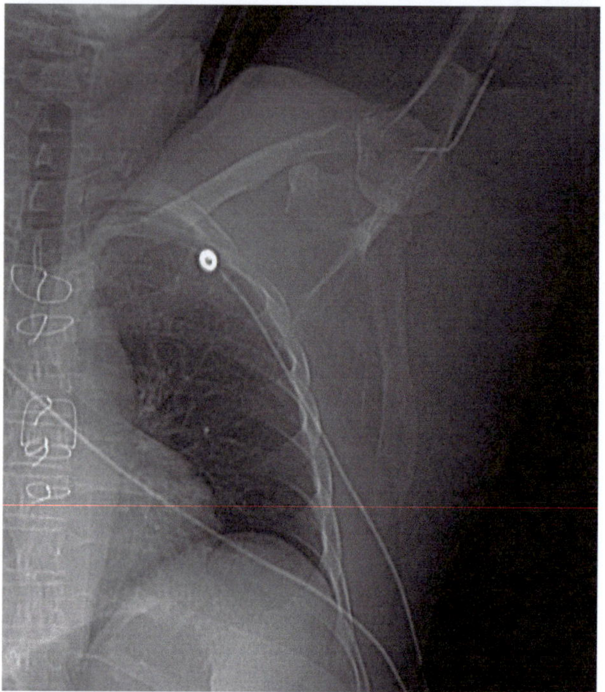

Fig. 9.4 Bending of a 68 mm left humeral IO catheter (upper right portion of the image) in a subject who had arms raised above the head during CT imaging of the thorax. (*Image courtesy of the authors*)

channel for retrograde fluid extrusion around the catheter, leading to fluid accumulation in direct correlation to the degree to which the drainage system is overwhelmed. High intramedullary pressure from overexuberant fluid infusion through an IO catheter may also contribute to rupture of the bony drainage veins, which could cause extravasation of blood and infusates from the venous drainage system in the soft tissues near the bone surface. In the absence of an obvious cause of cortical disruption (e.g., bone fracture) or catheter dislodgement, it may not be possible to know which of these mechanisms has led to the extravasation. However, since both leakage around the catheter and vein rupture are associated with overly aggressive fluid infusion, providers should monitor all patients receiving high-volume or high-pressure IO infusion for signs of extravasation, such as swelling around the IO insertion site and increased pain at the location.

Compartment syndrome is a potential complication of extravasation, resulting from dangerously increased compartmental pressure in soft tissue spaces tightly confined by fascial planes, especially those located in the anterior compartment of the lower extremity and the deep volar compartment of the forearm [14, 29–32]. Although this is a delayed complication, usually occurring hours or days after IO catheter insertion, it is highly associated with immediate complications such as bone fracture and extravasation. To minimize the risk of compartment syndrome, providers should monitor extremities cannulated with IO access frequently for signs of extravasation, including pain out of proportion to cannulation and extremity swelling. Intraosseous access should be replaced after more definitive access is obtained. Only one attempt should be made in a major bone to prevent fluid extravasation through the other cannulation sites [31]. Providers should avoid placing IO catheters into injured limbs or limbs with known fractured long bones as this increases risk of extravasation [29]. If there is evidence of fracture, edema, ecchymosis, or deformity, a radiograph should be obtained before IO catheter placement, although this may be challenging in urgent trauma cases. If compartment syndrome is suspected, arteriography may not improve clinical outcomes, as it can delay surgical decompression [32].

Confirmation of correct IO catheter placement with aspiration of marrow contents, loss of resistance as cortex is penetrated, and free flow of fluid into osseous cavity are recommended. When feasible, plain radiographs should be done to confirm that the catheter is well lodged within the bony cortex. Providers should stabilize the tubing and extremity (not just the catheter shaft) to minimize dislodgement. It is best to secure the IO line to the extremity using noncircumferential methods to avoid venous constriction. Providers should keep the catheter site visible, especially in the first 10–15 min after infusion has started. Document start and stop times, rate, and volume of fluid infused.

When utilizing IO catheters, infusion pumps should be set to a low-pressure limit when feasible to avoid infusing fluids under high pressures as this increases the risk of extravasation. Caution should also be taken when infusing certain medications, especially hypertonic solutions and other irritants [33]. Providers must monitor the infusion site both during and after removal of IO access to identify soft tissue injury due to extravasation as early as possible. Frequent neurovascular examinations (both motor and sensory) are important, as well as distal pulse assessment, repeated assessments of capillary refill, palpation of adjacent compartments, monitoring of the extremity circumference, and interval monitoring of vitals [34].

It is important to maintain a high index of suspicion for compartment syndrome in sedated or anesthetized children, as early signs of pain may be masked [35]. Alert patients will complain of pain out of proportion with passive stretch of muscles, followed by paresthesias, paralysis, and pulselessness [36]. It can be difficult to assess for compartment syndrome signs among preverbal pediatric patients, or any patient who is under sedation, on pain medication, or critically ill [32]. Secondary surveys in trauma patients (especially those who are unconscious) are necessary to evaluate for evolving pathology or previously missed injuries [37].

Dermal Injury

In addition to the potential for soft tissue ischemia due to excessive pressure on the skin surface, other dermal injuries such as skin abrasions and lacerations can also occur during IO catheter placement. Overbey and Kon reported two pediatric cases of circular dermal abrasion around the IO insertion site attributed to the use of the EZ-IO® semiautomatic device [38]. The first patient was noted to have a "doubled-red ring with a red center point lesion" that was treated daily and healed without any complications at 11 months post-injury. The second patient was noted to have a

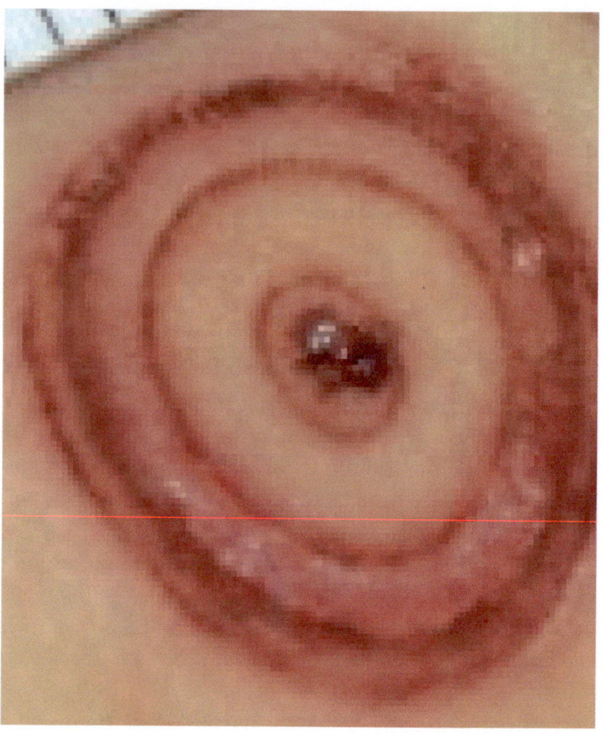

Fig. 9.5 Dermal abrasion due to excessive force and depth of insertion during semiautomatic IO catheter placement. (*Image courtesy of the authors*)

"target-shaped lesion" around the tibial insertion site that also healed uneventfully [38]. Such circular dermal lesions have only been reported with the EZ-IO® drill-assisted device and are likely friction burns due to spinning abrasion by the catheter hub on the skin surface during the insertion process. This is likely due to inappropriate over-advancement of the catheter with excessive hub contact with the skin surface. As noted above, optimal placement of an EZ-IO® catheter results in the hub barely contacting the skin or seated just above the skin surface. As these cases illustrate, excessive contact between the catheter hub and the skin surface during or after catheter placement introduces a higher risk of dermal injury. Figure 9.5 shows a characteristic dermal abrasion sustained during IO catheter placement with a drill driver.

Bone Injury

Bone injury during IO catheter placement and use is a rare but potentially serious complication of this procedure. One retrospective study including 143 pediatric patients cited a 1% rate of target bone fracture [39], although another larger study reporting on 291 pediatric patients found no incidents of fracture [40]. The latter study also included long-term outcome data for 51 of these patients, with no reports of delayed bone injury or growth plate disruption. It has been speculated that bone fracture with IO catheter placement is more common among neonates and very young patients due to excessive force of insertion relative to bone strength [41]. Alteration in local blood flow is one hypothetical mechanism for IO-induced bony injury, but there is no evidence that such injuries occur or have a clinical effect. Kim et al. showed in a porcine animal model that induced ischemia at the femoral neck and head did not cause any significant damage to the epiphyseal growth plate or disruption in subsequent leg growth [42]. One study in which radiographs were performed on 23 pediatric patients at a mean 29.2 months following intraosseous catheter placement showed no effects on bone growth. Other authors have found similar results [43]. Modern IO devices are believed to be relatively atraumatic, with fracture and bony injury due to excessive force with placement attempts rarely reported among adult subjects.

Sternal Perforation

Penetration through both tables of the sternum during sternal IO catheter placement could potentially result in cardiac injury or extravasation of fluid into the mediastinum. Although this complication was reported occasionally in the early IO literature, improvements to modern devices and decreased use of the sternal insertion site have made this complication exceedingly rare in the modern literature. Reported instances of sternal perforation with therapeutic IO catheter insertion (recorded in Table 9.2) are primarily from the 10-year period from 1944 to 1954, when sternal IO catheter use was at the height of its popularity in the USA and Europe.

All but one of the reported cases of trans-sternal perforation led to the death of the patient. In the single instance of patient survival, misplacement of the IO catheter led to massive hemomediastinum (due to subsequent infusion blood and resuscitative fluids), but the heart was not injured [51]. At least one author of an early report speculated that the cause of death was due to "apprehension [during the IO insertion process that] caused holding of the breath and this in turn led to stretching

Table 9.2 Reported cases of sternal perforation during IO catheter insertion

Author (year)	Patient age (years)	Patient gender
Meyer and Halpern (1944) [44]	51	Male
Scherer and Howe (1945) [45]	31	Male
Bardhan (1947) [46]	n/a	n/a
Bardhan (1947) [46]	n/a	n/a
Fortner and Moss (1951) [47]	23	Female
Fortner and Moss (1951) [47]	68	Male
Mathieu (1951)[a] [48]	13	n/a
Olmer and Knebelmann (1952) [49]	17	Female
Marrill (1954) [50]	5	Male
Bakir (1962) [48]	15	Female
Plancade (2013) [51]	45	Female

Note: *n/a* not available

[a] Reported in Bakir (1962) [48]

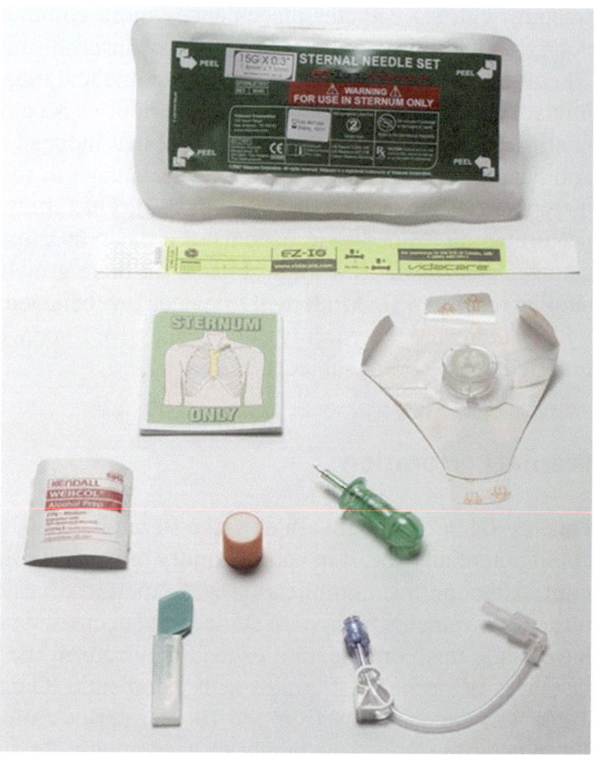

Fig. 9.6 Sternal 8 mm IO catheter (green hub) previously marketed by Vidacare for use with the EZ-IO® system. (*Image courtesy of the authors*)

of the heart and its approximation to the sternum" [46]. In this case, the clinician felt that forward movement of the heart, in combination with over-penetration through the deep sternal plate, led to right ventricular laceration and fatal pericardial tamponade [46].

Most IO devices are not recommended for sternal placement, and those devices that have been approved for sternal placement are highly specialized. The EZ-IO® system previously featured an 8 mm (green hub) sternal IO catheter that has since been discontinued, although the manufacturers continue to market the 38.5 mm long EZ-IO® T.A.L.O.N.™ catheter for military use at the sternal site. Other devices, such as the FAST-1™ and FAST-R™ devices, are only approved for the sternal insertion site and cannot be used at other locations. Figure 9.6 shows the EZ-IO® 8 mm catheter previously marketed for sternal infusion, which has since been discontinued by the manufacturer.

Pain

Pain, as the human brain experiences it, appears to become increasingly complex as more research is completed in the neuroscience field. Although we have yet to uncover all the mechanisms and mysteries of how pain is perceived and impacts our human experience and behavior, it is clear that pain is a highly subjective experience that varies greatly between individuals. Various studies have correlated an individual's previous experiences and their expectations of pain as two important factors shaping how one perceives painful experiences [52]. Studying pain is therefore a highly subjective task, which is further complicated by the lack of reliable, objective, methods for pain measurement [53]. Within the IO literature, the visual analog scale (VAS) is commonly used. This method asks patients to indicate their pain score by drawing a line on a 100 mm line, with scores ranging from "no pain at all" to "worst pain imaginable" [54]. Pain ratings using the VAS have been found not to vary significantly by gender or age [55].

The pain caused by intraosseous infusion is largely due to increased intramedullary pressure associated with sudden influx of non-physiologic fluid into the marrow cavity. The increase in pressure within the marrow space induces the activation of medullary pain receptors, prompting a pain response by the nervous system. Although it has been suggested that the pain from an IO insertion is comparable to that associated with an 18-gauge needle being inserted into a peripheral vein [56], little data exist on pain perception from IO insertion. This is largely because only about 15% of patients who have received IO infusion in the existing medical literature are likely conscious enough to communicate their pain score to providers. Dental studies exploring the use of IO injection of medications during oral surgery have found mixed results when comparing the pain associated with IO infusion to conventional anesthetic methods [57, 58]. One dental study performed by Nillus et al. found a direct correlation between increasing bone length and density and increasing residual pain after IO injection [59].

For those patients responsive to the pain caused by IO catheter placement and infusion, IO infusion of 2% lidocaine solution has been suggested to anesthetize the marrow space before infusion begins [56]. Insertion site selection may also influence the amount of pain perceived by the patient, as humeral IO infusion appears to be less painful than tibial placement for some patients [60]. The humerus is able to accommodate a much higher flow rate (6.3 L/h) compared to that of the tibia (1 L/h) [60]. Therefore, a high-flow injection may be better tolerated by patients when the humerus is used [60].

Delayed Complications

Infectious Complications

Osteomyelitis, defined as inflammation of bone or the bone marrow, is an exceedingly rare complication of IO infusion. Although the inflammation of osteomyelitis is often attributed to infection, it is likely that the presence of any foreign body will induce some degree of inflammation at the site in bone. Bone marrow is a highly vascularized space, with an abundance of leukocytes and other inflammatory mediators that contribute to a vigorous immune response to infection and other irritants. Rosetti and colleagues first reported that osteomyelitis occurs in 0.6% of all IO insertions in 1985, and this figure has been widely referenced [1]. Unfortunately, the data sources informing this meta-analysis were largely culled from the medical literature of the 1940s and 1950s, before modern sterilization techniques were available and in an era when IO devices were commonly reused between patients. One more recent (2013) study reported a 0.4% rate of osteomyelitis among 1802 clinical uses of IO devices [2]. Unfortunately, because IO catheters are often used in critically ill patients with an inherently poor prognosis, most patients treated with IO cannulation do not survive long enough after catheter use for the risk of osteomyelitis and other long-term complications to be accurately assessed.

Specific risk factors for osteomyelitis following IO catheter insertion have been suggested, including extended catheter dwell times, presence of preexisting bacteremia, inadequate asepsis with insertion, and infusion of hypertonic fluids [1, 61]. Although IO catheter-associated osteomyelitis is usually responsive to IO or IV antibiotic infusion alone, at least one severe refractory case has resulted in above-knee amputation [62]. Most cases of osteomyelitis are due to bacterial infection, although fungal osteomyelitis after IO infusion has also been reported [63].

In addition to sepsis, other preexisting patient medical conditions may increase the risk or severity of osteomyelitis, including malnutrition [63], diabetes mellitus [64], peripheral vascular disease, and intravenous drug abusers [65, 66]. Of course, all of these medical conditions are risk factors for other types of infection as well. Considering that IO catheters have traditionally been reserved for patients who are too dehydrated and hypovolemic to receive peripheral venous access, patients with sepsis are likely overrepresented among IO patients when compared to the general population of patients requiring vascular access for their care. A listing of reported cases of osteomyelitis attributed to IO catheter use is provided in Table 9.3.

The duration of infusion and type of fluid infused likely contribute to a patient's risk of osteomyelitis. Early clinician-investigators believed that osteomyelitis occurred "only if an infusion remained in place for a prolonged period or was placed in a bacteremic patient" [1]. Heinild, Sondergaard, and Tudvad all found that strong alkaline and/or hypertonic IO infusions were associated with an increased incidence of osteomyelitis when compared to hypotonic or isotonic solutions [67]. This finding suggests that the dilution of alkaline substances prior to infusion may reduce the risk of subsequent osteomyelitis [68]. However, the precise mechanism by which hypertonic fluids damage the marrow space or otherwise contribute to infection susceptibility remains unclear. Although direct cell lysis and death, ultimately contributing to reduced localized blood flow and tissue necrosis, is one likely mechanism by which hypertonic solutions may promote localized infection, other effects may exist that have not yet been elucidated.

In a study performed by Chalopin et al., most cases of osteomyelitis were attributed to the infiltration of pyogenic bacteria [65]. Preexisting sepsis is thought to be a risk factor for the development of osteomyelitis with IO placement. Of course, this makes sense on a clinical level because of the intersection of hematologically circulating bacteria and the extensive vascular meshwork in the bone marrow. However, little research exists to confirm the clinical correlation between sepsis status and IO-associated osteomyelitis. In some cases, it is unclear whether the

Table 9.3 Summary of case reports citing IO catheter-related osteomyelitis

Author (publication year)	Age	Sex	Medical condition	Septic at time of IO?	Time elapsed
Arakawa 2021 [62]	69 years	M	Factor VIII deficiency Massive GI bleed	n/a	2 months
Barron 1994 [69]	20 months	F	Seizure disorder	Yes	"Several days"
Behr 1944 [70]	"Infant"	n/a	n/a	n/a	3 days
Chalopin 2018 [65]	40 years	M	IV drug use	No	3 months
Clement 1947 [71]	2 months	F	Diarrhea	n/a	n/a
Clement 1947 [71]	n/a	n/a	n/a	n/a	n/a
Clement 1947 [71]	n/a	n/a	n/a	n/a	n/a
Dogan 2004 [72]	5 months	F	Chronic gastroenteritis Metabolic disease (not otherwise specified)	Yes	10 days
Ellison 1945 [73]	n/a	n/a	Gastroenteritis Other NOS	n/a	n/a
Gunz 1945 [74]	8 years	n/a	Pyloric stenosis	n/a	n/a
Heinild 1947 [67]	1 months	M	Gastroenteritis	Yes	12 days
Heinild 1947 [67]	16 days	M	Gastroenteritis	Yes	1 week
Henson 2011 [64]	62 years	M	Diabetes type 2 MGUS MRSA	n/a	6 months
Massey 1950 [75]	n/a	n/a	n/a	n/a	n/a
Platt 1993 [63]	10 weeks	M	Dehydration Malnutrition	No	22 days
Rooney 1944 [76]	15 months	n/a	Gastroenteritis Malnutrition	n/a	4 days
Rooney 1944 [76]	3 months	n/a	Gastroenteritis	n/a	10 days
Rosovsky 1994 [77]	14 months	M	Giardiasis	n/a	3 days
Sondergaard 1946 [78]	8 days[a]	M	Gastroenteritis	n/a	5 days
Sondergaard 1946 [78]	38 years	M	Gastric ulcer with gastroenteroscopy Jejunostomy Parotitis	n/a	3 weeks
Sondergaard 1946 [78]	64 years	M	Gastric ulcer	n/a	5 days
Sondergaard 1946 [78]	4 days[a]	F	Gastroenteritis	n/a	8 days
Sondergaard 1946 [78]	6 weeks[a]	M	Seizures "Collapse"	n/a	4 days
Stoll 2002 [79]	3 months	M	Spastic tetraplegia Resuscitation following complicated respiratory infection	No	24 h
Texter 1948 [80]	n/a	n/a	Diarrhea Anemia	n/a	n/a

(continued)

Table 9.3 (continued)

Author (publication year)	Age	Sex	Medical condition	Septic at time of IO?	Time elapsed
Texter 1948 [80]	n/a	n/a	Pyloric stenosis Pyloroplasty Malnutrition	n/a	n/a
Tocantins and O'Neill 1945 [81]	25 years	F	Poorly controlled diabetes Unilateral nephrectomy	n/a	7 weeks
Williams and Lockhart 1948 [82]	n/a	F	Congenital syphilis Diarrhea	n/a	n/a
Yee 2017 [66]	29 years	M	IV drug use Rhabdomyolysis Acute kidney injury	No	6 weeks

Notes: *M* male; *F* female; *n/a* not available

"Time elapsed" is time from IO placement to osteomyelitis diagnosis

[a] Premature infant

IO catheterization truly caused the osteomyelitis, or if preexisting bacteremia may have seeded the location due to the presence of a foreign body at the site. Nevertheless, in order to prevent cutaneously transmitted infection to the bone, strict antiseptic conditions must be utilized during the IO catheter placement itself and maintained for the duration of the catheter's use [62].

Case reports detailing IO catheter-related cases of osteomyelitis are provided in Table 9.3, including the subject's age at the time of IO catheter placement, associated medical conditions, and time elapsed before identification of the osteomyelitis infection.

It should be noted that the cases of osteomyelitis outlined in Table 9.3 were published as case reports, supporting the rarity of this complication. However, the presence of these reports in the existing literature also underscores the fact that this complication is important enough to merit publication and is an area in need of further study. These case reports demonstrate high variability in the time from catheter placement to recognition of the infection, which may help to elucidate its underlying cause. For example, a new infection caused by IO infusion would not be expected to occur less than 2–3 days following catheter placement. Acute osteomyelitis typically takes 1–2 weeks to develop from any source. Consequently, it is likely that patients who had diagnosis of osteomyelitis made less than 3 days after IO insertion may have had a preexisting infection (e.g., bacteremia) for which the foreign body (i.e., IO catheter) merely served as a nidus for abscess formation.

Pulmonary Fat Embolism

Pulmonary fat embolism (PFE) has been proposed as a potential complication of IO catheter infusion, based largely on hypothetical concerns without a clear clinical basis. One recent cadaveric study showed that 8 of 13 pediatric patients who received IO infusion during cardiopulmonary resuscitation (CPR) following cardiac arrest were found to have PFE on autopsy [83]. Four (30.7%) of these 13 subjects had histology scores of Falzi 2 or greater, suggesting that the emboli were multiple and disseminated in all microscopic fields [83].

It has been well established that PFE is not universally fatal or even clinically relevant in all cases. Bone fracture (especially involving the long bones) is a common cause of PFE, but multiple other conditions can predispose to fat emboli including soft tissue crush injury, diabetes mellitus, sickle cell anemia, and hemorrhagic pancreatitis [84]. The presence of PFE on autopsy among trauma victims ranges from 75 to 100% [85–88], and PFE has been found to be present in up to 70% of autopsies following CPR among non-trauma patients as well [89]. Thus, the finding of PFE on autopsy following CPR-associated IO placement is not conclusive evidence that IO infusion causes PFE or that a theoretical PFE so-produced would have any physiologic effect. While massive trauma is likely to cause fatal PFE, it remains unclear whether IO catheters cause clinically significant PFE, and no authors have ever reported a death shown to be caused by IO-associated PFE.

One author has suggested that IO catheter insertion may "lead to microscopic fractures of the metaphysis of the bone and vascular damage" [90], providing an opportunity for fat droplets to enter the venous circulation and accumulate in the pulmonary vasculature. **Air emboli** could be similarly introduced if the catheter and infusion tubing are not appropriately flushed, although the clinical significance of small air emboli is unknown [91]. Kristiansen et al. have found PFE to be universally present following aggressive IO fluid resuscitation in an anesthetized porcine hemorrhagic shock model [92]. However, these emboli are also universally subclinical and were not noted to cause any "major respiratory or cardiovascular deterioration" [92]. Orlowski and colleagues also found identical supporting evidence that fat and bone marrow emboli to the lungs were found in 30/30 canine and 2/2 pediatric resuscitations [93]. They found that the emboli varied in size according to the type of fluid infused, and "despite the universal occurrence of emboli, they do not appear to be of acute clinical importance" [93].

Hasan et al. measured the "pattern of fat droplets in the pulmonary blood," but found that "there was no consistent pattern of fat droplets" and decided that this was not a useful diagnostic tool for measuring pulmonary fat emboli [90], contradicting earlier studies by Adolph et al. [94]. Hasan concluded that the "risk of fat embolization is a concern," but its "clinical relevance is unclear" [90].

Soft Tissue Ischemia/Necrosis

Generally speaking, infused substances are categorized as either **vesicants** or non-vesicants. Vesicant substances are known to cause cellular injury (e.g., blistering) to soft tissues when they leak from an intravenous or intraosseous catheter into the adjacent soft tissues, while non-vesicant substances do not cause such injury and are generally more benign. **Irritants** are one category of non-vesicant medications that can cause localized inflammation and pain with infusion, but do not generally cause significant tissue damage. In the vascular access literature, **infiltration** is often defined as leakage of a non-vesicant substance from the vascular system into the surrounding soft tissue, while **extravasation** may be defined as similar leakage of a vesicant substance [95]. These definitions are not universal, however, and many sources consider these terms to be synonymous. Leakage of a vesicant substance should be expected to cause more significant injury to the soft tissues in the area surrounding the infusion site than leakage of a non-vesicant (e.g., irritant) substance. Vesicant substances often have a pH that is dramatically different than surrounding soft tissues (e.g., pH <5 or >9) or have a very high osmolarity (e.g., >600 mosmol/L). Examples of vesicant substances include antineoplastic agents, certain antibiotics, hypertonic saline, high-concentration dextrose solutions, epinephrine, and norepinephrine. It is currently unknown whether substances that have been shown to behave as vesicants when delivered via direct venous infusion have similar effects on local soft tissue when infused intraosseously, although this is generally assumed to be true. It is possible that some substances with minimal toxic effects when infused through a peripheral IV may have more clinically adverse effects when delivered through the intramedullary space. It is similarly possible that some medications assumed to require central venous infusion due to their potential for vascular injury may be safely delivered via IO access, as their concentrations may be diluted by the presence of other marrow contents and a vast network of smaller draining venous channels. Further study is needed to determine whether the potential toxicities ascribed to specific IV medications should be assumed when assessing the potential risks of IO infusion.

Ischemia and necrosis of the soft tissues in the area of the IO catheter insertion site can be related to a variety of patient-specific, drug-specific, and device-specific factors. Cannulation through areas of burned, cellulitic, or otherwise damaged skin should be avoided as this may increase the risk of soft tissue damage and infection [96]. Certain drugs, when infused through an IO catheter, may also increase the risk of soft tissue necrosis due to extravasation or local drug effects on the soft tissues. Infusion of 7.5% hypertonic saline, for example, has been shown to be associated with increased risk of soft tissue necrosis and/or bone necrosis in a porcine model of hemorrhagic shock [97]. This complication generally occurs 2–5 days post-infusion [97] and is likely due to the extravasation of hypertonic saline into the soft tissues following catheter malplacement or dislodgement. Despite the risk of extravasation-related injury, several studies have shown that IO infusion of 3 and 7.5% hypertonic saline can be performed safely [98–100]. Farrokh et al. reported a case series of six patients who received 23.4% hypertonic saline through an IO catheter without complications, although four of the six patients died prior to hospital discharge [101]. Local injection of **hyaluronic acid** into the soft tissues can be used to reverse the effects of hypertonic saline extravasation when this complication is identified early in the course of disease [102].

The rate of soft tissue necrosis after IO infusion appears to be quite low, although necrosis can lead to subsequent soft tissue infection as devitalized tissues may be prone to infection. Infection rates after IO infusion have been shown to be low, with one major study including 4270 children receiving IO insertions at the proximal tibial or sternal sites reporting an infection rate of only 0.6% [61]. Scheman et al.

reported two cases of localized inflammation at the IO site following high-dose IO adrenaline infusion resulting in cutaneous necrosis and subsequent osteomyelitis [103]. However, reports of this complication remain rare. Close monitoring of soft tissues surrounding the site of IO infusion can help clinicians to identify any potential complications early enough to avoid significant injury [104].

Compartment Syndrome

Compartment syndrome (CS) is a rare complication of intraosseous access [102] that can occur when a large quantity of fluid has extravasated or infiltrated from the site of IO injection into the muscle and other surrounding soft tissues. This accumulation of fluid can cause pressure to build up in the soft tissue compartment to dangerously high levels, leading to decreased blood flow and eventually ischemic injury. If the pressure is not relieved quickly, compartment syndrome can cause permanent disability and tissue death in the affected area [39]. This syndrome is characterized by **pain, paresthesia** (i.e., abnormal tingling due to nerve damage), **poikilothermia** (i.e., coolness of the extremity), **pallor, paralysis** (i.e., weakness of the extremity), and **pulselessness** in the affected extremity [14]. Pain is often the first presenting sign of compartment syndrome and generally involves the entire compartment (not just the insertion site), but may be difficult to distinguish from more benign discomfort typically associated with active IO infusion. The anterior compartment of the leg is located on the **lateral** side of the tibia, between the tibia and the fibula. Considering that the recommended IO catheter insertion site at the proximal tibia is on the **medial** side of the tibia, significant extravasation into the anterior compartment is rare if proper insertion technique is followed. However, **fracture of the tibia during IO catheter placement, or transcortical (i.e., through both the superficial and deep cortices) penetration due to excessive depth of insertion, is a significant risk factor for compartment syndrome**, especially in neonates or young children. Compartment syndrome in the setting of IO catheter infusion has been associated with catheter malposition or dislodgement, multiple cortical breaches, excessive rate or volume of fluid infusion, and extravasation [29]. A summary of reported cases of compartment syndrome following IO catheter placement is provided in Table 9.4.

Most cases of compartment syndrome in the existing literature appear to be associated with distal femoral or proximal tibial IO insertions, although cases of deltoid compartment syndrome have recently been reported [30]. Most cases follow a predictable clinical course. Within hours or days of IO infusion, the extremity receiving IO access begins to appear cyanotic and swollen, feels cool, and progressively loses palpable or Doppler-detectable pulses. Capillary refill decreases. The skin gradually becomes tense and the muscle firm, with decreased range of motion. Diagnosis of compartment syndrome is achieved by clinical examination, usually confirmed by measurement of compartment pressures using a specialized manometer transcutaneously inserted into the compartment of interest. The management of compartment syndrome includes immediate discontinuation of infusion and removal of the IO

Table 9.4 Case reports describing compartment syndrome after IO catheter placement

Author (year)	Age	Sex	Extremity	Indication for IO	IO device	Fasciotomy/ amputation?	Time elapsed (h)	Death?
Moscati, 1990 [31]	3 months	M	Left LE	Cardiopulmonary arrest, unsuccessful PIV access	18G spinal needle	Y/Y	2.5	N
Galpin, 1991 [106]	3 years	F	LE (both)	Hypovolemic shock, unsuccessful PIV access	16G manual needle	Y/N	12	N
Ribeiro, 1993 [36]	Case 1: 3 months	M	Right LE	Cardiopulmonary arrest	n/a	Y/N	2.75	N
Ribeiro, 1993 [36]	Case 2: 19 months	M	Right LE	Unsuccessful PIV access	n/a	Y/N	5.2	N
Vidal, 1993 [32]	1 months	M	Right LE	Unspecified	18G manual needle	Y/Y	72	N
Gayle, 1994 [107]	1 months	n/a	Right LE	Unspecified	18G manual needle	Y/Y	72	N
Wright, 1994 [33]	11 months	M	Left LE	Unsuccessful PIV access	n/a	Y/N	53	N
Launay, 2003 [108]	7 months	M	Left LE	PIV access not achieved fast enough	n/a	Y/Y	15	N
Atanda, 2008 [34]	2 years	M	Right LE	Cardiopulmonary resuscitation	n/a	Y/N	10	N
Cotte, 2011 [109]	57 years	n/a	Right LE	Unsuccessful PIV access	15G EZ-IO®	Y/N	10	N
D'Heurle, 2013 [29]	49 years	M	Left LE	Cardiopulmonary resuscitation, unsuccessful PIV access	n/a	Y/N	4	Y (cause of death: brain herniation secondary to TBI)
Suominen 2015 [110]	Neonate	n/a	Right LE	Cardiopulmonary resuscitation, unsuccessful PIV access	15G EZ-IO®	Y/Y	n/a	N

Author (year)	Age	Sex	Extremity	Indication for IO	IO device	Fasciotomy/ amputation?	Time elapsed (h)	Death?
Malhotra, 2016 [37]	59 years	M	LE (both)	Cardiopulmonary resuscitation, unsuccessful PIV access	n/a	Y/N	n/a	N
Thadikonda, 2017 [30]	67 years	F	UE (both)	Hypoxic respiratory failure and hypotension	n/a	Y/N	312	N
Turner, 2018 [35]	1 years	M	Left LE	Cardiopulmonary resuscitation, unsuccessful PIV access	15G EZ-IO®	Y/N	n/a	N
Abramson, 2018 [111]	63 years	M	Left LE	Obtunded from hypoglycemia, unsuccessful PIV access	15G EZ-IO®	Y/N	n/a	N
Kibrick, 2020 [112]	87 years	M	Right LE	Unsuccessful PIV access	n/a	Y/N	4	N
Arakawa, 2021 [62]	44 years	M	Right LE	Cardiopulmonary resuscitation, unsuccessful PIV access	n/a	Y/N	n/a	N
Chughtai, 2022 [113]	79 years	M	Right LE	Cardiopulmonary resuscitation, unsuccessful PIV access	n/a	Y/N	n/a	N
Singh, 2022 [114]	56 years	F	Right LE	Obtunded from hypoglycemia, unsuccessful PIV access	n/a	Y/N	n/a	N

Notes: *M* male; *F* female; *n/a* not available; *Y* yes; *N* no; *Ex-Lap* exploratory laparotomy; *LE* lower extremity (leg); *PIV* peripheral intravenous catheter; *MVA* motor vehicle accident; *UE* upper extremity (arm); *IO* intraosseous; *OR* operating room; *ROM* range of motion; *TTP* tender to palpation; *G* gauge. *Time elapsed* time elapsed from IO catheter placement to identification of compartment syndrome catheter, followed often by surgical fasciotomy. If recognition or fasciotomy is delayed, irreversible ischemic muscle damage can occur leading to amputation of the involved extremity.

Although dual-IO access (i.e., the insertion of two IO catheters into the same bone) has been shown to be feasible for large bones under controlled conditions in a swine animal model [105], multiple IO attempts at the same bone are discouraged. Per manufacturer recommendations, only one IO catheter should be inserted per bone. If an IO was previously inserted or attempted, that same bone should generally not be used within 48 h for subsequent IO insertion attempts. It is worth noting that this recommendation to wait 48 h before additional attempts on the target bone does not appear to be supported by data from clinical studies, and is speculative at best. Given that bone fractures usually take several months to fully heal, the time required to close an osteotomy due to failed IO access may take considerably longer than 48 h to close. Although the osteotomy may clot within hours or days, subsequent high infusion pressures within the medullary space might be expected to dislodge such a clot during active infusion.

Rates of Complications

Many published studies have attempted to quantify the rates of various IO-associated complications, yet the actual rates of most complications remain unknown. There are many reasons for this difficulty in quantifying complication rates, including both methodological and pragmatic challenges. For example, it is highly probable that different IO catheters have different rates of complications relatable to unique placement methods required for different catheters as well as device-specific design and performance characteristics. Despite this, most reports of IO complications fail to disclose the manufacturer or type of IO catheter implicated in the event. It is also likely that some complications (e.g., compartment syndrome, amputation) are more common among pediatric subjects than adult subjects, but subject age is often not disclosed in published reports. Perhaps the greatest challenge to predicting the likelihood of delayed complications following IO catheter placement is the high rate of death following IO catheter insertion. One recent review of adult complications after IO placement suggested that (among studies that report the cause of illness for IO infusion recipients) 92.2% of IO catheters are placed on cardiac arrest victims, with the remainder used to treat respiratory failure or hypovolemic shock [8]. Given the low rate of survival following cardiac arrest, the vast majority of patients who receive an IO catheter likely do not live long enough to develop delayed complications. Thus, the finding that IO infusion is generally safe and well tolerated is based primarily upon limited data describing reported **immediate** complications of IO insertion, with very few patients surviving to provide accurate data on more serious, usually **delayed** complications such as compartment syndrome and infection.

The most commonly cited reference for IO complication rates is a systematic review published in *Annals of Emergency Medicine* in 1985 by Rosetti and colleagues [1]. In this review, the authors identified only 37 complications (including

27 cases of osteomyelitis and 10 "other" complications) and only 89 (2.0%) failed placements among 4359 attempted IO infusions [1]. This review included 30 original reports, but 4307 (99.0%) of the subjects included in this review were treated during the 1940s by experienced providers using manually inserted IO catheters, and more than 90% were children [8]. The most common insertion site in the Rosetti review was the sternum, which is rarely used in modern clinical practice, and many patients received prophylactic IO infusion of antibiotics to prevent infection. Based upon the Rosetti review, the complication rate for IO catheters has been cited to be 0.6%, although Rosetti's own data suggests that the rate is closer to 1.1% in their own dataset [1].

Greenstein et al. attempted to quantify the rate of complications among adult ($\geq$14 years old) subjects receiving IO infusion and found that IO placement was successful in 91% of insertion attempts at the proximal tibia or humerus and 76% at the sternum [4]. They identified only five "serious" complications among 2106 attempted insertions (i.e., retained needle tip, tendon tear, skin necrosis, osteomyelitis), yielding a complication rate of 0.3% [4]. However, the authors did not consider extravasation or infiltration to be a complication unless it led to infection or tissue loss, and they did not identify any cases of compartment syndrome or bone fracture in adults. One recent review of complications following IO infusion in pediatric subjects suggests that the complication rate among children may be much higher than in adults, perhaps as high as 9.7%, although this review included both minor and major complications in its calculations [7].

The wide variability in complication rates reported in the existing medical literature raises the question of what should be considered to be a "serious" complication, and there is no clear consensus of opinion on this matter. As mentioned at the beginning of this chapter, we suggest that complications may be categorized as major, moderate, or minor depending upon the need for intervention and the risk to the patient. However, it could be argued that IO catheters are generally only used for patients who are unable to receive other forms of vascular access promptly. Thus, device failure or dislodgement preventing use of the catheter might be justifiably considered to be life-threatening if other forms of vascular access are not possible, as the inability to rapidly and reliably establish IO access might place the patient at substantial risk of death or injury due to the inability to administer lifesaving or stabilizing medications.

Eighty years ago, when alternative modalities for intravenous infusion (i.e., ultrasound-guided peripheral intravenous catheterization, central venous catheterization) were not available, it was far more common for clinicians to publish their experiences with IO infusion in the medical literature, including long-term follow-up to detect delayed complications. In the modern era, complications of IO catheter use are generally published as case reports (if at all), rather than case series or large cohort studies. Unfortunately, this lack of long-term data upon which to build a case for the safety of modern IO devices has led to an unconscionable situation in which clinical decisions on safety are based on outdated information from a bygone era in which sterility and the appropriateness of antibiotic use were defined differently. To date, no large, long-term studies on the safety of modern IO devices have been conducted or published. Consequently, **it is unlikely that the medical community will have reliable modern data on the safety and complication risk associated with IO infusion until the use of IO catheters is more widespread within the medical community** and clinicians resume careful monitoring and reporting of long-term safety outcomes such as infection and the effects of IO infusion on bone growth and development.

Additional prospective research is needed to provide modern data about the relative risks of IO infusion. Areas of suggested further research include:

- Examination of the relationship between anatomic insertion site (e.g., proximal tibia, humerus, sternum) and the incidence and severity of specific complication rates
- Examination of the relationship between the efficacy and duration of analgesic medication and proximity of the IO access site to a known area of traumatic injury
- Examination of the relationship between prehospital IO insertion in a septic patient and osteomyelitis at the IO placement site

Conclusion

Evidence provided in the existing medical literature suggests that IO complication rates are generally low. However, increased risk of complications is associated with pediatric status, high BMI, history of concurrent peripheral vascular diseases, diseases of bone integrity, and preexisting bacteremia. Very few of these complications present an immediate life threat to the patient. Early complications appear to be associated with improper device placement technique and are typically low in severity. However, most moderate or severe complications are associated with delayed recognition and/or delayed management of the condition. This dichotomy underscores the importance of early recognition of complications associated with IO infusion and the need for additional well-designed research to determine the true rate of complications associated with IO catheter use. Our modern appreciation for the complications associated with IO infusion is built upon historical data that are barely relevant to modern practice, and the medical community has not yet adopted a uniform method for reporting the safety and risk of IO catheter-associated complications. It is clear that clinicians need data on all patients who benefit from IO catheterization, not just those who experience a complication from its use. It is impossible to assess the safety of IO catheters without accounting for those patients who may be silently suffering from complications that are either not recognized or not reported. The significance of these complications is undermined by the lack of robust data from which to build a true understanding of the risk-benefit ratio for IO catheter use, and this knowledge gap represents a real obstacle to increased use of this modality to treat patients who may otherwise benefit from rapid IO access but are not deemed sick enough to warrant its consideration. Our review of the existing literature on complications also reveals wide variation in the reporting standards for IO catheter-associated complications, including what qualifies as a complication, leading to important questions about how those complications should ideally be reported to the medical community at large, given the subjective nature of an individual clinician's decision to publish (or not publish) on the topic. Broadly speaking, the medical community needs large, well-designed observational studies to truly assess the actual risk of the complications that we have described in this chapter.

Communication barriers may contribute to delayed or failed recognition of complications. Among patients who are sedated, anesthetized, or intubated, it is unclear whether complications would have manifested similarly if the patients were able to communicate pain or other symptoms. The lack of verbal skills among pediatric subjects receiving IO catheter placement suggests that preverbal status may be a risk factor for advanced complications following IO catheter placement. Although some complications have been shown to occur in both adult and pediatric patients, outcomes for some conditions (e.g., compartment syndrome) may be worse for pediatric patients when they do occur. Bony injuries, including epiphyseal growth plate injury and long bone fracture, are unique concerns within the pediatric population and are not commonly reported within the adult population.

Providers should consider the ideal insertion site to reduce discomfort when multiple insertion sites are possible. The risk of iatrogenic complications may be mitigated by monitoring infusion volume, rate, and pH of administered fluids or medications.

Overall, the rate of complications following IO placement is low, but the potential for complications related to IO catheter placement depends upon a number of factors that may be discernible to the cautious provider. Providers should carefully monitor the IO insertion site for evidence of complications and consider the risk of complications when deciding upon the need for IO catheter placement in appropriate patients.

Key Concepts
- Complications can occur at any time during the process of IO catheter insertion, use, and removal.
- Complications following intraosseous catheter placement can range widely in severity, although they are rarely life-threatening.
- Despite recommendations from emergency medicine experts to utilize IO devices when peripheral intravenous access is not feasible under emergent conditions, many barriers exist to appropriate IO catheter placement.
- Proper training in the placement, management, and monitoring of IO catheters may help to avoid many complications of IO catheter placement.
- Accurate data on the complication rates due to IO catheter use are lacking, and most evidence on this topic is antiquated and inapplicable to the modern patient population. Additional study is needed to determine modern complication rates with IO catheter insertion and infusion.

References

1. Rosetti VA, Thompson BM, Miller J, Mateer JR, Aprahamian C. Intraosseous infusion: an alternative route of pediatric intravascular access. Ann Emerg Med. 1985;14(9):885–8. https://doi.org/10.1016/s0196-0644(85)80639-9.
2. Hallas P, Brabrand M, Folkestad L. Complication with intraosseous access: Scandinavian users' experience. West J Emerg Med. 2013;14(5):440–3. https://doi.org/10.5811/westjem.2013.1.12000.
3. Barlow B, Kuhn K. Orthopedic management of complications of using intraosseous catheters. Am J Orthop (Belle Mead NJ). 2014;43(4):186–90.
4. Greenstein YY, Koenig SJ, Mayo PH, Narasimhan M. A serious adult intraosseous catheter complication and review of the literature. Crit Care Med. 2016;44(9):e904–9. https://doi.org/10.1097/CCM.0000000000001714.
5. Petitpas F, Guenezan J, Vendeuvre T, Scepi M, Oriot D, Mimoz O. Use of intra-osseous access in adults: a systematic review. Crit Care. 2016;20:102. https://doi.org/10.1186/s13054-016-1277-6.
6. Garside J, Prescott S, Shaw S. Intraosseous vascular access in critically ill adults—a review of the literature. Nurs Crit Care. 2016;21(3):167–77. https://doi.org/10.1111/nicc.12163. Epub 2015 Feb 17.
7. Bouhamdan J, Polsinelli G, Akers KG, Paxton JH. A systematic review of complications from pediatric intraosseous cannulation. Curr Emerg Hosp Med Rep. 2022;10:116–24. https://doi.org/10.1007/s40138-022-00256-x.
8. Palazzolo A, Akers KG, Paxton JH. Complications of intraosseous catheterization in adult patients: a review of the literature. Curr Emerg Hosp Med Rep. 2023;11:35–48. https://doi.org/10.1007/s40138-023-00261-8.
9. Kvist O, Luiza Dallora A, Nilsson O, et al. A cross-sectional magnetic resonance imaging study of factors influencing growth plate closure in adolescents and young adults. Acta Paediatr. 2021;110(4):1249–56. https://doi.org/10.1111/apa.15617. Epub 2020 Nov 1.
10. Brickman KR, Rega P, Koltz M, Guinness M. Analysis of growth plate abnormalities following intraosseous infusion through the proximal tibial epiphysis in pigs. Ann Emerg Med. 1988;17(2):121–3. https://doi.org/10.1016/s0196-0644(88)80294-4.
11. Boon JM, Gorry DL, Meiring JH. Finding an ideal site for intraosseous infusion of the tibia: an anatomical study. Clin Anat. 2003;16(1):15–8. https://doi.org/10.1002/ca.10071.
12. Venous access: intraosseous infusion. In: Gomella TL, et al., editors. Neonatology: management, procedures, on-call problems, diseases, and drugs. 7th ed. McGraw Hill; 2013. https://accesspediatrics.mhmedical.com/content.aspx?bookid=1303§ionid=79661971. Accessed 10 June 2023.
13. Barnes D, Yoon J. Intraosseous line extravasation in a pediatric trauma patient. PSNet: Patient Safety Network; 2022. https://psnet.ahrq.gov/web-mm/intraosseous-line-extravasation-pediatric-trauma-patient. Accessed 10 June 2023.
14. Torlincasi AM, Lopez RA, Waseem M. Acute compartment syndrome. In: StatPearls. Treasure Island, FL: StatPearls Publishing; 2023. https://www.ncbi.nlm.nih.gov/books/NBK448124/. Accessed 10 June 2023.
15. Kehrl T, Becker BA, Simmons DE, Broderick EK, Jones RA. Intraosseous access in the obese patient: assessing the need for extended needle length. Am J Emerg Med. 2016;34(9):1831–4. https://doi.org/10.1016/j.ajem.2016.06.055. Epub 2016 Jun 15.
16. Wampler D, Schwartz D, Shumaker J, Bolleter S, Beckett R, Manifold C. Paramedics successfully perform humeral EZ-IO intraosseous access in adult out-of-hospital cardiac arrest patients. Am J Emerg Med. 2012;30(7):1095–9. https://doi.org/10.1016/j.ajem.2011.07.010. Epub 2011 Oct 24.
17. Nutbeam T, Fergusson A. Intraosseous access in osteogenesis imperfecta (IO in OI). Resuscitation. 2009;80(12):1442–3. https://doi.org/10.1016/j.resuscitation.2009.08.016. Epub 2009 Oct 4.

18. Hafner JW, Bryant A, Huang F, Swisher K. Effectiveness of a drill-assisted intraosseous catheter versus manual intraosseous catheter by resident physicians in a swine model. West J Emerg Med. 2013;14(6):629–32. https://doi.org/10.5811/westjem.2013.4.13361.

19. Brenner T, Bernhard M, Helm M, Doll S, Völkl A, Ganion N, Friedmann C, Sikinger M, Knapp J, Martin E, Gries A. Comparison of two intraosseous infusion systems for adult emergency medical use. Resuscitation. 2008;78(3):314–9. https://doi.org/10.1016/j.resuscitation.2008.04.004. Epub 2008 Jun 24.

20. Sørgjerd R, Sunde GA, Heltne JK. Comparison of two different intraosseous access methods in a physician-staffed helicopter emergency medical service—a quality assurance study. Scand J Trauma Resusc Emerg Med. 2019;27(1):15. https://doi.org/10.1186/s13049-019-0594-6.

21. Hammer N, Möbius R, Gries A, Hossfeld B, Bechmann I, Bernhard M. Comparison of the fluid resuscitation rate with and without external pressure using two intraosseous infusion systems for adult emergencies, the CITRIN (Comparison of InTRaosseous infusion systems in emergency medicINe)-study. PLoS One. 2015;10(12):e0143726. https://doi.org/10.1371/journal.pone.0143726.

22. Hodgetts JM, Johnston A, Kendrew J. Long-term follow-up of two patients with retained intraosseous sternal needles. J R Army Med Corps. 2017;163(3):221–2. https://doi.org/10.1136/jramc-2016-000699. Epub 2017 Mar 1.

23. Fenton P, Bali N, Sargeant I, Jeffrey SL. A complication of the use of an intra-osseous needle. J R Army Med Corps. 2009;155(2):110–1. https://doi.org/10.1136/jramc-155-02-06.

24. Taylor DM, Bailey MS. A complication of the use of an intra-osseous needle. J R Army Med Corps. 2010;156(2):132.

25. Liu YY, Wang YP, Zu LY, Zheng K, Ma QB, Zheng YA, Gao W. Comparison of intraosseous access and central venous catheterization in Chinese adult emergency patients: a prospective, multicenter, and randomized study. World J Emerg Med. 2021;12(2):105–10. https://doi.org/10.5847/wjem.j.1920-8642.2021.02.004.

26. Harcke HT, Curtin RN, Harty MP, Gould SW, Vershvovsky J, Collins GL, Murphy S. Tibial intraosseous insertion in pediatric emergency care: a review based upon postmortem computed tomography. Prehosp Emerg Care. 2020;24(5):665–71. https://doi.org/10.1080/10903127.2019.1698682. Epub 2020 Jan 7.

27. Baker TW, King W, Soto W, Asher C, Stolfi A, Rowin ME. The efficacy of pediatric advanced life support training in emergency medical service providers. Pediatr Emerg Care. 2009;25(8):508–12. https://doi.org/10.1097/PEC.0b013e3181b0a0da.

28. Paxton JH, Knuth TE, Klausner HA. Proximal humerus intraosseous infusion: a preferred emergency venous access. J Trauma. 2009;67(3):606–11. https://doi.org/10.1097/TA.0b013e3181b16f42.

29. d'Heurle A, Archdeacon MT. Compartment syndrome after intraosseous infusion associated with a fracture of the tibia: a case report. JBJS Case Connect. 2013;3(1):e20. https://doi.org/10.2106/JBJS.CC.L.00231.

30. Thadikonda KM, Egro FM, Ma I, Spiess AM. Deltoid compartment syndrome: a rare complication after humeral intraosseous access. Plast Reconstr Surg Glob Open. 2017;5(1):e1208. https://doi.org/10.1097/GOX.0000000000001208.

31. Moscati R, Moore GP. Compartment syndrome with resultant amputation following intraosseous infusion. Am J Emerg Med. 1990;8(5):470–1. https://doi.org/10.1016/0735-6757(90)90247-w.

32. Vidal R, Kissoon N, Gayle M. Compartment syndrome following intraosseous infusion. Pediatrics. 1993;91(6):1201–2.

33. Wright R, Reynolds SL, Nachtsheim B. Compartment syndrome secondary to prolonged intraosseous infusion. Pediatr Emerg Care. 1994;10(3):157–9. https://doi.org/10.1097/00006565-199406000-00008.

34. Atanda A Jr, Statter MB. Compartment syndrome of the leg after intraosseous infusion: guidelines for prevention, early detection, and treatment. Am J Orthop (Belle Mead NJ). 2008;37(12):E198–200.

35. Turner J, Thies KC. Intra-osseous-access-associated lower limb compartment syndrome in a critically injured paediatric patient. Eur J Anaesthesiol. 2018;35(12):981–3. https://doi.org/10.1097/EJA.0000000000000873.

36. Ribeiro JA, Price CT, Knapp DR Jr. Compartment syndrome of the lower extremity after intraosseous infusion of fluid. A report of two cases. J Bone Joint Surg Am. 1993;75(3):430–3. https://doi.org/10.2106/00004623-199303000-00016.

37. Malhotra R, Chua WL, O'Neill G. Calf compartment syndrome associated with the use of an intra-osseous line in an adult patient: a case report. Malays Orthop J. 2016;10(3):49–51. https://doi.org/10.5704/MOJ.1611.014.

38. Overbey JK, Kon AA. Dermal abrasion experienced as an adverse effect of the EZ-IO®. J Emerg Med. 2016;50(1):e7–10. https://doi.org/10.1016/j.jemermed.2015.09.003. Epub 2015 Oct 24.

39. Reuter-Rice K, Patrick D, Kantor E, Nolin C, Foley J. Characteristics of children who undergo intraosseous needle placement. Adv Emerg Nurs J. 2015;37(4):301–7. https://doi.org/10.1097/TME.0000000000000077.

40. Hansen M, Meckler G, Spiro D, Newgard C. Intraosseous line use, complications, and outcomes among a population-based cohort of children presenting to California hospitals. Pediatr Emerg Care. 2011;27(10):928–32. https://doi.org/10.1097/PEC.0b013e3182307a2f.

41. Neuhaus D. Intraosseous infusion in elective and emergency pediatric anesthesia: when should we use it? Curr Opin Anaesthesiol. 2014;27(3):282–7. https://doi.org/10.1097/ACO.0000000000000069.

42. Kim HK, Stephenson N, Garces A, Aya-ay J, Bian H. Effects of disruption of epiphyseal vasculature on the proximal femoral growth plate. J Bone Joint Surg Am. 2009;91(5):1149–58. https://doi.org/10.2106/JBJS.H.00654.

43. Fiser RT, Walker WM, Seibert JJ, McCarthy R, Fiser DH. Tibial length following intraosseous infusion: a prospective, radiographic analysis. Pediatr Emerg Care. 1997;13(3):186–8. https://doi.org/10.1097/00006565-199706000-00003.

44. Meyer LM, Halpern J. Death following sternal puncture. Am J Clin Path. 1944;14:247.

45. Scherer JH, Howe JS. Fatal cardiac tamponade following sternal puncture. J Lab Clin Med. 1945;30:450.

46. Bardhan PN. Death from sternal puncture. Indian Med Gaz. 1947;82:459.

47. Fortner JG, Moss ES. Death following sternal puncture: report of two cases. Ann Int Med. 1951;34:809.

48. Bakir F. Fatal sternal puncture. Dis Chest. 1963;44(4):435–9.

49. Olmer J, Knebelmann G. Fatal accidents following sternal puncture. Presse Médicale (Paris). 1952;60:882. (cited in Foreign Letters (France). Fatal Sternal Puncture. JAMA. 1952; 150(8): 831.)

50. Marrill MF-G. Ponction sternal mortelle. Bull Mem Soc Med Des Hasp. 1954:9–10. (cited in Foreign Letters (France). Death from Sternal Punctures. JAMA. 1954; 155(14): 1276).

51. Plancade D, Millot I, Fétissof H, Landy C, Schaeffer E, Perez JP, Nadaud J. Sternal perforation with an intraosseous device and hemomediastinum infusion. Ann Fr Anesth Reanim. 2013;32(3):e69–70. https://doi.org/10.1016/j.annfar.2013.01.009. Epub 2013 Feb 28.

52. Koyama T, McHaffie JG, Laurienti PJ, Coghill RC. The subjective experience of pain: where expectations become reality. Proc Natl Acad Sci USA. 2005;102(36):12950–5. https://doi.org/10.1073/pnas.0408576102. Epub 2005 Sep 6.

53. McGuire DB. The measurement of clinical pain. Nurs Res. 1984;33(3):152–6. https://doi.org/10.1097/00006199-198405000-00007.

54. Bodian CA, Freedman G, Hossain S, Eisenkraft JB, Beilin Y. The visual analog scale for pain: clinical significance in postoperative patients. Anesthesiology. 2001;95(6):1356–61. https://doi.org/10.1097/00000542-200112000-00013.

55. Kelly AM. Does the clinically significant difference in visual analog scale pain scores vary with gender, age, or cause of pain? Acad Emerg Med. 1998;5(11):1086–90. https://doi.org/10.1111/j.1553-2712.1998.tb02667.x.

56. Miller L, Kramer GC, Bolleter S. Rescue access made easy. JEMS. 2005;30(10):suppl 8–18; quiz suppl 19.
57. Peñarrocha-Oltra D, Ata-Ali J, Oltra-Moscardó MJ, Peñarrocha-Diago M, Peñarrocha M. Side effects and complications of intraosseous anesthesia and conventional oral anesthesia. Med Oral Patol Oral Cir Bucal. 2012;17(3):e430–4. https://doi.org/10.4317/medoral.17512.
58. Özer S, Yaltirik M, Kirli I, Yargic I. A comparative evaluation of pain and anxiety levels in 2 different anesthesia techniques: locoregional anesthesia using conventional syringe versus intraosseous anesthesia using a computer-controlled system (Quicksleeper). Oral Surg Oral Med Oral Pathol Oral Radiol. 2012;114(5 Suppl):S132–9. https://doi.org/10.1016/j.oooo.2011.09.021. Epub 2012 May 6.
59. Nilius M, Mueller C, Nilius MH, Haim D, Leonhardt H, Lauer G. Intraosseous anesthesia in symptomatic irreversible pulpitis: impact of bone thickness on perception and duration of pain. J Dent Anesth Pain Med. 2020;20(6):367–75. https://doi.org/10.17245/jdapm.2020.20.6.367. Epub 2020 Dec 28.
60. Philbeck TE, Miller LJ, Montez D, Puga T, Hurts so good. Easing IO pain and pressure. JEMS. 2010;35(9):58–62, 65–6, 68; quiz 69. https://doi.org/10.1016/S0197-2510(10)70232-1.
61. Leidel BA, Kirchhoff C, Bogner V, Stegmaier J, Mutschler W, Kanz KG, Braunstein V. Is the intraosseous access route fast and efficacious compared to conventional central venous catheterization in adult patients under resuscitation in the emergency department? A prospective observational pilot study. Patient Saf Surg. 2009;3(1):24. https://doi.org/10.1186/1754-9493-3-24.
62. Arakawa J, Woelber E, Working Z, Meeker J, Friess D. Complications of intraosseous access: two case reports from a single center JBJS Case Connect. 2021;11(2). https://doi.org/10.2106/JBJS.CC.19.00382.
63. Platt SL, Notterman DA, Winchester P. Fungal osteomyelitis and sepsis from intraosseous infusion. Pediatr Emerg Care. 1993;9(3):149–50. https://doi.org/10.1097/00006565-199306000-00008.
64. Henson NL, Payan JM, Terk MR. Tibial subacute osteomyelitis with intraosseous abscess: an unusual complication of intraosseous infusion. Skeletal Radiol. 2011;40(2):239–42. https://doi.org/10.1007/s00256-010-1027-9. Epub 2010 Sep 14.
65. Chalopin T, Lemaignen A, Guillon A, Geffray A, Derot G, Bahuaud O, Agout C, Rosset P, Castellier C, De Pinieux G, Valentin AS, Bernard L, Bastides F, Centre De Référence Des Infections Ostéo-Articulaires Du Grand-Ouest (CRIOGO) Study Team. Acute tibial osteomyelitis caused by intraosseous access during initial resuscitation: a case report and literature review. BMC Infect Dis. 2018;18(1):665. https://doi.org/10.1186/s12879-018-3577-8.
66. Yee D, Deolankar R, Marcantoni J, Liang SY. Tibial osteomyelitis following prehospital intraosseous access. Clin Pract Cases Emerg Med. 2017;1(4):391–4. https://doi.org/10.5811/cpcem.2017.9.35256.
67. Heinild S, Sondergaard T, Tudvad F. Bone marrow infusion in childhood; experiences from a thousand infusions. J Pediatr. 1947;30(4):400–12. https://doi.org/10.1016/s0022-3476(47)80080-0.
68. Tobias JD, Ross AK. Intraosseous infusions: a review for the anesthesiologist with a focus on pediatric use. Anesth Analg. 2010;110(2):391–401. https://doi.org/10.1213/ANE.0b013e3181c03c7f. Epub 2009 Nov 6.
69. Barron BJ, Tran HD, Lamki LM. Scintigraphic findings of osteomyelitis after intraosseous infusion in a child. Clin Nucl Med. 1994;19(4):307–8. https://doi.org/10.1097/00003072-199404000-00006.
70. Behr G. Bone-marrow infusions. Br Med J. 1944;1(4338):305.
71. Clement R, Gerbeaux J, Bouveau. Bone marrow perfusion in infants according to 65 observations. Society of Pediatrics of Paris; 1947. p. 531–4.
72. Doğan A, Irmak H, Harman M, Ceylan A, Akpinar F, Tosun N. Kemik içi infüzyonuna bağli tibia osteomiyeliti: Olgu sunumu [Tibial osteomyelitis following intraosseous infusion: a case report]. Acta Orthop Traumatol Turc. 2004;38(5):357–60. Turkish.

73. Ellison JB. Osteomyelitis after bone-marrow transfusion. Br Med J. 1945;4392:342–3. https://doi.org/10.1136/bmj.1.4392.342-a.
74. Gunz FW, Dean RF. Tibial bone-marrow transfusions in infants. Br Med J. 1945;1(4389):220–1. https://doi.org/10.1136/bmj.1.4389.220.
75. Massey LW. Bone-marrow infusions: intratibial and intravenous routes compared. Br Med J. 1950;2(4672):197–8. https://doi.org/10.1136/bmj.2.4672.197.
76. Rooney EF. Bone marrow infusion with two cases of localized osteomyelitis. Arch Pediatr. 1944;64:611–6.
77. Rosovsky M, FitzPatrick M, Goldfarb CR, Finestone H. Bilateral osteomyelitis due to intraosseous infusion: case report and review of the English-language literature. Pediatr Radiol. 1994;24(1):72–3. https://doi.org/10.1007/BF02017671.
78. Sondergaard R. Osteomyelitis after intraosseous infusion. Hosp J. 1946:1094–6.
79. Stoll E, Golej J, Burda G, Hermon M, Boigner H, Trittenwein G. Osteomyelitis at the injection site of adrenalin through an intraosseous needle in a 3-month-old infant. Resuscitation. 2002;53(3):315–8. https://doi.org/10.1016/s0300-9572(02)00039-4.
80. Texter EC, Kaump DH. Intraosseous infusions in infants. J Mich State Med Soc. 1948;47(9):1002–7.
81. Tocantins LM, O'neill JF. Complications of intra-osseous therapy. Ann Surg. 1945;122(2):266–77. https://doi.org/10.1097/00000658-194508000-00011.
82. Williams JC, Lockhart J. Bone marrow infusions in infancy. Pa Med J. 1948;51(7):767–70.
83. Castiglioni C, Carminati A, Fracasso T. Fat embolism after intraosseous catheters in pediatric forensic autopsies. Int J Legal Med. 2023;137(3):787–91. https://doi.org/10.1007/s00414-022-02848-4. Epub 2022 Jun 30.
84. Milroy CM, Parai JL. Fat embolism, fat embolism syndrome and the autopsy. Acad Forensic Pathol. 2019;9(3–4):136–54. https://doi.org/10.1177/1925362119896351. Epub 2020 Jan 31.
85. Vance BM. The significance of fat embolism. Arch Surg. 1931;23(3):426–65. https://doi.org/10.1001/archsurg.1931.01160090071002.
86. Scully RE. Fat embolism in Korean battle casualties: its incidence, clinical significance, and pathologic aspects. Am J Pathol. 1956;32(3):379–403.
87. Wyatt JP, Khoo P. Fat embolism in trauma. Am J Clin Pathol. 1950;20(7):637–40. https://doi.org/10.1093/ajcp/20.7.637.
88. Robb-Smith AH. Pulmonary fat-embolism. Lancet. 1941;237(6127):135–41. https://doi.org/10.1016/s0140-6736(00)77494-0.
89. Eriksson EA, Pellegrini DC, Vanderkolk WE, et al. Incidence of pulmonary fat embolism at autopsy: an undiagnosed epidemic. J Trauma. 2011;71(2):312–5. https://doi.org/10.1097/TA.0b013e3182208280.
90. Hasan MY, Kissoon N, Khan TM, Saldajeno V, Goldstein J, Murphy SP. Intraosseous infusion and pulmonary fat embolism. Pediatr Crit Care Med. 2001;2(2):133–8. https://doi.org/10.1097/00130478-200104000-00007.
91. Azan B, Teran F, Nelson BP, Andrus P. Point-of-care ultrasound diagnosis of intravascular air after lower extremity intraosseous Access. J Emerg Med. 2016;51(6):680–3. https://doi.org/10.1016/j.jemermed.2016.05.064. Epub 2016 Sep 9.
92. Kristiansen S, Storm B, Dahle D, Domaas Josefsen T, Dybwik K, Nilsen BA, Waage-Nielsen E. Intraosseous fluid resuscitation causes systemic fat emboli in a porcine hemorrhagic shock model. Scand J Trauma Resusc Emerg Med. 2021;29(1):172. https://doi.org/10.1186/s13049-021-00986-z.
93. Orlowski JP, Julius CJ, Petras RE, Porembka DT, Gallagher JM. The safety of intraosseous infusions: risks of fat and bone marrow emboli to the lungs. Ann Emerg Med. 1989;18(10):1062–7. https://doi.org/10.1016/s0196-0644(89)80932-1.
94. Adolph MD, Fabian HF, el-Khairi SM, Thornton JC, Oliver AM. The pulmonary artery catheter: a diagnostic adjunct for fat embolism syndrome. J Orthop Trauma. 1994;8(2):173–6. https://doi.org/10.1097/00005131-199404000-00016.

95. Johnson M, Inaba K, Byerly S, Falsgraf E, Lam L, Benjamin E, Strumwasser A, David JS, Demetriades D. Intraosseous infusion as a bridge to definitive access. Am Surg. 2016;82(10):876–80.

96. Fuhrman B, Zimmerman J, Clarck R, Rotta A, Tobias J, Kudchadkar S. Pediatric vascular access and centeses. In: Fuhrman and Zimmerman's pediatric critical care. 6th ed. Philadelphia, PA: Elsevier - Health Sciences Division; 2021. p. 94–5.

97. Alam HB, Punzalan CM, Koustova E, Bowyer MW, Rhee P. Hypertonic saline: intraosseous infusion causes myonecrosis in a dehydrated swine model of uncontrolled hemorrhagic shock. J Trauma. 2002;52(1):18–25. https://doi.org/10.1097/00005373-200201000-00006.

98. Bebarta VS, Vargas TE, Castaneda M, Boudreau S. Evaluation of extremity tissue and bone injury after intraosseous hypertonic saline infusion in proximal tibia and proximal humerus in adult swine. Prehosp Emerg Care. 2014;18(4):505–10. https://doi.org/10.3109/1090312 7.2014.912704. Epub 2014 May 15.

99. Lawson T, Hussein O, Nasir M, Hinduja A, Torbey MT. Intraosseous administration of hypertonic saline in acute brain-injured patients: a prospective case series and literature review. Neurologist. 2019;24(6):176–9. https://doi.org/10.1097/NRL.0000000000000248.

100. Dubick MA, Kramer GC. Hypertonic saline dextran (HSD) and intraosseous vascular access for the treatment of haemorrhagic hypotension in the far-forward combat arena. Ann Acad Med Singap. 1997;26(1):64–9.

101. Farrokh S, Cho SM, Lefebvre AT, Zink EK, Schiavi A, Puttgen HA. Use of intraosseous hypertonic saline in critically ill patients. J Vasc Access. 2019;20(4):427–32. https://doi.org/10.1177/1129729818805958. Epub 2018 Oct 17.

102. Fenchel DD, Myers LA, Arteaga GM, Russi CS. Chart analysis of frequency and complications from intraosseous infusion in out-of-hospital pediatric and adult populations. Ann Emerg Med. 2013;62(4):S104. https://doi.org/10.1016/j.annemergmed.2013.07.112.

103. Scheman L, Janota M, Lewin P. The production of experimental osteomyelitis: preliminary report. JAMA J Am Med Assoc. 1941;117(18):1525. https://doi.org/10.1001/jama.1941.02820440033008.

104. Zimmet SE. The prevention of cutaneous necrosis following extravasation of hypertonic saline and sodium tetradecyl sulfate. J Dermatol Surg Oncol. 1993;19(7):641–6. https://doi.org/10.1111/j.1524-4725.1993.tb00404.x.

105. Douma MJ, Bara GS, O'Dochartaigh D, Brindley PG. Double-barrelled resuscitation: a feasibility and simulation study of dual-intraosseous needles into a single humerus. Injury. 2015;46(11):2239–42. https://doi.org/10.1016/j.injury.2015.08.029. Epub 2015 Sep 11.

106. Galpin RD, Kronick JB, Willis RB, Frewen TC. Bilateral lower extremity compartment syndromes secondary to intraosseous fluid resuscitation. J Pediatr Orthop. 1991;11(6):773–6. https://doi.org/10.1097/01241398-199111000-00014.

107. Gayle M, Kissoon N. A case of compartment syndrome following intraosseous infusions. Pediatr Emerg Care. 1994;10(6):378.

108. Launay F, Paut O, Katchburian M, Bourelle S, Jouve JL, Bollini G. Leg amputation after intraosseous infusion in a 7-month-old infant: a case report. J Trauma. 2003;55(4):788–90. https://doi.org/10.1097/01.TA.0000025875.18050.A4.

109. Cotte J, Prunet B, d'Aranda E, Asencio Y, Kaiser E. Un syndrome des loges secondaire à la pose d'un cathéter intra-osseux [A compartment syndrome secondary to intraosseous infusion]. Ann Fr Anesth Reanim. 2011;30(1):90–1. French. https://doi.org/10.1016/j.annfar.2010.05.038. Epub 2010 Nov 30.

110. Suominen PK, Nurmi E, Lauerma K. Intraosseous access in neonates and infants: risk of severe complications—a case report. Acta Anaesthesiol Scand. 2015;59(10):1389–93. https://doi.org/10.1111/aas.12602. Epub 2015 Aug 24.

111. Abramson TM, Alreshaid L, Kang T, Mailhot T, Omer T. FasclOtomy: ultrasound evaluation of an intraosseous needle causing compartment Syndrome. Clin Pract Cases Emerg Med. 2018;2(4):323–5. https://doi.org/10.5811/cpcem.2018.8.38854.

112. Kibrik P, Alsheekh A, Rajaee S, Marks N, Hingorani A, Ascher E. Compartment Syndrome of the leg after intraosseous (IO) needle insertion. Ann Vasc Surg. 2020;65:282.e9–282.e11. https://doi.org/10.1016/j.avsg.2019.10.066. Epub 2019 Oct 30.
113. Chughtai M, Pang A, Khan T, Cantrell WA, Mesko NW, Kamath AF. Compartment syndrome secondary to intraosseous access abutting tibial stem cement mantle of a total knee Arthroplasty: a case report. JBJS Case Connect. 2022;12(1). Erratum in: JBJS Case Connect. 2022;12(2). https://doi.org/10.2106/JBJS.CC.21.00655.
114. Singh A, Singh D. A case of compartment Syndrome due to out-of-hospital intraosseous misplacement during cardiopulmonary resuscitation. Cureus. 2022;14(6):e26228. https://doi.org/10.7759/cureus.26228.

Pain with Intraosseous Infusion

10

Bobak Ossareh, Aaron J. Wilke, and James H. Paxton

Introduction

Pain is among the most commonly listed drawbacks to the use of intraosseous (IO) infusion devices, relating to both initial device insertion and subsequent infusion of fluids or medications [1–3]. Pain perception may especially limit the use of IO access for aggressive bolus fluid or blood infusion due to the high infusion pressure required to advance large volumes of fluid into the constrained intramedullary space. While veins can stretch within certain limits to accommodate a sudden influx of additional volume, the medullary space cannot expand. Thus, increased infusion pressures and volumes are transmitted differently with IO infusion than with intravenous (IV) infusion. These differences must be considered when planning rapid high-pressure IO infusion, especially in awake patients due to various normal physiologic mechanisms that serve to identify areas of abnormally high pressure within the IO space.

Despite recent technological advances in the ability of providers to quickly and reliably insert IO devices [1, 4–6], the modern experience with IO infusion techniques appears to be largely limited to patients who are either seemingly insensate (e.g., cardiac arrest) or so clinically unstable that the need for immediate vascular access outweighs the risk of pain with IO infusion (e.g., respiratory failure, profound hemodynamic instability) [7–9]. In one recent review and meta-analysis of complications associated with adult IO catheter placement, 92.2% (4257 of 4609 subjects) of all included subjects for which data were available were categorized as cardiac arrest patients [10]. Consequently, most studies reporting quantitative data on pain perception with intraosseous infusion are small, industry-sponsored studies of healthy adult volunteers.

B. Ossareh (✉) · A. J. Wilke · J. H. Paxton
Department of Emergency Medicine, Wayne State University School of Medicine, Detroit, MI, USA
e-mail: ft8702@wayne.edu; ajwilke@wayne.edu; james.paxton@wayne.edu

J. H. Paxton (ed.), *Intraosseous Vascular Access*,
https://doi.org/10.1007/978-3-031-61201-5_10

The subjective nature of pain reporting also places additional limitations on our current understanding of IO infusion-related pain. A few reports have anecdotally suggested that the pain associated with IO infusion is less than that associated with other pain-inducing medical experiences, such as Foley catheter insertion [1], or the patient's underlying injuries [11]. However, data on pain perception collected from critically ill patients under emergent conditions may be subject to reporting biases and other confounders. Patients may also be distracted from appropriately experiencing IO insertion pain by other aspects of emergent care, including the use of spine boards and cervical collars, movement during transport, catecholamine release due to physical and psychological stressors, concomitant drug or alcohol intoxication, medical treatment with sedative or analgesic medications, or distracting events at the emergency scene [3].

Ultimately, the speed and success with which IO catheters can be placed make these devices an extremely valuable tool for fluid resuscitation and medication administration for all age groups (including neonates) in situations where traditional vascular access (e.g., peripheral IVs, central venous catheters) cannot be obtained. Future advances in reducing or eliminating pain with IO infusion could substantially improve providers' ability to leverage the benefits of IO infusion from additional populations of patients, including those who remain sensate and conscious.

In this chapter, we will explore the mechanisms by which pain is perceived during intraosseous vascular access and infusion, including various anatomic and biochemical factors. The existing medical literature on pain associated with therapeutic intraosseous infusion will be reviewed, and general conclusions will be drawn relating to the current state of our understanding on this topic. Current methods for pain control will be discussed, with attention to their mechanisms for action and proven efficacy. Finally, we will describe nascent and emerging modalities for the control of IO infusion-related pain that may 1 day contribute to increased use and effectiveness of this important vascular access technique.

Anatomy of Skeletal Pain

Neurons are distributed throughout the skeletal system and are responsible for transmitting sensory information. Put simply, the neuron consists of a **soma** (i.e., cell body), **dendrites** (i.e., cell extensions receiving nerve impulses from other nerve cells), and **axons** (i.e., cell extensions sending nerve impulses to other nerve cells) [12]. These components of the neuron can vary in number and in their anatomical arrangement, giving rise to unipolar, pseudounipolar, bipolar, and multipolar neurons as illustrated in Fig. 10.1 [12]. The soma houses the nucleus and organelles of the neuron, while dendrites and axons are responsible for afferent and efferent signaling, respectively [12]. Signals are transmitted from one nerve to another at a junction called a **synapse**, where the terminal axons of one nerve lie adjacent to the dendrites of another nerve [12]. Axons are insulated by a **myelin sheath** to prevent degradation of the nerve impulse.

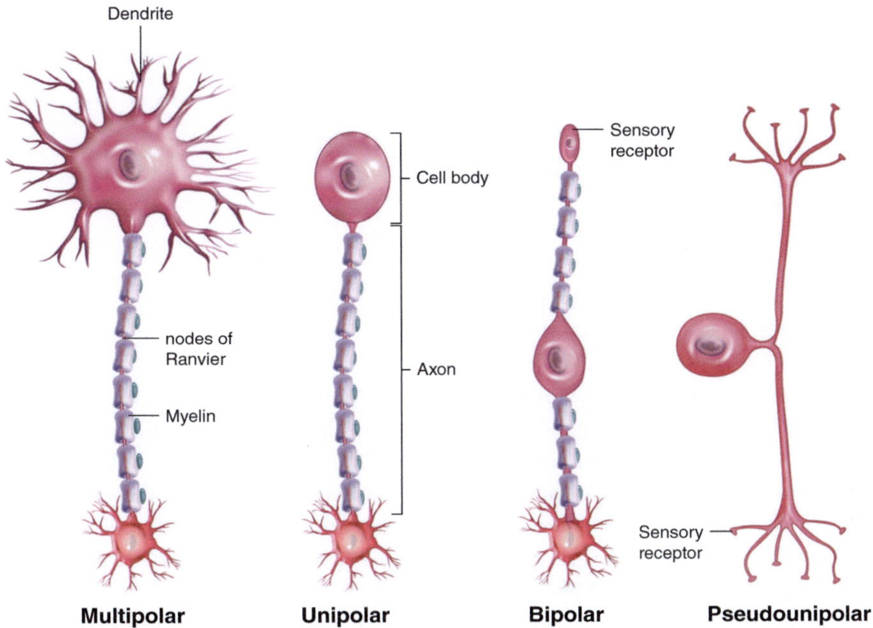

Fig. 10.1 Types of neurons

Nerve conduction is accomplished via **action potentials**, which are brief changes in the **membrane potential** of the nerve cell [13]. The resting membrane potential of the nerve cell is −70 mV, due to an imbalance between electrically charged ions creating a more negative environment at the interior of the nerve cell [13]. This electrical gradient is generated through the action of the **sodium-potassium pump**, which exchanges 3 sodium (Na^+) ions pumped outside of the cell for 2 potassium (K^+) ions pumped into the cell [13]. Upon receiving a signal, sodium channels along the nerve cell open, allowing for the influx of sodium ions and a resultant positive change in membrane potential [13]. Should the membrane potential reach the **threshold potential** of −55 mV, **depolarization** occurs as sodium channels along the length of the axon open and influx of sodium bringing membrane potential to +30 mV. Once the action potential reaches the terminal axon, it triggers the opening of **calcium** channels allowing for calcium ions (Ca^{+2}) to enter the cell and bind to the presynaptic membrane, leading to the release of neurotransmitters [13]. Very shortly after opening, sodium and terminal calcium channels will close and potassium channels will open leading to the efflux of potassium ions and the return of membrane potential to a resting −70 mV membrane potential [13].

The role of the **myelin sheath** is to increase the propagation speed of action potentials [13]. Myelin acts as an insulator along the length of the axon while also

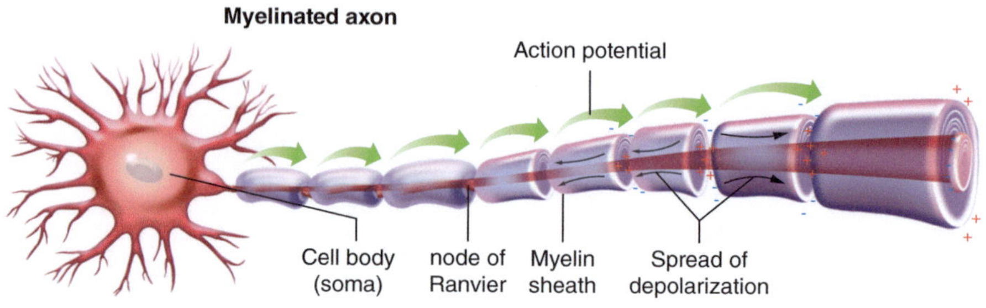

Fig. 10.2 Myelinated nerve conduction

leaving gaps called the **nodes of Ranvier** [13]. Action potentials occur only at the nodes of Ranvier, and the insulation provided by the myelin sheath facilitates the movement of ions along the length of the axon, leading to depolarization at the next node [14]. This generation of action potentials along the length of the axon at the nodes of Ranvier is termed **saltatory conduction** and results in an increased speed of propagation as compared to unmyelinated nerves [14]. An illustration of action potential propagation is depicted in Fig. 10.2.

Long bones, particularly the proximal tibia and fibula, have been traditionally considered to be preferred sites for intraosseous vascular access [15]. Long bones can be divided into three parts: the **epiphyses, metaphyses**, and **diaphysis** [15]. The epiphyses are located at the proximal and distal ends of the bone, bookending the diaphysis of the bone, which constitutes the majority of the bone shaft [15]. The metaphyses is situated between the epiphyses and diaphysis, in the region formerly occupied by the growth plate in adults [15]. On their exterior, long bones are covered by a thin, cellular, and fibrous tissue known as the **periosteum**, which overlies all portions of the bone lacking articular cartilage [15]. The periosteum overlies the bony **cortex,** underneath which lies the interior portion of the bone known as the **medullary cavity** [15]. The medullary cavity is the location of intraosseous vasculature as well as red and yellow marrow [15]. Hematopoietic **red marrow** is the primary marrow type in pediatric patients, but is gradually replaced by atrophic **yellow marrow** (i.e., adipose tissue) as humans age [15]. The yellow marrow contains a higher proportion of fatty tissue and is relatively lacking in hematopoietic capacity [15]. The anatomy of the femur, as an example of typical long bone anatomy, is shown in Fig. 10.3.

Regarding sensory innervation, the periosteum is the most densely innervated compartment of bone, while the **bone marrow** carries the largest absolute number of sensory fibers considering its total constituent volume [16–18]. The periosteum contains a meshwork of sensory afferent nerves responsible for carrying the sharp, localized pain experienced with insertion of the IO catheter [19, 20]. During subsequent infusion, pressure-sensing receptors within the medullary space are activated, causing pain perception with infusion [15].

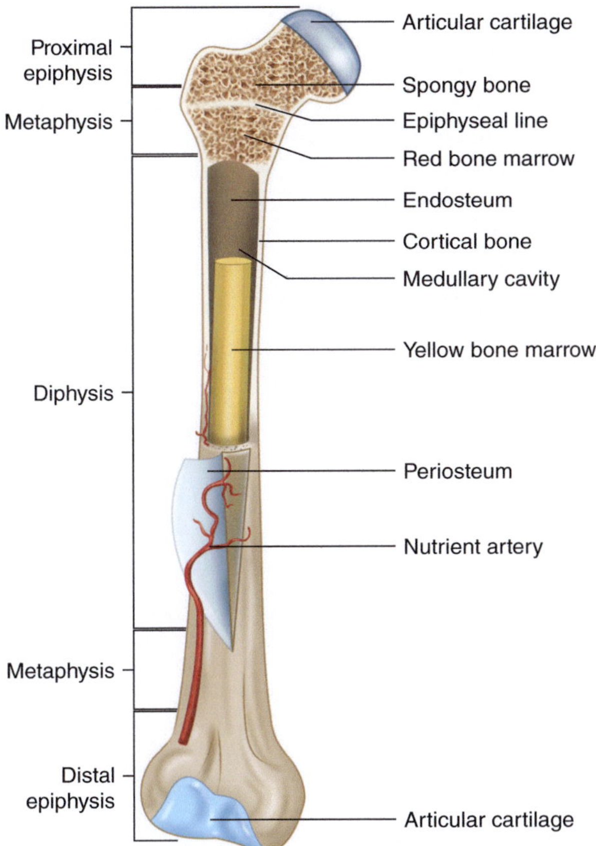

Fig. 10.3 Anatomy of a long bone

Pathophysiology of Skeletal Pain

A wide variety of medical conditions are known to cause skeletal pain in humans and other vertebrates, ranging from bone fracture to bone marrow-infiltrating diseases [16]. Although the precise mechanisms are not completely understood, much work has already been done to identify the nervous system components responsible for **nociception** (i.e., the encoding and processing of noxious stimuli by the nervous system) within the skeletal system. Several mammalian studies have demonstrated that the predominant fibers transmitting afferent sensory information from the bone are **A∂-fibers** and **C-fibers** [16, 20–24]. The A∂-fibers are fast-conducting (5–40 m/s), small-diameter (1–6 μm) myelinated primarily afferent fibers responsive to mechanical and thermal stimuli [17]. In contrast, C-fibers are slow-conducting (0.5–2 m/s), smaller diameter (1 μm) unmyelinated primarily afferent fibers responsive to thermal, mechanical, and chemical noxious stimuli [17]. Both fibers contain peptidergic nociceptors such as substance P (SP), calcitonin gene-related peptide (CGRP), tropomyosin receptor kinase A (TrkA), and transient receptor potential cation channel subfamily V member 1 (TRPV1) [21, 25]. The cell bodies of these nerve fibers are located in a dorsal root ganglion and synapse in the superficial dorsal horn of the spinal cord where information is carried via the lateral spinothalamic tract to the ventral-posterolateral nuclei of the thalamus and ultimately sent to the somatosensory cortices of the brain [25–27]. The information carried by these fibers can be topographically mapped within the somatosensory cortices in a fashion similar to that of skin, allowing for localization of pain [26]. A schematic representation of this neural pathway is illustrated in Fig. 10.4. As this figure shows, A∂-fibers

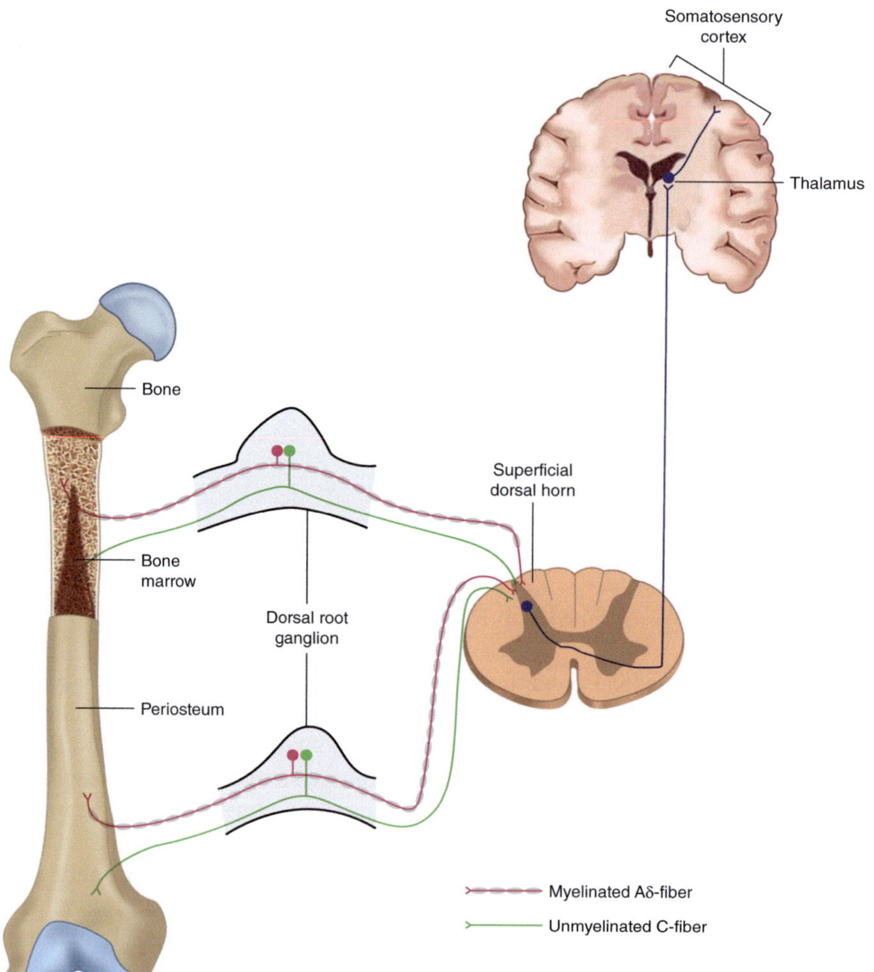

Fig. 10.4 Schematic representation of skeletal pain transmission

(magenta) and C-fibers (green) are shown innervating both the periosteum and bone marrow with their cell bodies housed within a dorsal root ganglion. The roots of these nerve fibers then continue to the spinal cord where they synapse with a second-order neuron (blue) in the superficial dorsal horn. This neuron then ascends to the brain via the lateral spinothalamic tract where it synapses on a final neuron located within the somatosensory cortex.

Periosteal Bone Pain

The **periosteum** is a thin, cellular, and fibrous tissue that tightly adheres to the outer surface of all but the articulated surfaces of bones and is the most densely innervated portion of the bone [16–18]. Pain induced by mechanical distortion of the periosteal layer has been well studied and described in rat models. Immunohistochemical labeling techniques have demonstrated that the Aδ-fibers and C-fibers innervating the periosteum are arranged in a mesh-like network (Fig. 10.5), allowing for the detection of even subtle alterations in bony architecture [19, 20]. This arrangement helps to explain the pain associated with bone fracture. When a bone is fractured, the resultant acute sharp, stabbing pain is thought to be carried by the displaced network of fast-conducting Aδ-fibers [28, 29]. When the fracture is then stabilized via reduction (restoring the spatial orientation of the bone and the network of sensory afferents), there is an immediate reduction in perceived

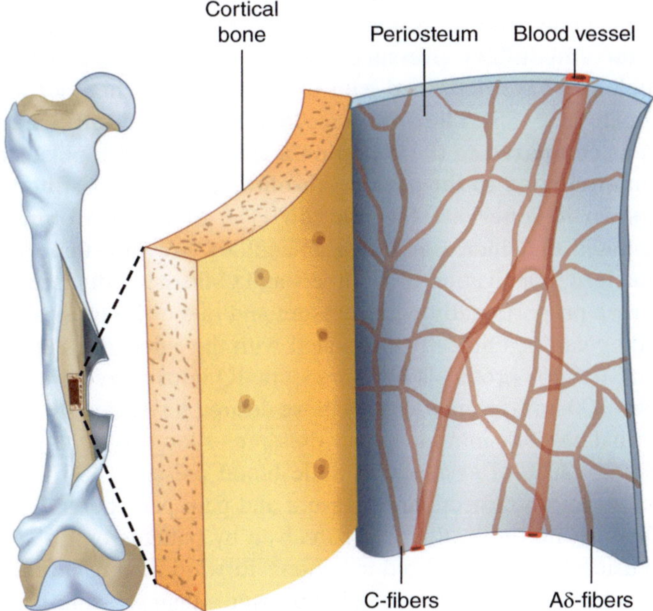

Fig. 10.5 Sensory nerve distribution within the periosteum

pain [28, 29]. In contrast, dull persistent pain following fracture stabilization is likely transmitted by slow-conducting C-fibers [28, 29].

In addition to mechanical stimulation, Aδ-fibers and C-fibers may become sensitized in response to **inflammatory mediators** released in the setting of a fracture or other trauma. In response to trauma, osteoblasts, osteoclasts, and immune cells secrete inflammatory factors such as bradykinin, prostaglandin E2, serotonin, TNF-α, colony-stimulating factors, nerve growth factor (NGF), and protease-activated receptor 2 [30]. There are several mechanisms by which these inflammatory mediators sensitize sensory afferent nerve endings. Histamine, serotonin, bradykinin, and prostaglandin E2 lead to increased mechanoreceptor sensitivity via a decrease in threshold depolarization [31]. Meanwhile, NGF increases sensory nerve sensitivity via promoting the phosphorylation of various ion channels and cytokine receptors, as well as by increasing the transcription of nociceptive genes [30]. These chemically induced changes ultimately work in concert to modulate pain signaling and are thought to contribute to the dull pain that persists following fracture stabilization [28, 29].

Medullary Bone Pain

While the periosteum is the most densely innervated compartment of bone, the **bone marrow** carries the largest absolute number of sensory fibers based upon total constituent volume [19]. Nerve fibers enter the bone marrow by either traversing the periosteum or entering through the **nutrient foramina** of the bone [21]. Like the periosteum, the bone marrow is responsive to mechanical stimuli, particularly increases in **intramedullary pressure**. Anecdotal reports of patients with bone marrow pathologies have described pain originating from this location to have a dull, aching quality [32–35]. **The difference in the quality of dull, aching marrow-related pain as compared to the sharp pain associated with periosteal disruption has been attributed to the greater absolute number of C-fibers relative to Aδ-fibers known to innervate the marrow** [18]. Studies performed in rodents have demonstrated that increases in intramedullary pressure three to five times above baseline lead to activation of Aδ-fibers and C-fibers, with discharge frequencies that increase proportionally with pressure and rate of IO pressure change [34, 35]. This finding can be clinically correlated with the subjective experience of IO infusion pain. Common protocols for therapeutic IO infusion require infusion pressures of at least 300 mmHg in order to achieve desired flow rates [1, 3]. This is well above the normal baseline intramedullary pressure of long bones in mammals (i.e., approximately 25–30% of systemic systolic blood pressure) [36, 37]. Given the relationship between intramedullary pressure and pain perception during IO infusion, providers can minimize the pain perceived by patients by utilizing only the minimum infusion pressure required to achieve forward flow of infusates. Syringe injection can achieve much higher infusion pressures than pressure-bag infusion or gravity infusion, which may equate to greater pain with infusion. In general, a slow syringe infusion should be preferred over a rapid syringe infusion, and gravity infusion (generating the lowest infusion pressure of these techniques) should be employed when adequate. The size of the medullary cavity and the speed with which infusates are removed from the medullary cavity may also influence intramedullary pressure and resultant pain perception. Consequently, IO insertion sites associated with a larger medullary cavity and more rapid medullary drainage should be preferred over smaller, more congested insertion sites. Trabecular density, which is greater in weight-bearing bones (e.g., proximal and distal tibia) may also contribute to intramedullary resistance to flow and increase intramedullary pressure. Thus, the optimal IO insertion site should have a large medullary cavity with exceptional venous drainage and low trabecular density. Although the proximal tibia site is most often used in published reports on IO infusion, it is likely that the sternal and proximal humerus insertion sites will have a more favorable profile along these lines than lower extremity targets. Additional research is needed to determine whether and how pain perception with IO infusion differs according to different IO insertion sites, and the degree to which these anatomic considerations can be optimized to reduce pain perception.

Acid-Base Disturbances

Localized tissue **acidosis** is known to contribute to increased pain perception. Serum acidosis is characterized by a serum pH <7.35, often due to a fall in the serum bicarbonate and/or a rise in the partial pressure of carbon dioxide within the bloodstream. Conversely, serum **alkalosis** (pH >7.45) can be caused by increased serum bicarbonate or lowered partial pressure of carbon dioxide within the blood [38]. Under normal physiological conditions, the pH within the bone marrow closely approximates serum levels [39]. However, local factors within the bone can disrupt this equilibrium, leading to alterations in intramedullary pH and resultant changes in pain perception.

Pathologic processes associated with increased bone turnover are characterized by increased **osteoclast** activity, creating a localized acidic environment within the bone, which in turn activates both Aδ-fibers and C-fibers [40–42]. This change in pH is detected via acid-sensing ion channels such as acid-sensing ion channel-1 (ASIC-1), ASIC-3, and transient receptor potential channel vanilloid subfamily member 1 (TRVP1) [39, 43–46]. These channels are activated when local pH drops below a range of 6–4 [47–49]. Not surprisingly, acidosis-induced medullary pain can be improved with interventions to restore pH balance by increasing local pH. Bisphosphonates, for example, exert their ameliorating effects in part by inhibiting osteoclast activity, thus normalizing local pH and relieving pain associated with osteoporosis, Paget's disease, and various bone cancers associated with increased osteoclast activity [50–52].

In a similar manner, fluids and medications infused via the IO route have diverse pH values, which should be expected to produce transient localized changes in the intramedullary pH. Common IO infusates include 0.9% normal saline (pH 5.5), Ringer's lactate solution (pH 6.5), lidocaine (pH 6.1), morphine (pH 2.5–6.5), epinephrine (pH 2.3–3.5), and sodium bicarbonate (pH 8.5). Each of these substances can produce alterations in the intramedullary pH value commensurate with the volume of the substance infused, the degree to which the pH of the infusate differs from preexisting pH levels within the marrow, how quickly the infusate is transported out of the marrow space, and the degree to which the compound binds to other substances within the marrow cavity. Thus, it is likely that different fluids and substances infused via the IO route may exert their own unique pH-dependent nociceptive effects within the bone, leading to increased or decreased pain perception by the patient. In one study of IO pH during cardiopulmonary resuscitation in piglets, it was found that infusion of epinephrine resulted in a statistically significant decrease in IO pH as compared to central venous pH, while the infusion of bicarbonate led to a clinically relevant increase in IO pH as compared to central venous pH [53]. Epinephrine is a potent vasoconstrictor, which induces reduced blood flow to peripheral organs (including the bone marrow) whether introduced endogenously (e.g., with the physiologic stress response) or exogenously (e.g., with IO or IV infusion of epinephrine). Intraosseous infusion of epinephrine has been shown to reduce blood flow to the bone marrow space, which may be expected to reduce subsequent uptake of medications from the IO space due to increased local vasoconstriction [54]. However, other vasopressors (e.g., vasopressin) may not exert the same effect [54]. The cause of these divergent effects on bony blood flow between different vasopressors remains unclear.

Decreased perfusion of the bone marrow would be expected to lead to a lag in the response of marrow pH to changing serum pH values during prolonged shock states, although some studies suggest that the dissonance between arterial, venous, and IO lactate levels (for example) is not statistically significant early in resuscitation following cardiac arrest in the porcine model [39]. In any event, shock states invariably lead to increased serum lactic acid concentrations, due to compromised perfusion of peripheral tissues and organs. This elevation in serum lactate level persists for a variable time after the restoration of local blood flow, but may not correlate directly with measured IO lactate levels if marrow perfusion remains compromised by other factors.

While acidosis within the bone marrow space likely increases the experience of skeletal pain during IO infusion, this area of inquiry remains largely unexplored. Certain medical conditions, especially those associated with shock states, are associated with high serum levels of lactic acid and other metabolites, which may introduce a certain degree of acidosis within the circulating blood and organs. Considering that many patients receiving IO infusion may experience some degree of serum acidosis due to their underlying medical condition, the relationship between the pH of infusates and the intramedullary pH is thus further complicated. The degree of acidosis within the IO space has been shown to be similar to that seen in the central venous system with pH values approaching 7.0 as CPR is prolonged [53, 54]. However, the pH within the IO space is likely made more acidic by therapeutic infusion of IO epinephrine and more alkalotic with IO bicarbonate infusion [53]. Future study regarding the marrow pH of acidotic patients undergoing IO cannulation will be of great value in determining the role of infusate pH in pain perception associated with various substances infused via the IO route.

Local Anesthetics

Existing data suggest that the pain experienced by patients during IO *infusion* is generally greater than that experienced with *insertion* of the catheter [1–3, 11, 55, 56]. As a result, manufacturers do not universally recommend local anesthesia of the periosteum prior to IO insertion, although this can be done for sensate patients [57, 58]. Systemic analgesia and anxiolysis to alleviate the discomfort associated with IO catheter placement with IV fentanyl (12.5–100 mcg) or IV midazolam (1–3 mg) have been reported, and these medications may also be administered via the intramuscular (IM) route prior to IO device insertion [58].

Current recommendations for pain control with IO infusion focus upon the administration of 1–2 mL (20–40 mg) of **preservative-free 2% (20 mg/mL) lido-caine** without epinephrine through the IO catheter after placement but prior to any infusion attempts [1, 3, 4]. This lidocaine infusion is performed slowly over 120 s, with a recommended dwell time of 60 s prior to subsequent fluid or medication infu-sion [1, 3, 4, 59]. The onset of effect should be within 90 s. Dosing can be repeated as needed, although providers must take care to avoid exceeding the maximum safe dose of lidocaine (4 mg/kg/h, up to maximum 300 mg/h) [60]. In a pediatric popula-tion, some authors recommend adjusting the initial dose of lidocaine to 0.5 mg/kg, not to exceed 40 mg total dose [59]. Although no maximum safe daily dose of IV lidocaine has been established, it is not recommended to administer more than a total of 3 mg/kg of lidocaine in treatment of IO-catheter associated pain. As lido-caine has a half-life of 1.5–2.0 h, with 90% hepatic metabolism, liver dysfunction (whether acute or chronic) can prolong the drug's half-life up to 3.5 times. Patients experiencing shock, congestive heart failure, or cardiac arrest should likely not receive more than 1.2 mg/kg/h, as they likely have impaired drug clearance by the liver.

Lidocaine is an **amide-type** local anesthetic (LA) agent, which acts via inhi-bition of **voltage-gated sodium channels**, leading to membrane stabilization and slowing of membrane depolarization and repolarization [61]. Local anes-thetics have a greater effect on fast-conducting (Aδ) than on slow-conducting (C) fibers, so patients who have received these medications typically have less sharp, stabbing pain but retain the ability to perceive dull pain and pres-sure [62].

The **pKa**, or negative base-10 logarithm of the acid dissociation constant (Ka), is a measure of how weak or strong an acid is [63]. Functionally, the pKa is the **pH value at which the ionized and non-ionized forms of the drug are present in equal amounts**. This relationship is predicted by the **Henderson-Hasselbalch equation** [64], in which [A-] is the concentration of acid and [HA] is the concentra-tion of its conjugate base, as shown in Fig. 10.6.

Fig. 10.6 The Henderson-Hasselbalch equation

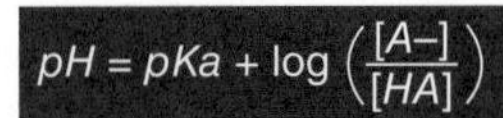

The pKa of lidocaine is known to be 7.9. Thus, when lidocaine is in a syringe (where ambient pH is approximately 6.0), 99% of the medication remains in its ionized form as the environment is far more acidic than the drug's pKa [65, 66]. However, when lidocaine is injected into the extracellular environment (where pH is approximately 7.4), a large number of lidocaine molecules give up hydrogen ions (which subsequently bind with chloride ions), resulting in the formation of hydrogen chloride and non-ionized lidocaine. The non-ionized lidocaine molecule is much more lipophilic and is therefore able to migrate across the cell membrane towards the more acidic (pH 7.1) intracellular environment. Once lidocaine enters the cell, the more acidic intracellular environment leads to preferential ionization of the lidocaine molecule. This ionized lidocaine molecule is drawn to the negative charge of the voltage-gated sodium channel, inhibitively binding the channel and preventing additional sodium influx. The mechanism for action for lidocaine, similar to most local anesthetics, is depicted in Fig. 10.7.

Ester-type LAs are also available, which differ from amide LAs in their chemical structure. However, ester-type local anesthetics are associated with increased risk of allergic reaction due to p-aminobenzoic acid (PABA) metabolite formation and are therefore less commonly used than amide-type local anesthetics [67]. In distinguishing amide from ester local anesthetics, it should be noted that all common amide local anesthetics have an "i" in the first half of their name (e.g., lidocaine, bupivacaine), while esters do not.

With a pKa of 7.9, approximately 24% of lidocaine in the bloodstream is non-ionized and therefore capable of entering the nerve cell and exerting its effects. When the local pH within the bloodstream or bone marrow becomes more acidic, the difference between the pH and the pKa of the local anesthetic increases and more of the drug becomes ionized. Since most local anesthetics are weak bases (i.e., they do not ionize fully in aqueous solution with drug pKa >7.4), **local anesthetics with a higher pKa generally have diminished magnitude of effect and increased latency** (i.e., delayed onset of analgesic effect) when compared to drugs with a pKa closer to 7.4. Many amide and ester local anesthetics have been developed, primarily for dental or topical dermal applications. Of these, benzocaine is the only local anesthetic that is strongly acidic, which results in a very low potency and presumably low rate of protein binding.

The **potency** (i.e., amount required to produce an effect of given intensity) of local anesthetics varies widely, generally from 0.1 to 4.0 times that of lidocaine. Potency is directly related to the degree to which a local anesthetic is lipid soluble and highly protein binding. Local anesthetics with a high percentage of protein binding will generally have a longer duration of action and lower bioavailability at any given time. Ester-type local anesthetics tend to be less protein bound than amide-type anesthetics.

The addition of 1:100,000 epinephrine significantly reduces the pH of 2% lidocaine solution, from 6.0 (in syringe) to approximately 3.9 [68]. Intraosseous injection of epinephrine can also contribute to increased arterial and venous vasoconstriction, potentially decreasing blood flow to and from the marrow space. Thus, **the addition of epinephrine to IO local anesthetics should be avoided** due

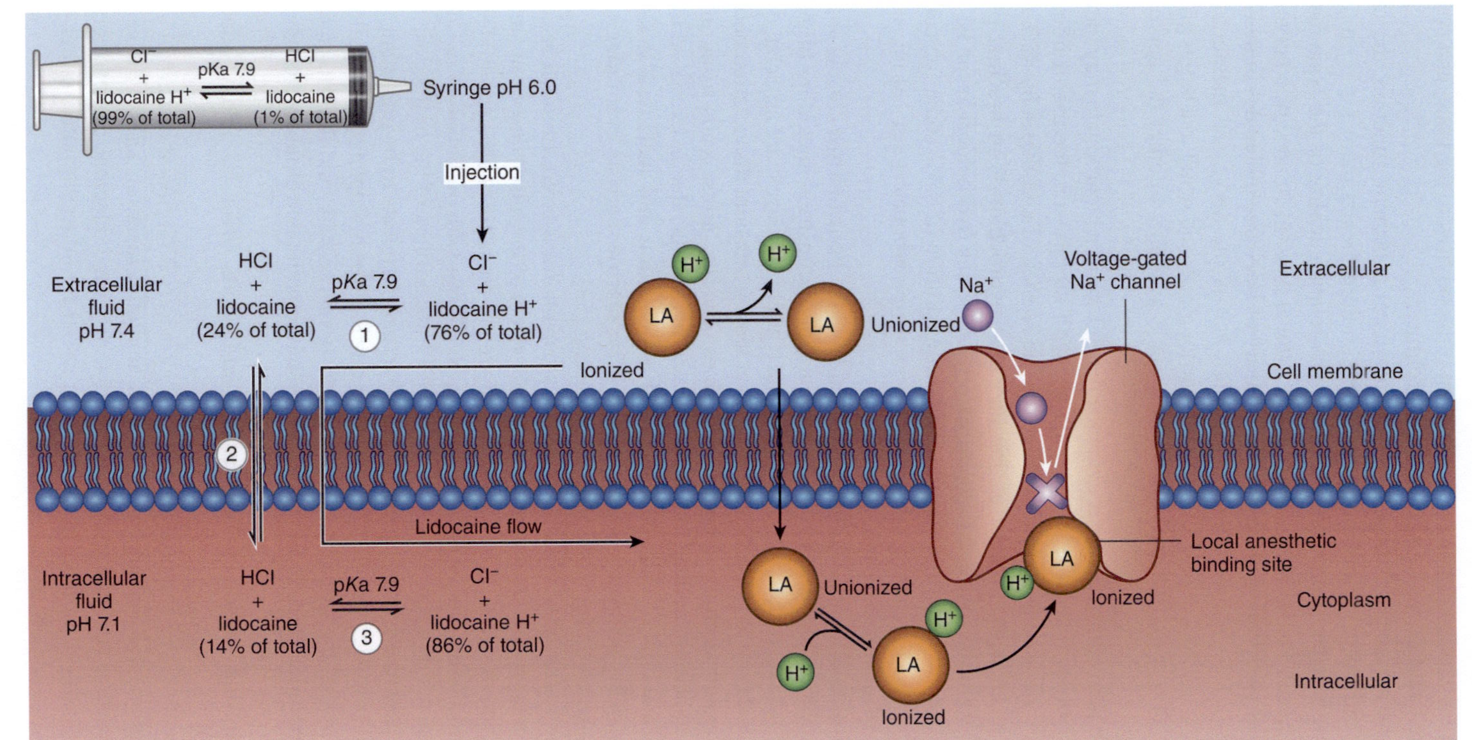

Fig. 10.7   Mechanism of action for lidocaine

to increased risk of pain, potential reduction of blood flow to the bone, and no clear physiologic benefit over LAs without epinephrine.

Given the acid-base mechanics governing local anesthetic function, the use of so-called "**buffered" lidocaine** (with added sodium bicarbonate) for IO infusion pain control may be of particular interest. The relative acidity of the bone marrow space along with the acidotic state of many critical patients in need of emergent IO infusion may contribute to keeping the majority of lidocaine molecules in their pro-tonated form, thus preventing their diffusion across the nerve cell membrane. In theory, buffering lidocaine with sodium bicarbonate should result in a larger propor-tion of the drug's non-ionized form being made available to enter the nerve cell. Although no published studies have been done on the use of IO buffered lidocaine for infusion pain control, there is evidence that IO sodium bicarbonate may increase the efficacy of local anesthetics. Though not with IO infusion, the use of lidocaine carbonate (1.1%) has been shown to reduce the latency of anesthesia by 45% when compared to an equal amount of 1% lidocaine hydrochloride in brachial plexus block, with a similar duration of therapy [69]. Lidocaine hydrochloride can be "car-bonated" to achieve near-physiologic pH by the addition of 8.4% sodium bicarbon-ate in a 10:1 ratio (e.g., 0.1 mL of 8.4% sodium bicarbonate with 1.0 mL of 1% lidocaine hydrochloride) [68].

In states of normal health, blood aspirated from the bone marrow closely approx-imates circulating blood in regard to most major chemistries, including blood pH [53, 70]. However, certain low-flow states such as cardiac arrest are associated with reduced blood flow to the bones, leading to at least a transient dissociation between intraosseous and central venous blood values. Cardiac arrest leads to an almost immediate concomitant drop in both serum and marrow pH due to increased lactate production associated with reduced blood oxygenation and increased anaerobic metabolism. This acidotic state within the bone marrow persists even after serum pH has recovered during continued resuscitation [53].

After the initial dose of IO lidocaine has been administered, frequent reassess-ment of pain is recommended as the analgesic effect of the initial dose is of variable magnitude and duration. While some authors recommend that subsequent lidocaine doses should be half the original IO dose (e.g., 20 mg with an initial 40 mg dose), this recommendation is not evidence based [59]. Regardless of the initial dose used, repeat lidocaine dosing during prolonged IO infusion appears to be important to the control of IO infusion pain [3]. This may be due to infusates opening new pathways within the medullary space that were previously inaccessible and thus not anesthe-tized by the initial dose of lidocaine [3]. Systemic pain control may be considered for patients requiring IO infusion who are not responsive to IO lidocaine. However, lidocaine dosing should not exceed 3 mg/kg in order to avoid lidocaine toxicity [60].

One recent study compared pain from continuous IO infusion of normal saline among healthy adult volunteers at various anatomic insertion sites with varying infusion pressures (ranging from 100 to 300 mmHg) and lidocaine dosing regimens [3]. In this study, all subjects were given an initial IO lidocaine bolus (either 40 or

80 mg) followed by a rapid saline flush and immediate additional 20 mg lidocaine dose. Most (8/10, or 80%) of the tibial IO patients required frequent additional 20 mg aliquots of IO lidocaine at regular intervals (mean 39 ± 20 min) during the 90-min observation period to maintain a pain visual analog scale (VAS) score < 5 [3]. Interestingly, none of the patients receiving humeral IO infusion required more than the initial two lidocaine boluses, and infusion at the humerus was consistently associated with less infusion pain than the tibia (4.4 ± 2.6 VAS for 40 mg initial bolus vs. 3.6 ± 2.3 VAS for 80 mg bolus at the tibia, 3.0 ± 1.5 VAS for 40 mg bolus at the humerus). Although the authors concluded that there was no difference in pain control between the 40 and 80 mg initial boluses, absolute pain scores were clearly lower in the 80 mg group. One clear conclusion that can be drawn from this study is the importance of additional (even planned) IO lidocaine administration after the flush following initial IO lidocaine bolus.

Tetracaine, another ester-type local anesthetic, is considerably more lipophilic than lidocaine, resulting in increased binding of the drug at the site of the injection, prolonged duration of effect, and less systemic uptake than lidocaine when administered topically [71]. A topical anesthetic patch with 70 mg each of lidocaine and tetracaine has been found to be at least as good as intradermal injection of lidocaine for analgesia with arterial catheter insertion [72], although it is unknown whether dermal application of local analgesics could improve pain related to periosteal or intramedullary stimuli associated with IO catheter use. While tetracaine has been administered intravenously [73], this drug is generally used as a topical anesthetic. Thus, the potential use of tetracaine for the treatment of IO infusion pain has not yet been explored.

Bupivacaine is an amide-type local anesthetic that may be of some value in providing IO analgesia. Widely used for obstetrical procedures, the primary risk of this drug is its potential cardiotoxicity [73]. **Levobupivacaine** (the pure S-enantiomer of bupivacaine) has recently been developed and may be safer than racemic bupivacaine with fewer adverse cardiac reactions [74]. The onset of action for bupivacaine is 5–10 min [73], considerably slower than that for lidocaine (<2 min), which may limit its utility for this indication [75]. In patients undergoing abdominal and thoracic surgery, 0.5% bupivacaine provides excellent sensory anesthesia with increased duration of action, reducing the need for postoperative analgesic medications [73]. When used for ulnar nerve block, 0.25% and 0.5% bupivacaine solutions provide excellent sensory and sympathetic anesthesia without complete motor paralysis [73]. In an intravenous regional anesthetic setting, bupivacaine is highly bound to non-albumin plasma proteins; when unbound, bupivacaine can induce toxic reactions [73]. However, this increased potential for bupivacaine toxicity is rarely achieved due to erythrocyte-binding sites readily absorbing the displaced drug [73].

As local anesthetics generally function by blocking voltage-gated sodium channels to abolish the propagation of action potentials in nerve cells, symptoms of toxicity predominantly arise in the central nervous and myocardial conduction systems [76]. Early neurological symptoms of LA toxicity include circumoral numbness, metallic taste, lightheadedness, dizziness, auditory and visual disturbances, disorientation, and drowsiness. More severe cardiovascular symptoms manifest as arrhythmias, bradycardia, hypotension, cardiac arrest, and respiratory arrest [77].

The potential for systemic toxicity with local anesthetics is increased with high plasma concentrations of these medications. When used in peripheral nerve blocks, the rate at which LAs enter the systemic circulation is dependent largely upon blood flow to the area of injection. With those applications, the potential for LA toxicity can be decreased by administering these medications with vasoconstrictors such as epinephrine that reduce blood flow to the injection site [76]. However, additional caution must be taken when injecting LAs into the medullary space during IO cannulation. Given direct communication of the intramedullary space with the systemic circulation, high plasma levels of LA are achieved at a much faster rate than with peripheral nerve blocks. As such, severe symptoms such as seizures, loss of consciousness, and rarely cardiovascular collapse can occur in the absence of more mild central nervous system symptoms listed earlier [78]. To avoid such symptoms, IO lidocaine infusion should not exceed safe limits, previously reported to be 300 mg/h in patients with uncompromised hepatic clearance [60].

Physicians are encouraged to inform patients of the possible toxic side effects of LA infusion through an IO device and to frequently monitor patients for neurologic changes such as dysarthria and altered mental status during and after infusion. Clinicians should also administer the lowest possible LA dose that is able to control the patient's pain. Additional caution should be taken in those patients with cardiovascular disease, liver disease, low body mass, or advanced age as all of these factors increase the risk for LA toxicity. Should complications arise, the administration of LA should be immediately discontinued, and efforts to secure the patient's airway and stabilize circulation should be initiated. For serious central nervous system manifestations such as seizures, the immediate administration of benzodiazepines is generally considered first-line abortive therapy [77].

When considering local anesthetic systemic toxicity (LAST), the **cardiovascular collapse:central nervous system (CC:CNS) ratio** is a commonly used value that compares the local anesthetic dose required to induce cardiac arrest to the dose required to induce seizures [79]. Drugs with a high CC:CNS ratio are generally safe, as evidence of early toxicity (e.g., seizures) occurs at much lower levels of overdose than cardiac arrest. Bupivacaine has among the lowest CC:CNS ratio of all local anesthetics, suggesting a relatively high risk of cardiotoxicity compared to lidocaine and most other commonly-used anesthetics [80]. However, a **combination of lidocaine and levobupivacaine** (or other local anesthetics) might provide rapid-onset and long-duration analgesia while avoiding toxic side effects from either drug [81]. Some characteristics of various local anesthetics are provided in Table 10.1.

Table 10.1 Characteristics of various commonly used local anesthetics [82–84]

Local anesthetic	Type	pKa	Potency	Protein binding (%)	Non-ionized fraction[a]	CC:CNS ratio
Benzocaine	Ester	2.5	0.1	n/a	n/a	n/a
Chloroprocaine	Ester	8.7	0.5	Low (n/a)	5	n/a
Cocaine	Ester	8.6	1	95	n/a	n/a
Procaine	Ester	8.9	0.5	6	3	n/a
Tetracaine	Ester	8.4	4	75	7	n/a
Articaine	Amide	7.8	1.5	70	n/a	n/a
Bupivacaine	Amide	8.1	4	95	17	2
Levobupivacaine	Amide	8.1	4	95	17	2
Lidocaine	Amide	7.9	1	70	25	7.1
Mepivacaine	Amide	7.7	1	77	39	7.1
Prilocaine	Amide	7.9	1	55	24	n/a
Ropivacaine	Amide	8.1	4	94	17	2

Notes: pKa provided is at 25 °C; potency is relative to lidocaine (1). *n/a* not available; *CC:CNS* cardiovascular collapse:central nervous system ratio
[a] Physiologic pH 7.4

Future Directions

Distraction Techniques

The use of **distraction techniques** has already been shown to be effective in reducing pain perception for pediatric subjects receiving peripheral IV insertion and immunization [85–87], although targeted studies on the use of these techniques for adults or those undergoing IO insertion have not yet been reported.

Distraction techniques can be used to reduce pain perception by reducing activity in the areas of the brain responsible for processing painful stimuli, including the insula, midcingulate, thalamus, and anterior cingulate gyrus [88, 89]. Increased cognitive engagement with distracting stimuli has been shown to inversely correlate with subjective pain ratings [88]. In order to maximize engagement, these techniques should be tailored to suit the age and maturity level of the patient. Previously reported techniques include interactive toys and games, music, and television [90]. In theory, **active** forms of distraction (e.g., toys and games) should result in better pain control than **passive** forms (e.g., music, television) as they involve higher levels of cognitive engagement [91, 92], but the results of comparative studies are inconsistent [90]. One recent study showed that an interactive storybook resulted in better pain control among pediatric patients undergoing Port-a-Cath® and Hickman line access procedures than watching movies [93]. In contrast, another group found that movies provided more effective pain control than interactive robots among children undergoing peripheral venipuncture [94].

In recent years, **virtual reality** (VR) has emerged as a promising candidate for the reduction of pain perception in both adult and pediatric populations. This technique can involve the use of a headset worn by the patient to create a virtual world in which the patient can interact. One VR application named SnowWorld™ (Imprint

Table 10.2 Distraction techniques, with associated benefits and drawbacks

Distraction technique	Benefits	Drawbacks
Music	Wide choice selection, quick implementation, patient choice	Passive technique
Movies	Wide choice selection, shown to perform well, quick implementation, patient choice	Passive technique
Interactive toys/games	Implemented quickly, interactive (visual, auditory, and tactile stimulation), patient choice	Weakest active technique
Virtual reality headset	Outperforms all other active techniques, fully immersive	Novel, limited literature, time intensive, costly

Interactive Technology, Seattle, Washington) allows patients to virtually enter an icy canyon and interact with penguins, snowmen, and other characters via the use of a one-handed controller [95]. Patients have the ability to choose a wide variety of different "worlds" and games to interact with. In one study, the use of VR was shown to decrease the average fear level associated with receiving an immunization by 77% as perceived by the child's parent. In the same study, average anticipated pain perceived by the parent was decreased by 83%, and overall pain score decreased by 77% [96]. The use of VR applications has also been shown to reduce mental stress and pain perception during dental treatments, chemotherapy, venipuncture, and long-term hospitalization [96–98] and may be more effective than other active distraction methods [99]. The use of eye-tracking software with VR applications may increase cognitive engagement, further augmenting this effect [100]. As IO infusion is often required for emergent conditions, clinicians must minimize the amount of time taken in choosing a distracting stimulus while maximizing its compatibility with a child's age and maturity level in order to ensure optimal cognitive engagement. Smartphones and other portable media devices may be of great use in this context as they allow for the use of multiple types of media such as movies, music, and interactive games. Parents, caregivers, and/or pediatric patients themselves should be involved in the selection of the distracting stimulus whenever possible in order to tailor treatment to individual preferences. Common pediatric distraction techniques as well as their associated benefits and drawbacks are listed in Table 10.2.

Regional Nerve Blocks to the Shoulder and Tibia

Peripheral nerve blocks are of particular interest in the management of IO catheter-related pain. Anatomically, the **popliteal** and **femoral nerve blocks** may be most applicable to tibial IO catheterization, while **brachial plexus nerve blocks** may be considered at the humeral insertion site. Nerve block procedures are already commonly used to provide procedural, intraoperative, and postoperative pain control in the upper and lower extremities, making this an enticing treatment modality for controlling IO catheter-related pain. While the efficacy of these procedures for the treatment of IO catheter-associated pain has not yet been studied, in this chapter, we will discuss current evidence regarding their analgesic efficacy as well as applications and techniques surrounding their use.

Peripheral nerve blocks are commonly utilized in the treatment of both acute and chronic pain. In comparison to simple local tissue infiltration by the anesthetic agent, peripheral nerve blocks are advantageous in that by injecting the agent directly adjacent to or into the **peripheral nerve sheath**, a large area of blockade is achieved corresponding to the distribution of nerve fibers distal to the site of injection. For example, a femoral nerve block will follow the distribution of its nerve supply, resulting in anesthesia of the entire anterior portion of the thigh as well as the medial upper and lower leg [101].

Once the local anesthetic has been injected adjacent to the peripheral nerve, certain factors affect the volume of anesthetic that is able to reach the site of action (i.e., the inner pore of the voltage-gated sodium channel). The first is **relative mass**, defined as the mass of the nerve in relation to the mass of the tissues surrounding the volume of the local anesthetic agent injected [102]. Local anesthetic must equilibrate between all tissues, and with the mass of other tissues ranging between five and ten times more than that of the nerve, only a small amount of injected anesthetic will actually reach the nerve [102]. Thus, when targeting a nerve within a larger space, a larger volume of anesthetic is required. Additionally, the thickness of the fascial sheath surrounding the nerve directly correlates with the amount of local anesthetic needed to provide an effective block [102]. This is because the local anesthetic must diffuse through the perineurium surrounding the nerve fascicles [102]. A visual depiction of the fascial layers associated with peripheral nerves is shown in Fig. 10.8. As this figure depicts, each individual nerve fiber is surrounded by a connective tissue layer (i.e., endoneurium). Bundles of these individual nerve fibers are then surrounded by another layer of connective tissue (i.e., perineurium), forming the nerve fascicle. Bundles of nerve fascicles are then encased by a final layer of connective tissue (i.e., the epineurium), which surrounds the entire nerve. Blood vessels providing nutrients to the nerve are found within the perineurial and epineurial layers, as illustrated in Fig. 10.8.

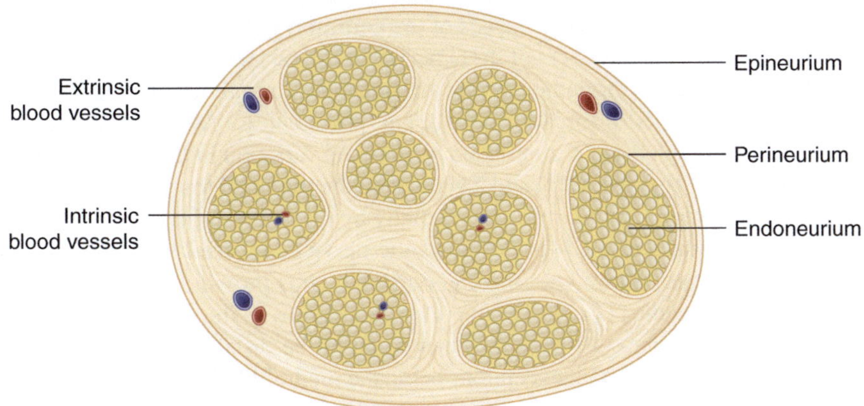

Fig. 10.8 Fascial layers of the peripheral nerve

Table 10.3 Comparison of various common local anesthetics used for peripheral nerve blockade

Anesthetic	Onset (min)	Duration of anesthesia (h)	Duration of analgesia (h)	Maximum dose (mg/kg without/ with epi)
Lidocaine (2%)	10–20 [105–107]	2–5 [105, 107]	3–8 [105]	4.5/7 [105]
Mepivacaine (1.5%)	10–20 [105, 108]	2–5 [105, 108]	3–10 [105, 108]	5/7 [105]
Ropivacaine (0.2%)	10–30 [105, 109]	4–6 [105]	5–16 [105, 109]	3/3.5 [105]
Ropivacaine (0.5%)	10–30 [105, 110]	4–12 [105, 110]	5–24 [105]	3/3.5 [105]
Bupivacaine (0.25%)	15–30 [105]	4–12 [111]	5–26 [105]	2.5/3 [105]
Bupivacaine (0.5%)	10–30 [110, 112]	4–20 [110, 112]	10–17 [112]	2.5/3 [105]
Bupivacaine (0.5%) with epinephrine	15–30 [105]	5–15 [105]	6–30 [105, 113]	2.5/3 [105]

The vascularity of the surrounding tissue also influences the amount of local anesthetic that ultimately reaches the nerve [102]. The more vascularized an area is, the faster the local anesthetic is absorbed and cleared from the area [102]. Although the use of epinephrine is not recommended for the IO infusion of local anesthetics, it is frequently employed in peripheral nerve blocks. As discussed above, epinephrine's vasoconstrictive effects reduce blood flow to the injection site, thus allowing more of the anesthetic to reach the nerve while reducing the risk of systemic toxicity [76]. In addition to the use of epinephrine, the effectiveness of peripheral nerve blockade may also be enhanced by combining multiple local anesthetics to achieve both immediate and long-lasting analgesia. Enhanced onset and duration of drug effect have been reported for combinations of lidocaine and bupivacaine over those associated with either anesthetic agent alone [103, 104]. The properties of various local anesthetics can be found in Table 10.3.

Popliteal and Femoral Nerve Blocks

The **popliteal nerve block** provides analgesia to the **sciatic nerve** at the level of the popliteal fossa, which is responsible for sensory and motor innervation to most of the lower leg. The sciatic nerve consists of the **common peroneal nerve** (CPN) and **tibial nerve** (TN) with the fibers of these nerves arranged laterally to medially [114, 115]. These fibers travel together in this arrangement throughout the course of the sciatic nerve until its bifurcation 6–10 cm proximal to the popliteal crease (Fig. 10.12), although there is significant anatomical variation in the location of this bifurcation [114, 116]. The CPN and TN traverse the popliteal fossa, bounded laterally by the **biceps femoris tendon** and medially by the **semitendinosus tendon** and **semimembranosus tendon** [114]. The sciatic nerve is encased by a **paraneural sheath** which divides along with the CPN and TN, thus providing them with their own paraneural sheaths [117, 118]. The relevant anatomy is illustrated in Fig. 10.9.

The sciatic nerve provides sensory innervation to the distal femur and all bones below the knee with important exceptions being the **medial tibial plateau** and medial malleolus, which are innervated by the **femoral nerve** (FN) (Fig. 10.10) [114]. This osteotomal distribution is of great significance to the placement of proximal tibial IO catheters as the insertion site is located 2 cm (i.e., two finger widths) inferior to the

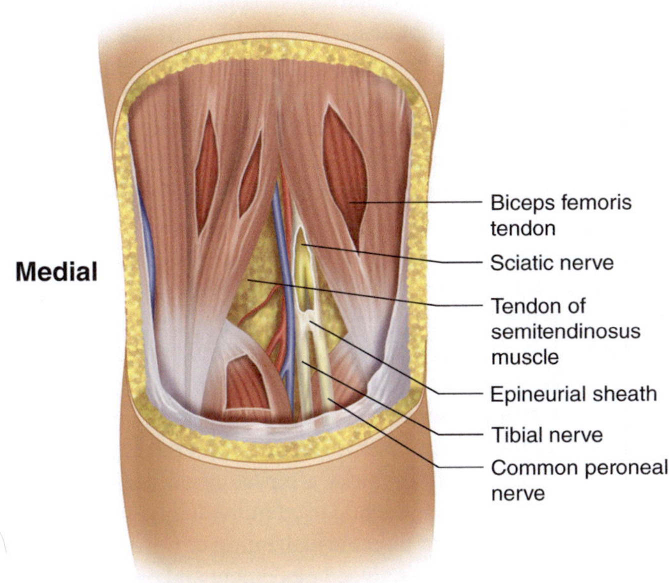

Fig. 10.9 Anatomy of the sciatic nerve at the level of the popliteal fossa

Fig. 10.10 Osteotomes of the distal lower extremity, with the proximal tibia IO insertion site marked with a red dot

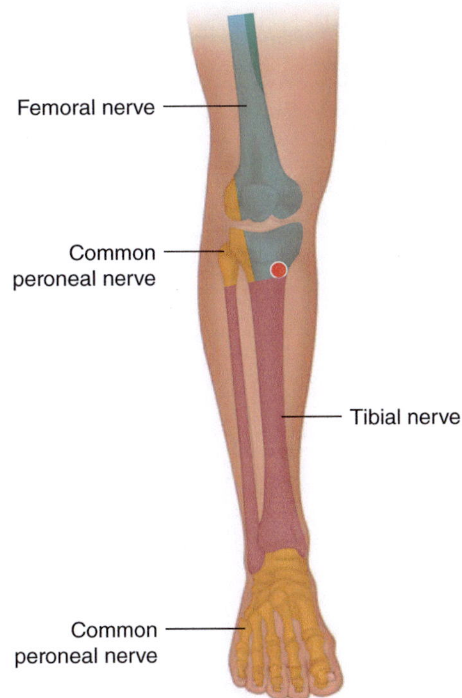

patella and 2 cm medial to the tibial tuberosity in adults, corresponding anatomically to the location of the medial tibial plateau (Fig. 10.13) [15]. As the proximal tibia IO insertion site lies at the junction between the common peroneal and femoral nerve osteotomes, both the popliteal and femoral nerve blocks could be considered to provide analgesia at this insertion site. Femoral nerve blocks can provide additional cutaneous pain control at the insertion site as its saphenous nerve branch provides cutaneous innervation over the anteromedial medial aspect of the lower leg [119].

The FN courses inferior to the inguinal ligament and enters the thigh via the **femoral triangle**, which is formed by the **sartorius muscle** (laterally), **adductor longus muscle** (medially), and **inguinal ligament** (superiorly) [119]. Blockade of the FN is achieved by ultrasound guidance with the ultrasound probe placed over the inguinal crease allowing for visualization of the FN within the femoral triangle (Fig. 10.11) [120]. As shown in the figure, after ultrasound identification of the femoral nerve, the nerve block needle is introduced lateral to medial depositing the anesthetic just lateral to the femoral nerve (identified in the Figure with an X).

Both femoral and popliteal nerve blocks are performed using guidance by **ultrasound** or **nerve stimulation**, which may be used individually or in combination [114, 120]. Because ultrasound allows for direct visualization of the target nerve, it is associated with higher block success rates, reduced placement and onset time, and decreased risk of vascular puncture [118, 121]. Nerve stimulation can be used to confirm the success of an ultrasound-guided block or used if the desired nerve is poorly visible on ultrasound. Both the femoral triangle and popliteal fossa are readily accessible with the

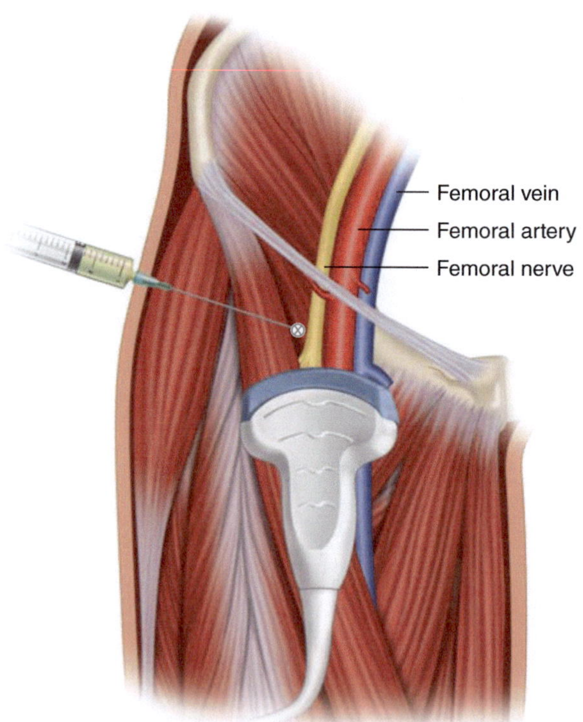

Fig. 10.11 Femoral triangle with ultrasound probe and needle placement for femoral nerve block

patient in the supine position and the leg elevated and slightly flexed at the knee [114]. The choice of local anesthetic used for the block is based upon the desired onset of action and duration of sensory and/or motor blockade. For continuous block, a catheter infusing local anesthetic may be placed to extend block duration.

Popliteal and femoral nerve blocks are commonly utilized procedures that provide considerable pain relief in the lower extremity for surgical procedures, fractures, and severe pain associated with conditions such as critical limb ischemia and complex regional pain syndrome [122–125]. The effectiveness of these peripheral nerve blocks across a wide range of painful conditions makes them promising candidates for treating IO catheter-related pain. Moreover, this approach to pain relief has considerable potential advantages over IO lidocaine infusion such as long durations of analgesia with a single injection that cannot be "washed out" of the intramedullary space during continuous fluid infusion, as well as the potential for motor blockade which limits lower extremity movement that can lead to painful dislodgment of the IO catheter. Future studies are needed to formally assess the clinical efficacy and utility of peripheral nerve blocks with tibial IO cannulation.

Brachial Plexus Nerve Block

Sensory and motor innervation of the upper extremity is provided by the **brachial plexus**, which is anatomically divided into **roots, trunks, divisions, cords**, and **branches** [126]. The nerve roots are located adjacent to the transverse processes of the cervical spine and posterior to the vertebral artery [126]. The nerve roots continue as the superior (C5, C6), middle (C7), and inferior trunks (C8, T1) as they pass between the middle and anterior scalene muscles [126]. Behind the clavicle, each trunk divides into anterior and posterior divisions, which correspond to the ventral and dorsal aspects of the upper extremity, respectively [126]. As these trunks pass over the first rib, they form the anterior, posterior, and lateral cords corresponding to their positions relative to the axillary artery [126]. The terminal nerve branches that arise from the cords mainly responsible for innervation of the humerus are the axillary nerve (C5, C6), suprascapular nerve (C5, C6), radial nerve (C5–T1), and musculocutaneous nerve (C5–C7) [127].

There are several levels at which the brachial plexus may be blocked. Approaches include **interscalene block, supraclavicular block, infraclavicular block**, and **axillary block** [127]. Each of these approaches targets different anatomical portions of the brachial plexus, which correspond to different distributions of nerve block. As it pertains to IO catheter-related pain, interscalene, supraclavicular, and infraclavicular blocks are the most appropriate candidates for pain control as they target both the IO insertion site and diaphysis of the humerus. While axillary block provides analgesia to the proximal diaphysis and distal humerus, the IO insertion site at the proximal humerus is spared making it ineffective for use in this application. This is because the axillary approach introduces anesthetic at the level of the brachial plexus nerve branches, distal to where the axillary nerve branches off from the posterior cord. Various potential sites for a brachial plexus block are illustrated in Fig. 10.12. In the figure, the portions highlighted in red, purple, green, and blue

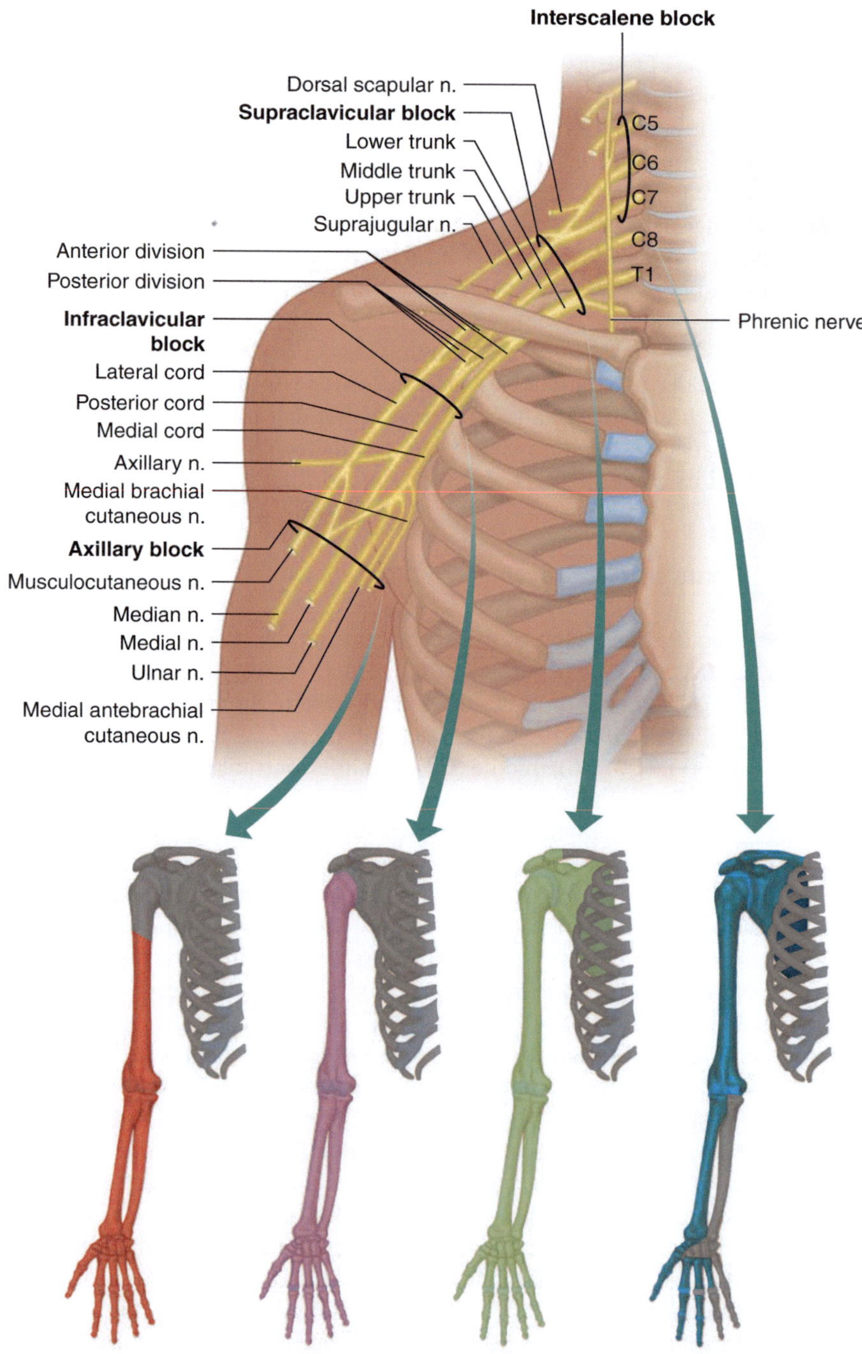

Fig. 10.12 Various approaches to brachial plexus block

represent the bony structures that are anesthetized with axillary, infraclavicular, supraclavicular, and interscalene nerve blocks, respectively.

The osteotomal distribution of these nerves along the humerus is shown in Fig. 10.13. The **axillary nerve** innervates the proximal humerus down to the surgical neck [127]. The (anterior) proximal and distal midshaft of the humerus are innervated by the **radial** and **musculocutaneous nerves**, respectively [127]. The IO insertion site at the greater tuberosity of the proximal humerus is located 1–2 cm above the surgical neck of the humerus, at the most prominent aspect of the greater tubercle [121]. Thus, anesthetization at the insertion site correlates to blockade of the axillary nerve, while intramedullary infusion pain is accomplished via block of the radial and musculocutaneous nerves.

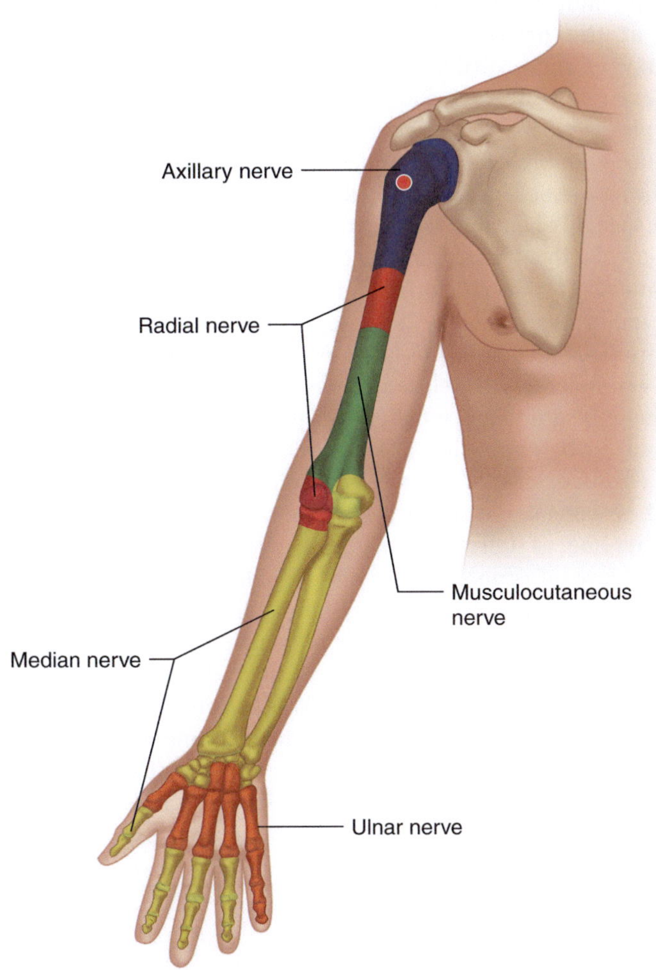

Fig. 10.13 Osteotomes of the upper extremity

Systematic reviews comparing interscalene and periclavicular blocks have shown comparable efficacy in pain control between these approaches [128, 129]. Consequently, factors such as complications, desired duration of block, and degree of technical difficulty may be more pertinent in choosing the best approach for IO catheter-related pain. Current data shows that the rate of complications such as hemidiaphragmatic paresis (due to unintended anesthetization of the phrenic nerve) and Horner's syndrome is significantly lower when using a periclavicular (as opposed to an interscalene) approach [128]. Because of the proximity to the lung cupula and pleura in the supraclavicular and infraclavicular approaches, respectively, there is a significant risk of puncturing the lung and producing a pneumothorax using either technique if needle insertion during the blockade attempt is not precisely controlled [129]. **Current complications data support the use of the periclavicular (specifically, the infraclavicular) approach rather than the interscalene approach for regional anesthesia at the proximal humerus** [129]. However, the infraclavicular approach may be more difficult to administer in patients with large pectoral muscles or excessive breast tissue [129].

Brachial plexus blocks may be performed using either ultrasound or nerve stimulation guidance with higher success rates and decreased complication rates associated with the combined use of both techniques [130]. The inclusion of motor blockade is especially beneficial for proximal humeral IO catheters, as this insertion site is associated with an increased risk of bending or dislodgement of the IO catheter if the patient lifts the catheterized arm over their head. Isolated sensory blockade without motor blockade may increase this risk as patients may not experience pain as the inserted catheter begins to be levered out of the bone.

Table 10.4 summarizes the relevant nerve blocks that may be used to control pain from IO catheter insertion and infusion in sensate patients.

To conclude, when choosing a peripheral nerve block for IO analgesia, the distribution of block, ease of access to the injection site, and potential complications should be considered. For tibial analgesia, popliteal nerve block may be considered first line, as it provides analgesia to the tibial shaft, thus reducing pain from high-pressure infusion. Femoral nerve block can be considered as an adjunct as it provides analgesia to the medial tibial plateau, where the proximal tibia IO catheter is inserted. Femoral nerve block may also provide motor paralysis at the quadriceps muscles, reducing the risk for catheter dislodgement with movement of the knee joint. For humeral IO analgesia, a periclavicular (supra- or infraclavicular) approach may be preferred given its lower complication rate compared to interscalene blocks and analgesia of the humeral head that is not accomplished with axillary blocks [128]. Additionally, the clavicle serves as a prominent bony landmark that is more easily found and may be more accessible than the sternocleidomastoid muscle and axillary fossa in interscalene and axillary nerve blocks, respectively.

Table 10.4 Summary of nerve blocks relevant to analgesia for intraosseous catheter insertion

Nerve block	Insertion site	Sensory/motor blockade	Benefits	Drawbacks
Popliteal nerve	Popliteal fossa, midway between the tendons of the biceps femoris and semitendinosus muscles [131]	**Sensory**: Entire distal two-thirds of the lower extremity with the notable exception of the medial tibial plateau [131] **Motor**: Most of the entire lower leg [131]	Proven effective modality for anesthesia and analgesia for a wide variety of surgical procedures below the knee	Medial tibial plateau remains unanesthetized with isolated popliteal nerve block. Patient at risk for falls due to motor blockade
Femoral nerve	Just below the inguinal crease, 1–2 cm lateral to the pulse of the femoral artery [101]	**Sensory**: Anterior and medial thigh, medial lower leg, medial foot, femur, and proximal medial tibia [101] **Motor**: Quadriceps muscles [101]	Motor blockade at the knee joint helps prevent dislodgement of IO catheter due to patient movement	Tibial shaft remains unanesthetized. Patient at risk for falls due to motor blockade
Interscalene nerve	Interscalene groove, located between the anterior and middle scalene muscles [132]	**Sensory**: Lateral aspect of the upper and lower arm (cutaneous), humerus, and radius [132] **Motor**: Deltoid, teres major, rotator cuff muscles [132]	Motor blockade at shoulder joint helps prevent dislodgement of the IO catheter with patient movement	Complications include spinal, epidural, and/or vertebral artery injection; pneumothorax; Horner's syndrome
Supraclavicular nerve	Just above the midpoint of the clavicle, 2.5 cm lateral to the insertion of the sternocleidomastoid muscle to the mid-clavicle [133]	**Sensory**: Entire upper extremity [133] **Motor**: Entire upper extremity [133]	Rate of complications lower than interscalene approach. Motor blockade helps prevent dislodgement of IO catheter due to patient movement	Complications include phrenic nerve block with diaphragmatic paralysis, pneumothorax, and Horner's syndrome
Infraclavicular nerve	3 cm below the midpoint of the clavicle [134]	**Sensory**: The entire upper extremity [134] **Motor**: Entire upper extremity [134]	Rate of complications lower than interscalene approach. Motor blockade helps prevent dislodgement of the IO catheter due to patient movement	Complications include phrenic nerve block with diaphragmatic paralysis, pneumothorax, and Horner's syndrome
Axillary nerve	Above and/or below the axillary artery [135]	**Sensory**: From mid-arm down to and including hand [135] **Motor**: Entire upper extremity except deltoid and teres minor [135]	Avoidance of major structures encountered in interscalene and periclavicular nerve blocks	No blockade provided to IO insertion site at the proximal humerus. Note that the name of the block is due to the location of its approach, rather than blockade of the axillary nerve itself

Systemic Analgesia and Anxiolysis

Patients who require intraosseous vascular access often have painful or anxiety-provoking medical conditions that may benefit from systemic analgesic or anxiolytic medication administration. When administered through the IO catheter, it is likely that these medications will have specific local effects on the intramedullary environment as well.

The only prospective, randomized crossover pharmacokinetic study done to date studying IO infusion of a medication in human subjects was published in 2008 [136]. In this crossover study, subjects were randomized to either IO or peripheral IV infusion of a 5 mg bolus of morphine sulfate, followed 24 h later by an equal infusion of medication through the other route. The authors found that most pharmacokinetic parameters were equal between access routes, although there was a statistically significant difference in the volume of distribution in the central compartment [136]. This difference was attributed by the authors to a local deposition effect near the intraosseous access port or within the bone marrow. However, volume of distribution at steady state had no statistical difference indicating that the amount of residual morphine was minimal [136].

Within usual therapeutic dosing range, only 20–35% of circulating morphine binds to plasma proteins [137], as morphine (and the related drug, hydromorphone) is hydrophilic without a high affinity for lipid binding [150]. In contrast, fentanyl and related derivative opioids are more lipophilic [138], which may lead to a larger depot effect when infused directly into the lipid-rich intraosseous environment. Whether this increased IO lipid binding may provide some analgesic effect relating to pain experienced with subsequent IO infusion is unknown, and speculation about a potentially diminished systemic effect for IO fentanyl compared to IV infusion is currently without any scientific basis.

Morphine has previously been shown to vasodilate both veins and arteries when administered through the IV route [138, 139], although it is not clear to what degree this effect may influence egress from the intramedullary space. This vasodilatory effect appears to be mediated by histamine and nitric oxide [140], which introduces the possibility that administration of other IO drugs affecting local concentrations of these intermediaries may further influence any local effect on IO blood flow. It appears likely that fentanyl has a similar ability to induce local vasodilation [141], although the relative degree to which various opioids influence local vascular tone remains unclear. Naloxone, a potent opioid antagonist commonly used to reverse opiate toxicity, has been shown to be effective when administered by the IO route [142], although this drug is highly lipophilic [143]. This high degree of lipid binding gives naloxone a brain-to-serum ratio 12–15 times greater than morphine, but may theoretically contribute to a depot effect when administered via IO infusion requiring higher doses to achieve a desired plasma concentration [143]. Some studies have suggested that naloxone may interfere to some degree with granulocytopoiesis within the bone marrow [144], although subsequent animal studies have suggested that this effect is likely minimal [145].

One double-blind, randomized controlled trial of intraoperative IO versus IV infusion of a 10 mg morphine bolus during total knee arthroplasty demonstrated an average decrease of two points on the Visual Analog Scale (VAS) pain score in favor of patients who received the IO morphine infusion, with reduced opioid requirements up to 2 weeks postoperatively and improved functional and other clinical outcomes [146]. This study also showed lower serum morphine concentrations at 15 min and 10 h post-infusion in the IO group, supporting the conclusion that IO-infused morphine may be less bioavailable within the bloodstream than IV-infused morphine despite these favorable clinical effects [146]. This finding suggests that IO morphine may be more efficacious in the treatment of locally induced painful stimuli at or near the IO insertion site (e.g., IO infusion pain) than IV morphine.

The infusion of local anesthetics at doses higher than those currently recommended for local IO insertion analgesia may have beneficial effects for both local and nonlocal pain. Due to its favorable safety profile, lidocaine infusion for the treatment of acute and chronic pain has been extensively studied and found to significantly reduce pain from chronic daily headaches, fibromyalgia, and lumbago in doses ranging from 0.5 to 3.0 mg/kg/h [147]. Long-term follow-up of patients experiencing daily headaches indicated that their pain was less severe and 51% of patients no longer experienced chronic daily headaches [147]. Pain control with IV lidocaine was found to be greater than that provided by standard-of-care interventions, including high-flow oxygen therapy, corticosteroids, and triptans [147]. Rare side effects including nausea and mild hypotension did not lead to discontinuation of treatment. Due to toxicity concerns, advocates for IV lidocaine therapy recommend avoidance of cumulative doses in excess of a plasma concentration of 5–8 mcg/mL or 4.5 mg/kg [148]. Postoperative IV lidocaine administration following bowel surgery has been shown to improve postoperative bowel function, decrease opioid consumption, reduce hyperalgesia, and provide an anti-inflammatory effect by reducing the concentration of circulating cytokines [149, 150].

Conclusions

Pain control remains a major limitation to the use of intraosseous infusion in clinical practice, especially for awake, sensate patients. Unfortunately, most published reports of IO use have focused primarily on user-centered outcomes such as ease of use and rates of successful placement, with very limited attention paid to patient-centered outcomes such as pain perception and success with strategies to mitigate pain associated with IO infusion. Despite recent advances in IO catheter design and improved placement success rates, research into pain control with IO infusion predominantly relates to the use of IO lidocaine, which has been shown to be variably effective with awake patients. Future directions for research into more effective pain control methods may include exploration of alternative local analgesics, increased use of morphine or other systemic analgesics with potential local analgesic advantages, and non-pharmacologic methods. More research is needed to describe the efficacy of current pain control techniques, with a focus on the local effects of various medications infused through the IO route. The potential for depot effect of certain medications should be studied, especially how these drug characteristics may influence factors modulating pain perception in human subjects.

Key Concepts

- Pain is a major drawback to the use of IO devices for pressurized infusion, largely limiting its use in sensate patients.
- Mechanical disruption of the periosteal nerve meshwork is primarily responsible for the acute, sharp, stabbing pain associated with initial IO catheter insertion. By contrast, pressure-sensing nerve endings within the medullary space are responsible for the dull, aching pain associated with subsequent IO infusion.
- The injection of 2% lidocaine (preservative free and epinephrine free) through the IO catheter after placement remains standard practice for pain control with IO infusion. However, providers must be cautious to avoid toxicity associated with excessive IO doses of local anesthetics.
- As pediatric populations are particularly susceptible to pain, the utilization of distraction techniques and other non-pharmacologic methods may be beneficial to improving the quality of analgesia during IO catheter insertion and infusion.
- While the proximal tibia is the most commonly utilized IO insertion site, other sites (especially the sternum and proximal humerus) may be associated with a more favorable pain profile.
- Experimental modalities yet to be fully explored for use with IO infusion pain may include the use of alternative local anesthetic agents, peripheral nerve blocks, and use of bicarbonate-buffered or viscous lidocaine formulations.

References

1. Paxton JH, Knuth TE, Klausner HA. Proximal humerus intraosseous infusion: a preferred emergency venous access. J Trauma. 2009;67(3):606–11. https://doi.org/10.1097/TA.0b013e3181b16f42.
2. Horton MA, Beamer C. Powered intraosseous insertion provides safe and effective vascular access for pediatric emergency patients. Pediatr Emerg Care. 2008;24(6):347–50. https://doi.org/10.1097/PEC.0b013e318177a6fe.
3. Philbeck TE, Miller LJ, Montez D, Puga T. Hurts so good. Easing IO pain and pressure. JEMS. 2010;35(9):58–69. https://doi.org/10.1016/S0197-2510(10)70232-1.
4. Chreiman KM, Dumas RP, Seamon MJ, et al. The intraosseous have it: a prospective observational study of vascular access success rates in patients in extremis using video review. J Trauma Acute Care Surg. 2018;84(4):558–63. https://doi.org/10.1097/TA.0000000000001795.
5. Feldman O, Nasrallah N, Bitterman Y, et al. Pediatric intraosseous access performed by emergency department nurses using semiautomatic devices: a randomized crossover simulation study. Pediatr Emerg Care. 2021;37(9):442–6. https://doi.org/10.1097/PEC.0000000000001621.
6. Ngo AS, Oh JJ, Chen Y, Yong D, Ong ME. Intraosseous vascular access in adults using the EZ-IO in an emergency department. Int J Emerg Med. 2009;2(3):155–60. https://doi.org/10.1007/s12245-009-0116-9.

7. Link MS, Berkow LC, Kudenchuk PJ, et al. Part 7: Adult advanced cardiovascular life support: 2015 American Heart Association guidelines update for cardiopulmonary resuscitation and emergency cardiovascular care [published correction appears in circulation. 2015 Dec 15;132(24):e385]. Circulation. 2015;132(18 Suppl 2):S444–64. https://doi.org/10.1161/CIR.0000000000000261.

8. Panchal AR, Berg KM, Kudenchuk PJ, et al. 2018 American Heart Association focused update on advanced cardiovascular life support use of antiarrhythmic drugs during and immediately after cardiac arrest: an update to the American Heart Association guidelines for cardiopulmonary resuscitation and emergency cardiovascular care. Circulation. 2018;138(23):e740–9. https://doi.org/10.1161/CIR.0000000000000613.

9. Subcommittee on Advanced Trauma Life Support (ATLS), American College of Surgeons (ACS), Committee on Trauma, 2017–2018. Advanced trauma life support course for physicians, vol. 2018. Chicago: Committee on Trauma, American College of Surgeons. p. 52.

10. Palazzolo A, Akers K, Paxton J. Complications of intraosseous catheterization in adult patients: a review of the literature. Curr Emerg Hosp Med Rep. 2023;11:1–14. https://doi.org/10.1007/s40138-023-00261-8.

11. Cooper BR, Mahoney PF, Hodgetts TJ, Mellor A. Intra-osseous access (EZ-IO) for resuscitation: UK military combat experience. J R Army Med Corps. 2007;153(4):314–6.

12. Ludwig PE, Reddy V, Varacallo M. Neuroanatomy, neurons. In: StatPearls. Treasure Island, FL: StatPearls Publishing; 2022. https://www.ncbi.nlm.nih.gov/books/NBK441977/. Accessed 10 July 2023.

13. Ashley K, Lui F. Physiology, nerve. In: StatPearls. Treasure Island, FL: StatPearls Publishing; 2022. https://www.ncbi.nlm.nih.gov/books/NBK551652/. Accessed 10 July 2023.

14. Morell P, Quarles RH. The myelin sheath. In: Siegel GJ, Agranoff BW, Albers RW, et al., editors. Basic neurochemistry: molecular, cellular and medical aspects. 6th ed. Philadelphia: Lippincott-Raven; 1999. https://www.ncbi.nlm.nih.gov/books/NBK27954/. Accessed 10 July 2023.

15. Kenney C, Paxton JH. Chapter 7: Intraosseous catheters. In: Paxton JH, editor. Emergent vascular access. Springer; 2021. p. 133–75.

16. Mach DB, Rogers SD, Sabino MC, et al. Origins of skeletal pain: sensory and sympathetic innervation of the mouse femur. Neuroscience. 2002;113(1):155–66. https://doi.org/10.1016/s0306-4522(02)00165-3.

17. Basbaum AI. Chapter 3. Basic mechanisms. In: Charles E, Argoff, McCleane G, editors. Pain management secrets. 3rd ed. Mosby; 2009. p. 19–26, ISBN 9780323040198. https://doi.org/10.1016/B978-0-323-04019-8.00003-2.

18. Steverink JG, Oostinga D, van Tol FR, et al. Sensory innervation of human bone: an immunohistochemical study to further understand bone pain. J Pain. 2021;22(11):1385–95. https://doi.org/10.1016/j.jpain.2021.04.006.

19. Martin CD, Jimenez-Andrade JM, Ghilardi JR, Mantyh PW. Organization of a unique net-like meshwork of CGRP+ sensory fibers in the mouse periosteum: implications for the generation and maintenance of bone fracture pain. Neurosci Lett. 2007;427(3):148–52. https://doi.org/10.1016/j.neulet.2007.08.055.

20. Jimenez-Andrade JM, Bloom AP, Mantyh WG, et al. Capsaicin-sensitive sensory nerve fibers contribute to the generation and maintenance of skeletal fracture pain. Neuroscience. 2009;162(4):1244–54. https://doi.org/10.1016/j.neuroscience.2009.05.065.

21. Thai J, Kyloh M, Travis L, Spencer NJ, Ivanusic JJ. Identifying spinal afferent (sensory) nerve endings that innervate the marrow cavity and periosteum using anterograde tracing. J Comp Neurol. 2020;528(11):1903–16. https://doi.org/10.1002/cne.24862.

22. Ivanusic JJ. Size, neurochemistry, and segmental distribution of sensory neurons innervating the rat tibia. J Comp Neurol. 2009;517(3):276–83. https://doi.org/10.1002/cne.22160.

23. Castañeda-Corral G, Jimenez-Andrade JM, Bloom AP, et al. The majority of myelinated and unmyelinated sensory nerve fibers that innervate bone express the tropomyosin receptor kinase a. Neuroscience. 2011;178:196–207. https://doi.org/10.1016/j.neuroscience.2011.01.039.

24. Jimenez-Andrade JM, Mantyh WG, Bloom AP, et al. A phenotypically restricted set of primary afferent nerve fibers innervate the bone versus skin: therapeutic opportunity for treating skeletal pain [published correction appears in Bone. 2010;46(6):1670-1]. Bone. 2010;46(2):306–13. https://doi.org/10.1016/j.bone.2009.09.013.

25. Zhen G, Fu Y, Zhang C, et al. Mechanisms of bone pain: progress in research from bench to bedside. Bone Res. 2022;10(1):44. https://doi.org/10.1038/s41413-022-00217-w.

26. Ivanusic JJ, Sahai V, Mahns DA. The cortical representation of sensory inputs arising from bone. Brain Res. 2009;1269:47–53. https://doi.org/10.1016/j.brainres.2009.03.001.

27. Haegerstam GA. Pathophysiology of bone pain: a review. Acta Orthop Scand. 2001;72:308–17.

28. Santy J, Mackintosh C. A phenomenological study of pain following fractured shaft of femur. J Clin Nurs. 2001;10(4):521–7. https://doi.org/10.1046/j.1365-2702.2001.00506.x.

29. Mahns DA, Ivanusic JJ, Sahai V, Rowe MJ. An intact peripheral nerve preparation for monitoring the activity of single, periosteal afferent nerve fibres. J Neurosci Methods. 2006;156(1–2):140–4. https://doi.org/10.1016/j.jneumeth.2006.02.019.

30. Oostinga D, Steverink JG, van Wijck AJM, Verlaan JJ. An understanding of bone pain: a narrative review. Bone. 2020;134:115272. https://doi.org/10.1016/j.bone.2020.115272.

31. Zhao J, Levy D. The sensory innervation of the calvarial periosteum is nociceptive and contributes to headache-like behavior. Pain. 2014;155(7):1392–400. https://doi.org/10.1016/j.pain.2014.04.019.

32. Ivanusic JJ. Molecular mechanisms that contribute to bone marrow pain. Front Neurol. 2017;8:458. https://doi.org/10.3389/fneur.2017.00458.

33. Luger NM, Mach DB, Sevcik MA, Mantyh PW. Bone cancer pain: from model to mechanism to therapy. J Pain Symptom Manag. 2005;29(5 Suppl):S32–46. https://doi.org/10.1016/j.jpainsymman.2005.01.008.

34. Nencini S, Ivanusic J. Mechanically sensitive Aδ nociceptors that innervate bone marrow respond to changes in intra-osseous pressure. J Physiol. 2017;595(13):4399–415. https://doi.org/10.1113/JP273877.

35. Nencini S, Ivanusic JJ. The physiology of bone pain. How much do we really know? Front Physiol. 2016;7:157. https://doi.org/10.3389/fphys.2016.00157.

36. De Lorenzo RA, Ward JA, Jordan BS, et al. Relationships of intraosseous and systemic pressure waveforms in a swine model. Acad Emerg Med. 2014;21(8):899–904.

37. Gurkan UA, Akkus O. The mechanical environment of bone marrow: a review. Ann Biomed Eng. 2008;36(12):1978–91. https://doi.org/10.1007/s10439-008-9577-x.

38. Hamilton PK, Morgan NA, Connolly GM, Maxwell AP. Understanding acid-base disorders. Ulster Med J. 2017;86(3):161–6. Epub 2017 Sep 12.

39. Jousi M, Saikko S, Nurmi J. Intraosseous blood samples for point-of-care analysis: agreement between intraosseous and arterial analyses. Scand J Trauma Resusc Emerg Med. 2017;25(1):92. https://doi.org/10.1186/s13049-017-0435-4.

40. Yoneda T, Hiasa M, Nagata Y, Okui T, White F. Contribution of acidic extracellular microenvironment of cancer-colonized bone to bone pain. Biochim Biophys Acta. 2015;1848(10 Pt B):2677–84. https://doi.org/10.1016/j.bbamem.2015.02.004.

41. Nagae M, Hiraga T, Yoneda T. Acidic microenvironment created by osteoclasts causes bone pain associated with tumor colonization. J Bone Miner Metab. 2007;25(2):99–104. https://doi.org/10.1007/s00774-006-0734-8.

42. Julius D, Basbaum AI. Molecular mechanisms of nociception. Nature. 2001;413(6852):203–10. https://doi.org/10.1038/35093019.

43. Hiasa M, Okui T, Allette YM, et al. Bone pain induced by multiple myeloma is reduced by targeting V-ATPase and ASIC3. Cancer Res. 2017;77(6):1283–95. https://doi.org/10.1158/0008-5472.CAN-15-3545.

44. Ikeuchi M, Kolker SJ, Sluka KA. Acid-sensing ion channel 3 expression in mouse knee joint afferents and effects of carrageenan-induced arthritis. J Pain. 2009;10(3):336–42. https://doi.org/10.1016/j.jpain.2008.10.010.

45. Olson TH, Riedl MS, Vulchanova L, Ortiz-Gonzalez XR, Elde R. An acid sensing ion channel (ASIC) localizes to small primary afferent neurons in rats. Neuroreport. 1998;9(6):1109–13. https://doi.org/10.1097/00001756-199804200-00028.

46. Morgan M, Nencini S, Thai J, Ivanusic JJ. TRPV1 activation alters the function of Aδ and C fiber sensory neurons that innervate bone. Bone. 2019;123:168–75. https://doi.org/10.1016/j.bone.2019.03.040.

47. Waldmann R. Proton-gated cation channels—neuronal acid sensors in the central and peripheral nervous system. Adv Exp Med Biol. 2001;502:293–304. https://doi.org/10.1007/978-1-4757-3401-0_19.

48. Lingueglia E. Acid-sensing ion channels in sensory perception. J Biol Chem. 2007;282(24):17325–9. https://doi.org/10.1074/jbc.R700011200.

49. Jimenez-Andrade JM, Mantyh WG, Bloom AP, Ferng AS, Geffre CP, Mantyh PW. Bone cancer pain. Ann N Y Acad Sci. 2010;1198:173–81. https://doi.org/10.1111/j.1749-6632.2009.05429.x.

50. Ringe JD, Body JJ. A review of bone pain relief with ibandronate and other bisphosphonates in disorders of increased bone turnover. Clin Exp Rheumatol. 2007;25(5):766–74.

51. Sevcik MA, Luger NM, Mach DB, et al. Bone cancer pain: the effects of the bisphosphonate alendronate on pain, skeletal remodeling, tumor growth and tumor necrosis. Pain. 2004;111(1–2):169–80. https://doi.org/10.1016/j.pain.2004.06.015.

52. Body JJ, Diel IJ, Bell R, et al. Oral ibandronate improves bone pain and preserves quality of life in patients with skeletal metastases due to breast cancer. Pain. 2004;111(3):306–12. https://doi.org/10.1016/j.pain.2004.07.011.

53. Abdelmoneim T, Kissoon N, Johnson L, Fiallos M, Murphy S. Acid-base status of blood from intraosseous and mixed venous sites during prolonged cardiopulmonary resuscitation and drug infusions. Crit Care Med. 1999;27(9):1923–8.

54. Voelckel WG, Lindner KH, Wenzel V, et al. Intraosseous blood gases during hypothermia: correlation with arterial, mixed venous, and sagittal sinus blood. Crit Care Med. 2000;28(8):2915–20. https://doi.org/10.1097/00003246-200008000-00038.

55. Schalk R, Schweigkofler U, Lotz G, Zacharowski K, Latasch L, Byhahn C. Efficacy of the EZ-IO needle driver for out-of-hospital intraosseous access—a preliminary, observational, multicenter study. Scand J Trauma Resusc Emerg Med. 2011;19:65. https://doi.org/10.1186/1757-7241-19-65.

56. Davidoff J, Fowler R, Gordon D, et al. Clinical evaluation of a novel intraosseous device for adults: prospective, 250-patient, multi-center trial. JEMS. 2005;30(10):20–3.

57. Mattera CJ. Take aim—hit your IO target. A comprehensive approach to pediatric intraosseous infusion, including site selection, needle insertion & ongoing assessment. Part 2. JEMS. 2000;25(4):38–48.

58. Philbeck TE, Puga TA, Montez DF, Davlantes C, DeNoia EP, Miller LJ. Intraosseous vascular access using the EZ-IO can be safely maintained in the adult proximal humerus and proximal tibia for up to 48 h: report of a clinical study. J Vasc Access. 2022;23(3):339–47. https://doi.org/10.1177/1129729821992667.

59. Teleflex.com. Pain Management | US | Teleflex. 2022. https://www.teleflex.com/usa/en/product-areas/emergency-medicine/intraosseous-access/arrow-ez-io-system/pain-management/index.html. Accessed 30 June 2022.

60. Hospira Inc. Lidocaine hydrochloride injection, USP. Package Insert EN-0118. Hospira Inc.; 2004.

61. Beecham GB, Nessel TA, Goyal A. Lidocaine. In: StatPearls. Treasure Island, FL: StatPearls Publishing; 2022. https://www.ncbi.nlm.nih.gov/books/NBK539881/. Accessed 10 July 2023.

62. Berde CB, Strichartz GR. Local anesthetics. In: Miller RD, Eriksson LI, Fleisher LA, et al., editors. Miller's anesthesia. 7th ed. Philadelphia, PA: Elsevier, Churchill Livingstone; 2009.

63. 6.1: pKa. Biology LibreTexts. 2017. https://bio.libretexts.org/Courses/University_of_California_Davis/BIS_2A%3A_Introductory_Biology_(Easlon)/Readings/06.1%3A_pKa. Accessed 10 July 2023.

64. Hills AG. pH and the Henderson-Hasselbalch equation. Am J Med. 1973;55(2):131–3. https://doi.org/10.1016/0002-9343(73)90160-5.

65. Collins JB, Song J, Mahabir RC. Onset and duration of intradermal mixtures of bupivacaine and lidocaine with epinephrine. Can J Plast Surg. 2013;21(1):51–3. https://doi.org/10.1177/229255031302100112.

66. Brummett CM, Williams BA. Additives to local anesthetics for peripheral nerve blockade. Int Anesthesiol Clin. 2011;49(4):104–16. https://doi.org/10.1097/AIA.0b013e31820e4a49.

67. Eggleston ST, Lush LW. Understanding allergic reactions to local anesthetics. Ann Pharmacother. 1996;30(7–8):851–7. https://doi.org/10.1177/106002809603000724.

68. Frank SG, Lalonde DH. How acidic is the lidocaine we are injecting, and how much bicarbonate should we add? Can J Plast Surg. 2012;20(2):71–3. https://doi.org/10.1177/229255031202000207.

69. Sukhani R, Winnie AP. Clinical pharmacokinetics of carbonated local anesthetics. I: Subclavian perivascular brachial block model. Anesth Analg. 1987;66(8):739–45.

70. Ummenhofer W, Frei FJ, Urwyler A, Drewe J. Are laboratory values in bone marrow aspirate predictable for venous blood in paediatric patients? Resuscitation. 1994;27(2):123–8.

71. Russell SC, Doyle E. A risk-benefit assessment of topical percutaneous local anesthetics in children. Drug Saf. 1997;16:279–87.

72. Ruetzler K, Sima B, Mayer L, et al. Lidocaine/tetracaine patch (Rapydan) for topical anaesthesia before arterial access: a double-blind, randomized trial. Br J Anaesth. 2012;109:790–6.

73. Babst CR, Gilling BN. Bupivacaine: a review. Anesth Prog. 1978;25(3):87–91.

74. Burlacu CL, Buggy DJ. Update on local anesthetics: focus on levobupivacaine. Ther Clin Risk Manag. 2008;4(2):381–92. https://doi.org/10.2147/tcrm.s1433.

75. Gagliardi AR, Yip CYY, Irish J, et al. The psychological burden of waiting for procedures and patient-centred strategies that could support the mental health of wait-listed patients and caregivers during the COVID-19 pandemic: a scoping review. Health Expect. 2021;24(3):978–90. https://doi.org/10.1111/hex.13241.

76. Torp KD, Metheny E, Simon LV. Lidocaine toxicity. In: StatPearls. Treasure Island, FL: StatPearls Publishing; 2022. https://www.ncbi.nlm.nih.gov/books/NBK482479/?report=classic. Accessed 10 July 2023.

77. Mahajan A, Derian A. Local anesthetic toxicity. In: StatPearls. Treasure Island, FL: StatPearls Publishing; 2023. https://www.ncbi.nlm.nih.gov/books/NBK499964/. Accessed 10 July 2023.

78. Chapter 20: Lidocaine toxicity and drug interactions. Liposuction 101 Liposuction Training. 2022. https://liposuction101.com/liposuction-textbook/chapter-20-lidocaine-toxicity-and-drug-interactions/#:~:text=Toxic%20Effects%20and%20Treatment&text=With%20slow%20systemic%20absorption%20of. Accessed 10 July 2023.

79. El-Boghdadly K, Pawa A, Chin KJ. Local anesthetic systemic toxicity: current perspectives. Local Reg Anesth. 2018;11:35–44. https://doi.org/10.2147/LRA.S154512.

80. Groban L. Central nervous system and cardiac effects from long-acting amide local anesthetic toxicity in the intact animal model. Reg Anesth Pain Med. 2003;28(1):3–11. https://doi.org/10.1053/rapm.2003.50014.

81. Nasr YM, Waly SH, Morsy AA. Scalp block for awake craniotomy: lidocaine-bupivacaine versus lidocaine-bupivacaine with adjuvants. Egyptian Journal of Anaesthesia. 2020;36(1):7–15. https://doi.org/10.1080/11101849.2020.1719301.

82. Butterworth JF 4th. Models and mechanisms of local anesthetic cardiac toxicity: a review. Reg Anesth Pain Med. 2010;35(2):167–76. https://doi.org/10.1097/aap.0b013e3181d231b9.

83. Taylor A, McLeod G. Basic pharmacology of local anaesthetics. BJA Educ. 2020;20(2):34–41. https://doi.org/10.1016/j.bjae.2019.10.002.

84. Long B, Chavez S, Gottlieb M, Montrief T, Brady WJ. Local anesthetic systemic toxicity: a narrative review for emergency clinicians. Am J Emerg Med. 2022;59:42–8. https://doi.org/10.1016/j.ajem.2022.06.017. Epub 2022 Jun 13

85. Schechter NL, Zempsky WT, Cohen LL, McGrath PJ, McMurtry CM, Bright NS. Pain reduction during pediatric immunizations: evidence-based review and recommendations. Pediatrics. 2007;119(5):e1184–98. https://doi.org/10.1542/peds.2006-1107.

86. Blount RL, Piira T, Cohen LL. Management of pediatric pain and distress due to medical procedures. In: Roberts MC, editor. Handbook of pediatric psychology. The Guilford Press; 2003. p. 216–33.

87. DeMore M, Cohen LL. Distraction for pediatric immunization pain: a critical review. J Clin Psychol Med Settings. 2005;12:281–91. https://doi.org/10.1007/s10880-005-7813-1.

88. Bantick SJ, Wise RG, Ploghaus A, Clare S, Smith SM, Tracey I. Imaging how attention modulates pain in humans using functional MRI. Brain. 2002;125(Pt 2):310–9. https://doi.org/10.1093/brain/awf022.

89. Frankenstein UN, Richter W, McIntyre MC, Rémy F. Distraction modulates anterior cingulate gyrus activations during the cold pressor test. NeuroImage. 2001;14(4):827–36. https://doi.org/10.1006/nimg.2001.0883.

90. Koller D, Goldman RD. Distraction techniques for children undergoing procedures: a critical review of pediatric research. J Pediatr Nurs. 2012;27(6):652–81. https://doi.org/10.1016/j.pedn.2011.08.001.

91. Dahlquist LM, McKenna KD, Jones KK, Dillinger L, Weiss KE, Ackerman CS. Active and passive distraction using a head-mounted display helmet: effects on cold pressor pain in children. Health Psychol. 2007;26(6):794–801. https://doi.org/10.1037/0278-6133.26.6.794.

92. Dahlquist LM, Pendley JS, Landthrip DS, Jones CL, Steuber CP. Distraction intervention for preschoolers undergoing intramuscular injections and subcutaneous port access. Health Psychol. 2002;21(1):94–9.

93. Mason S, Johnson MH, Woolley C. A comparison of distractors for controlling distress in young children during medical procedures. J Clin Psychol Med Settings. 1999;6:239–48.

94. MacLaren JE, Cohen LL. A comparison of distraction strategies for venipuncture distress in children. J Pediatr Psychol. 2005;30(5):387–96. https://doi.org/10.1093/jpepsy/jsi062.

95. Atzori B, Hoffman HG, Vagnoli L, et al. Virtual reality analgesia during venipuncture in pediatric patients with onco-hematological diseases. Front Psychol. 2018;9:2508. https://doi.org/10.3389/fpsyg.2018.02508.

96. Chad R, Emaan S, Jillian O. Effect of virtual reality headset for pediatric fear and pain distraction during immunization. Pain Manag. 2018;8(3):175–9. https://doi.org/10.2217/pmt-2017-0040.

97. Aminabadi NA, Erfanparast L, Sohrabi A, Ghertasi Oskouei S, Naghili A. The impact of virtual reality distraction on pain and anxiety during dental treatment in 4-6 year-old children: a randomized controlled clinical trial. J Dent Res Dent Clin Dent Prospects. 2012;6(4):117–24. https://doi.org/10.5681/joddd.2012.025.

98. Gold JI, Mahrer NE. Is virtual reality ready for prime time in the medical space? A randomized control trial of pediatric virtual reality for acute procedural pain management. J Pediatr Psychol. 2018;43(3):266–75. https://doi.org/10.1093/jpepsy/jsx129.

99. Dahlquist LM, Weiss KE, Law EF, et al. Effects of videogame distraction and a virtual reality type head-mounted display helmet on cold pressor pain in young elementary school-aged children. J Pediatr Psychol. 2010;35(6):617–25. https://doi.org/10.1093/jpepsy/jsp082.

100. Al-Ghamdi NA, Meyer WJ, Atzori B, et al. Virtual reality analgesia with interactive eye tracking during brief thermal pain stimuli: a randomized controlled trial (crossover design). Front Hum Neurosci. 2019;13:467. https://doi.org/10.3389/fnhum.2019.00467.

101. Vlocka JD, Hadzic A, Gautier P. Femoral nerve block. New York School of Regional Anesthesia; 2002. https://www.nysora.com/techniques/lower-extremity/femoral/femoral-nerve-block/. Accessed 10 July 2023.

102. Vadhanan P, Tripaty DK, Adinarayanan S. Physiological and pharmacologic aspects of peripheral nerve blocks. J Anaesthesiol Clin Pharmacol. 2015;31(3):384–93. https://doi.org/10.4103/0970-9185.161679.

103. Lee-Elliott CE, Dundas D, Patel U. Randomized trial of lidocaine vs lidocaine/bupivacaine periprostatic injection on longitudinal pain scores after prostate biopsy. J Urol. 2004;171(1):247–50. https://doi.org/10.1097/01.ju.0000098688.12631.a0.

104. Seow LT, Lips FJ, Cousins MJ, Mather LE. Lidocaine and bupivacaine mixtures for epidural blockade. Anesthesiology. 1982;56(3):177–83. https://doi.org/10.1097/00000542-198203000-00004.

105. Gadsden J. Chapter 2. Local anesthetics: clinical pharmacology and rational selection. In: Hadzic A, editor. Hadzic's peripheral nerve blocks and anatomy for ultrasound-guided regional anesthesia. 2nd ed. McGraw Hill; 2012. https://accessanesthesiology.mhmedical.com/content.aspx?bookid=518§ionid=41534288. Accessed 10 July 2023.

106. Hull J, Heath J, Bishop W. Supraclavicular brachial plexus block for arteriovenous hemodialysis access procedures. J Vasc Interv Radiol. 2016;27(5):749–52. https://doi.org/10.1016/j.jvir.2016.02.003.

107. O'Donnell BD, Iohom G. An estimation of the minimum effective anesthetic volume of 2% lidocaine in ultrasound-guided axillary brachial plexus block. Anesthesiology. 2009;111(1):25–9. https://doi.org/10.1097/ALN.0b013e3181a915c7.

108. Marin R, Silva MG, Espinoza X, Lopez A, Pellegrini M, Sala-Blanch X. Minimum effective anaesthetic volume of 1.5% mepivacaine in ultrasound-guided popliteal block at sciatic nerve division: 8AP1-4. Eur J Anaesthesiol. 2013;30:117.

109. Christiansen CB, Madsen MH, Rothe C, Andreasen AM, Lundstrøm LH, Lange KHW. Volume of ropivacaine 0.2% and sciatic nerve block duration: a randomized, blinded trial in healthy volunteers. Acta Anaesthesiol Scand. 2020;64(2):238–44. https://doi.org/10.1111/aas.13489.

110. McGlade DP, Kalpokas MV, Mooney PH, Chamley D, Mark AH, Torda TA. A comparison of 0.5% ropivacaine and 0.5% bupivacaine for axillary brachial plexus anaesthesia. Anaesth Intensive Care. 1998;26(5):515–20. https://doi.org/10.1177/0310057X9802600507.

111. Baskan S, Taspinar V, Ozdogan L, et al. Comparison of 0.25% levobupivacaine and 0.25% bupivacaine for posterior approach interscalene brachial plexus block. J Anesth. 2010;24(1):38–42. https://doi.org/10.1007/s00540-009-0846-0.

112. Vaghadia H, Chan V, Ganapathy S, Lui A, McKenna J, Zimmer K. A multicentre trial of ropivacaine 7.5 mg x ml(−1) vs bupivacaine 5 mg x ml(−1) for supra clavicular brachial plexus anesthesia. Can J Anaesth. 1999;46(10):946–51. https://doi.org/10.1007/BF03013129.

113. Sagherian BH, Kile TA, Seamans DP, Misra L, Claridge RJ. Lateral popliteal block in foot and ankle surgery: comparing ultrasound guidance to nerve stimulation. A prospective randomized trial. Foot Ankle Surg. 2021;27(2):175–80. https://doi.org/10.1016/j.fas.2020.03.011.

114. Allen B, Statzer N. Popliteal block procedure guide. In: Post TW, editor. UpToDate. UpToDate; 2022. https://www.uptodate.com/contents/popliteal-block-procedure-guide?search=popliteal%20nerve%20block&source=search_result&selectedTitle=1~10&usage_type=default&display_rank=1#H2487582430. Accessed 10 July 2023.

115. Farag E, Mounir-Soliman L. Brown's atlas of regional Anaesthesia. Elsevier; 2017.

116. Vloka JD. The division of the sciatic nerve in the popliteal fossa: anatomical implications for popliteal nerve blockade. Anesth Analges. 2001;92(1):215.

117. Karmakar MJ. High-definition ultrasound imaging defines the paraneural sheath and the fascial compartments surrounding the sciatic nerve at the popliteal fossa. Reg Anesth Pain Med. 2013;38(5):447.

118. Perlas A. Ultrasound-guided popliteal block through a common paraneural sheath versus conventional injection: a prospective, randomized, double-blind study. Region Anesth Pain Med. 2013;38(3):218.

119. Refai NA, Tadi P. Anatomy, bony pelvis and lower limb, thigh femoral nerve. In: StatPearls. Treasure Island, FL: StatPearls Publishing; 2022. https://www.ncbi.nlm.nih.gov/books/NBK556065/?report=classic. Accessed 10 July 2023.

120. Jeng C, Rosenblatt M. Lower extremity nerve blocks: techniques. In: Post TW, editor. UpToDate. UpToDate; 2022. https://www.uptodate.com/contents/lower-extremity-nerve-blocks-techniques?search=femoral%20nerve%20anatomy§ionRank=1&usage_type=d

efault&anchor=H1413150737&source=machineLearning&selectedTitle=2~150&display_rank=2#H1413150737. Accessed 10 July 2023.

121. Danelli G, Fanelli A, Ghisi D, et al. Ultrasound vs nerve stimulation multiple injection technique for posterior popliteal sciatic nerve block. Anaesthesia. 2009;64(6):638–42. https://doi.org/10.1111/j.1365-2044.2009.05915.

122. Gottlieb M, Long B. Peripheral nerve block for hip fracture. Acad Emerg Med. 2021;28(10):1198–9. https://doi.org/10.1111/acem.14239.

123. Rongstad K, Mann RA, Prieskorn D, Nichelson S, Horton G. Popliteal sciatic nerve block for postoperative analgesia. Foot Ankle Int. 1996;17(7):378–82. https://doi.org/10.1177/107110079601700704.

124. Vinent PMS, Oliveira EJSG, Oliveira CMB, et al. Ultrasound-guided popliteal sciatic nerve block in a pediatric patient with complex regional pain syndrome: a case report. Braz J Anesthesiol. 2021:744233. https://doi.org/10.1016/j.bjane.2021.07.012.

125. Gedikoglu M, Eker HE. Ultrasound-guided popliteal sciatic nerve block: an effective alternative technique to control ischaemic severe rest pain during endovascular treatment of critical limb ischaemia. Pol J Radiol. 2019;84:e537–41. https://doi.org/10.5114/pjr.2019.91271.

126. Jeng C, Rosenblatt M. Upper extremity nerve blocks: techniques. In: Post TW, editor. UpToDate. UpToDate; 2022. https://www.uptodate.com/contents/upper-extremity-nerve-blocks-techniques?search=upper%20extremity%20nerve%20block&source=search_result&selectedTitle=1~150&usage_type=default&display_rank=1. Accessed 10 July 2023.

127. Tran D, Shubada D, Asenjo JF. Chapter 13: Upper extremity nerve blocks. In: Kaye AD, Urman RD, Vadivelu N, editors. Essentials of regional anesthesia. Springer; 2012. p. 339–83.

128. Kaye AD, Allampalli V, Fisher P, et al. Supraclavicular vs. infraclavicular brachial plexus nerve blocks: clinical, pharmacological, and anatomical considerations. Anesth Pain Med. 2021;11(5):e120658. https://doi.org/10.5812/aapm.120658.

129. Mian A, Chaudhry I, Huang R, Rizk E, Tubbs RS, Loukas M. Brachial plexus anesthesia: a review of the relevant anatomy, complications, and anatomical variations. Clin Anat. 2014;27(2):210–21. https://doi.org/10.1002/ca.22254.

130. Omoregbe OR, Idehen HO, Imarengiaye CO. Supraclavicular brachial plexus block for upper limb fracture fixation: a comparison of nerve stimulation, ultrasound-guided technique and a combination of both techniques. West Afr J Med. 2020;37(7):757–62.

131. Vlocka JD, Hadzic A. Popliteal sciatic nerve block—landmarks and nerve stimulator technique, NYSORA; 2022. https://www.nysora.com/topics/regional-anesthesia-for-specific-surgical-procedures/lower-extremity-regional-anesthesia-for-specific-surgical-procedures/foot-and-anckle/block-sciatic-nerve-popliteal-fossa/. Accessed 10 July 2023.

132. Gautier PE, Vandepitte C, Jeff G. Ultrasound-guided interscalene brachial plexus nerve block. NYSORA; 2023. https://www.nysora.com/techniques/upper-extremity/intescalene/ultrasound-guided-interscalene-brachial-plexus-block/. Accessed 10 July 2023.

133. Franco CD, Byloos B, Hasanbegovic I. Supraclavicular brachial plexus block—landmarks and nerve stimulator technique. NYSORA; 2022. https://www.nysora.com/topics/regional-anesthesia-for-specific-surgical-procedures/upper-extremity-regional-anesthesia-for-specific-surgical-procedures/anesthesia-and-analgesia-for-elbow-and-forearm-procedures/supraclavicular-brachial-plexus-block/#toc_COMPLICATIONS. Accessed 10 July 2023.

134. Clark L. Infraclavicular brachial plexus block—landmarks and nerve stimulator technique. NYSORA; 2022. https://www.nysora.com/topics/regional-anesthesia-for-specific-surgical-procedures/upper-extremity-regional-anesthesia-for-specific-surgical-procedures/anesthesia-and-analgesia-for-elbow-and-forearm-procedures/infraclavicular-brachial-plexus-block-2/. Accessed 10 July 2023.

135. Koscielniak-Nielsen ZJ, Golebiewski M. Axillary brachial plexus block—landmarks and nerve stimulator technique. NYSORA; 2022. https://www.nysora.com/techniques/upper-extremity/axillary/axillary-brachial-plexus-block/. Accessed 10 July 2023.

136. Von Hoff DD, Kuhn JG, Burris HA, Miller LJ. Does intraosseous equal intravenous? A pharmacokinetic study. Am J Emerg Med. 2008;26(1):31–8. https://doi.org/10.1016/j.ajem.2007.03.024.

137. Glare PA, Walsh TD. Clinical pharmacokinetics of morphine. Ther Drug Monit. 1991;13(1):1–23.
138. Bujedo BM. Spinal opioid bioavailability in postoperative pain. Pain Pract. 2014;14(4):350–64. https://doi.org/10.1111/papr.12099. Epub 2013 Jul 8
139. Grossman M, Abiose A, Tangphao O, Blaschke TF, Hoffman BB. Morphine-induced venodilation in humans. Clin Pharm Ther. 1996;60:554–60.
140. Afshari R, Maxwell SR, Webb DJ, Bateman DN. Morphine is an arteriolar vasodilator in man. Br J Clin Pharmacol. 2009;67(4):386–93. https://doi.org/10.1111/j.1365-2125.2009.03364.x.
141. Sahin AS, Duman A, Atalik EK, Ogün CO, Sahin TK, Erol A, Ozergin U. The mechanisms of the direct vascular effects of fentanyl on isolated human saphenous veins in vitro. J Cardiothorac Vasc Anesth. 2005;19(2):197–200. https://doi.org/10.1053/j.jvca.2005.01.031.
142. Larsson T, Strandberg G, Eriksson M, Bondesson U, Lipcsey M, Larsson A. Intraosseous samples can be used for opioid measurements—an experimental study in the anaesthetized pig. Scand J Clin Lab Invest. 2013;73(2):102–6. https://doi.org/10.3109/00365513.2012.744088.
143. Moss RB, Carlo DJ. Higher doses of naloxone are needed in the synthetic opioid era. Subst Abuse Treat Prev Policy. 2019;14(1):6. https://doi.org/10.1186/s13011-019-0195-4.
144. Krizanac-Bengez L, Boranić M, Testa NG, Kardum I. Naloxone interferes with granulocytopoiesis in long-term cultures of mouse bone marrow; buffering by the stromal layer. Res Exp Med (Berl). 1994;194(6):375–82. https://doi.org/10.1007/BF02576400.
145. Janas A, Folwarczna J. Opioid receptor agonists may favorably affect bone mechanical properties in rats with estrogen deficiency-induced osteoporosis. Naunyn Schmiedeberg's Arch Pharmacol. 2017;390(2):175–85. https://doi.org/10.1007/s00210-016-1295-6. Epub 2016 Nov 28
146. Brozovich AA, Incavo SJ, Lambert BS, et al. Intraosseous morphine decreases postoperative pain and pain medication use in total knee arthroplasty: a double-blind, randomized controlled trial. J Arthroplast. 2022;37(6S):S139–46. https://doi.org/10.1016/j.arth.2021.10.009.
147. Tully J, Jung JW, Patel A, et al. Utilization of intravenous lidocaine infusion for the treatment of refractory chronic pain. Anesth Pain Med. 2020;10(6):e112290. https://doi.org/10.5812/aapm.112290.
148. Estebe JP. Intravenous lidocaine. Best Pract Res Clin Anaesthesiol. 2017;31(4):513–21. https://doi.org/10.1016/j.bpa.2017.05.005.
149. Kaba A, Laurent SR, Detroz BJ, et al. Intravenous lidocaine infusion facilitates acute rehabilitation after laparoscopic colectomy. Anesthesiology. 2007;106(1):11–8; discussion 5. https://doi.org/10.1097/00000542-200701000-00007.
150. Kandil E, Melikman E, Adinoff B. Lidocaine infusion: a promising therapeutic approach for chronic pain. J Anesth Clin Res. 2017;8(1):697. https://doi.org/10.4172/2155-6148.1000697.

Decision-Making for Intraosseous Infusion

11

Zaid Mohsen and James H. Paxton

Introduction

Vascular access during emergent resuscitation is both critical and difficult in children and adults. Patient assessment, decision-making, and time management skills are crucial when choosing an appropriate route for emergent vascular access. Critically ill patients requiring the emergent administration of fluids and drugs often present with the most difficult vascular access, a vicious downward spiral. Timing is everything in medicine. To the neurologist, "time is brain" during a stroke code. To the cardiologist, "time is cardiac tissue" during a myocardial infarction. Thus, time to vascular access is an important consideration. Time to vascular access is one of many factors that clinicians must consider when making decisions during an emergent resuscitation. Other factors to consider include the patient's presenting condition, acuity of illness, need for immediate fluid or medication, clinical stability, and patient preferences. This chapter discusses the various factors that should be considered when deciding when and how to place an intraosseous (IO) catheter.

Decision-making during a resuscitation with limited information creates a stressful environment for patients and providers alike. Although providers hope to "rise to the occasion," we inevitably "fall to the level of our training." Lack of equipment and lack of training are frequently cited as the main reasons for avoiding IO access when it is otherwise clinically indicated [1]. In one recent study of American EM academic programs, 72% of programs reported experience using IO vascular access devices in adult subjects [2]. The most common device use in this study was the EZ-IO®, generally at the proximal tibia. However, for unstable patients requiring vascular access after failed **peripheral intravenous** (PIV) access, **central venous catheter** (CVC) placement was the predominant choice for a second attempt. In the

Z. Mohsen (✉) · J. H. Paxton
Department of Emergency Medicine, Wayne State University School of Medicine, Detroit, MI, USA
e-mail: zmm@wayne.edu; james.paxton@wayne.edu

J. H. Paxton (ed.), *Intraosseous Vascular Access*,
https://doi.org/10.1007/978-3-031-61201-5_11

event of a failed CVC attempt, another CVC attempt was the most common choice. If a fourth attempt was required, IO access became the technique of choice. Since IO access has been shown to be quick, safe, and easy to learn, why is it so underutilized? Among physicians, reported barriers to IO access include a lack of confidence in the indications and the belief that IO access is unfamiliar to nursing staff [3]. In this chapter, we will discuss how to approach vascular access in emergent situations, when to choose IO infusion, and how to select the appropriate IO vascular access device for a patient.

General Approach to Vascular Access

Under non-emergent conditions, the preferred route for achieving vascular access is through cannulation of a **peripheral vein in the upper extremity**. When selecting a candidate peripheral vein, providers generally start by visually inspecting the extremity to identify any veins that appear prominent and readily accessible. Veins are palpated to assess their depth, size, and direction before any cannulation attempt is made. A systematic approach to PIV insertion is generally used, with providers starting with consideration of distal peripheral veins on the upper extremity and working proximally. As a result, many hemodynamically stable patients will receive PIV insertion in the finger or dorsum of the hand, sites that are usually only able to accommodate a 20-gauge or 22-gauge cannula. Target veins in such cases include the **cephalic vein, basilic vein**, or contributories of the **dorsal venous network** (Fig. 11.1).

Fig. 11.1 Veins of the dorsal hand commonly used for PIV insertion in stable patients [4]

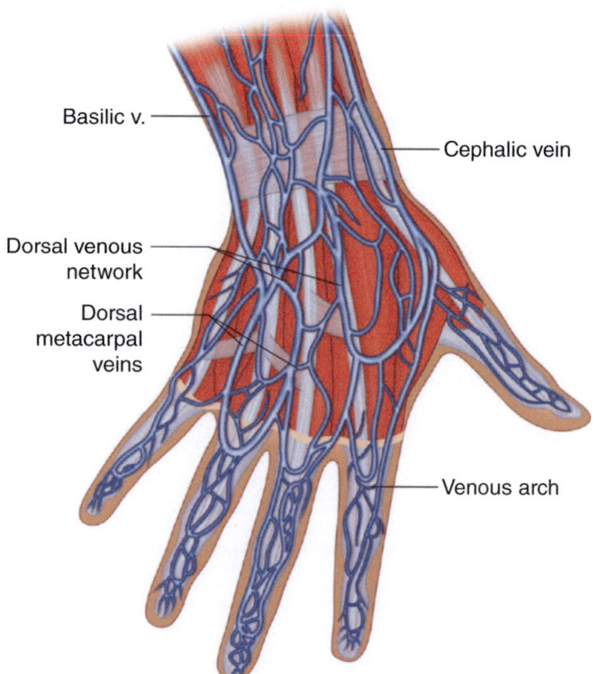

When dorsal hand or wrist veins are not available for PIV insertion, providers will begin to assess the more proximal, larger veins of the upper extremity. Preferred veins in this area include the **median antecubital vein, cephalic vein, and basilic vein** (Fig. 11.2). These vessels may be quite superficial in some patients and are often readily accessed in patients who are not intravascularly volume depleted. If no accessible veins are identified in the upper extremity, providers may look next to the **external jugular (EJ) vein** in adults and larger children, as this vessel is still considered a peripheral vein and is preferred over lower extremity venous targets. However, the use of ultrasound (US) guidance and other modalities for vein visualization can greatly increase the likelihood of successful PIV cannulation in the upper extremity, which usually limits the need to consider placement of an EJ line.

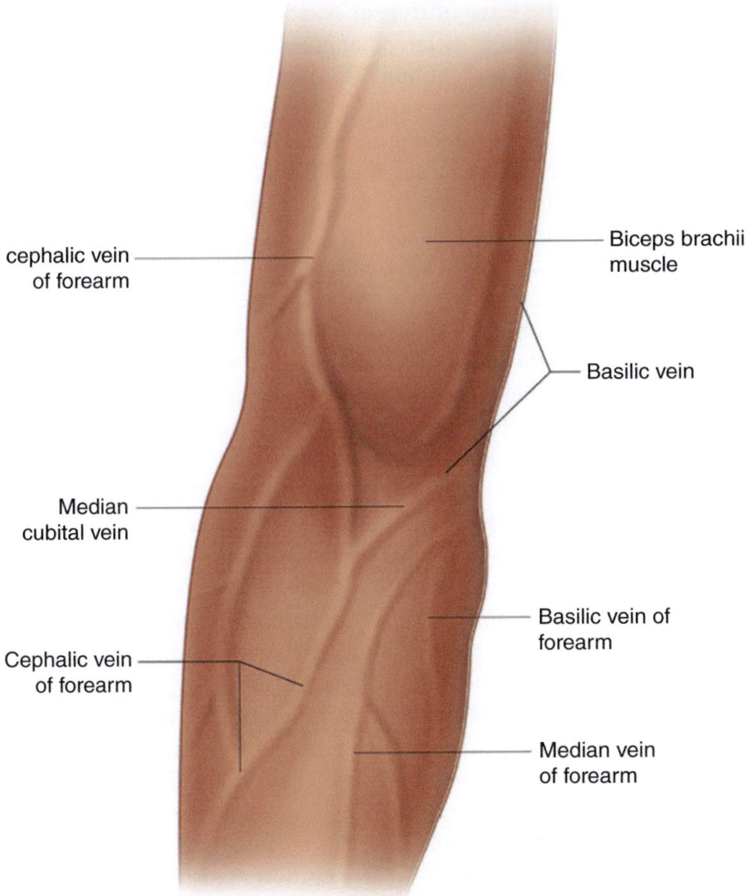

Fig. 11.2 Veins of the proximal upper extremity commonly used for PIV insertion [4]

While the catheterization of small veins in the hand and distal forearm may be appropriate for clinically stable patients, **patients who are critically ill often require rapid large-volume infusion of blood products or fluids**. Unfortunately, providers may not be able to achieve adequate resuscitative fluid infusion rates with small-bore catheters inserted at very distal peripheral venous sites. Consequently, patients who are likely to require high-volume infusion should have large-bore (e.g., 16 gauge, 18 gauge) PIV cannulae placed more proximally, at the **antecubital fossa** or above. Larger catheter diameter allows for greater flow rates, and more proximal locations also offer the advantage of lower intraluminal pressures (i.e., lower resistance to flow) and closer proximity to the central venous circulation. These factors combine to provide a superior alternative for high-volume infusion or infusion of medications that might otherwise irritate target veins as they are more quickly picked up by the circulation and less likely to produce untoward effects such as venous damage or local soft tissue damage when irritant medications are infused.

Critically ill patients have different vascular access needs than stable patients, which necessitates a different approach to securing emergent venous access. Beyond the need for high-volume fluid infusion, hypotensive patients may have reduced **systemic vascular resistance** (SVR) requiring the use of vasopressor infusion to temporarily increase blood pressure and restore perfusion to vital organs. Although short-term vasopressor infusion can be safely achieved via PIV infusion, these patients often require placement of a CVC when extended vasopressor infusion is indicated. Vasopressor medications can cause profound vasoconstriction, which can be deleterious when extravasated into the soft tissues, sometimes leading to soft tissue damage and necrosis.

Intraosseous catheters have the same limitations for medication infusion as PIV catheters, because the medications and fluids infused into the medullary space are transferred to the central circulation by the relatively small-caliber peripheral veins draining the bone. Thus, IO catheter infusion may be an appropriate surrogate for direct PIV infusion, but does not obviate the need for CVC placement in patients who would otherwise require a central line. **Clinically, it is best to think of an IO line as an indirect PIV line that is available with minimal delay**. Most medications compatible with PIV infusion have been administered safely via IO infusion, but medications normally infused via CVC should only be infused via IO cannulae when the delay associated with CVC insertion is considered to be clinically unacceptable. The best example of such a situation is with cardiac arrest, when bolus doses of epinephrine (a potent vasoconstrictor) are routinely given by PIV or IO line when attempting to achieve **return of spontaneous circulation** (ROSC). Once ROSC has been achieved, CVC access is recommended for extended vasopressor infusion, whether the initial peripheral venous access is via direct PIV or indirect IO infusion.

Most providers will attempt to place a PIV in critically ill patients before deciding to place an IO catheter. Consequently, **IO catheters are sometimes considered to be an approach of last resort**, only attempted after multiple failed PIV attempts or when the provider considers additional PIV catheter insertion attempts to be futile. This could be early, as when the provider is unable to identify a candidate peripheral vein on initial examination, or delayed as when multiple attempts at PIV cannula insertion have failed and the patient is deemed too unstable to tolerate additional delay. This bias towards delaying the decision to attempt IO access can lead to further deterioration of the patient's medical condition while the optimistic provider continues their fruitless search for an ultimately unavailable PIV insertion. Overconfidence and a lack of situational awareness undoubtedly contribute to this dilemma, which can be resolved with improved self-awareness and recognition by the provider that PIV access is not always possible.

There are many different types of factors contributing to difficulty in establishing vascular access, including **environmental**, **provider-specific**, **patient-specific**, and **device-specific** causes. **Environmental** causes can include poor lighting, austere circumstances, limited availability of different vascular access devices (VADs), and other factors that are attributable to the location of the access attempt and could theoretically be alleviated in a different care environment [5]. **Provider-specific** causes of difficult vascular access (DVA) include lack of adequate training, lack of familiarity with the device being used, and other factors that might be attributable to the provider's ability to place the VAD. **Patient-specific** factors contributing to DVA include obesity, patient comorbidities (e.g., diabetes mellitus, chronic steroid use, renal insufficiency, IV drug abuse, history of chemotherapy), noncompliance with vascular access attempts, history of DVA, hypovolemia or other causes of hypotension, and other factors that are attributable to the patient's specific medical condition [5, 6]. **Device-specific** causes can include device malfunction, limitations of the device being used, and other limitations imposed by the choice of VAD selected that may be avoided by use of a different IO access device.

The reported failure rates for peripheral IV access are between 10 and 40% [7]. In one study at an urban tertiary care hospital, nearly 1 in 10 adults presented with difficult venous access [8]. When looking at predictive factors, these researchers found that diabetes mellitus, sickle cell disease, and IV drug use were all correlated with difficult venous access. In another study looking at the relationship between body mass index (BMI) and venous access failure in the ED, a BMI >30 and a BMI <18.5 were both considered to be risk factors for difficult venous access [9].

In 2010, the American Heart Association (AHA) first recommended IO access as an alternative to direct venous access in the treatment of cardiac arrest. Since that time, the International Liaison Committee on Resuscitation (ILCOR) and other authoritative bodies have joined the AHA in supporting the use of IO cannulation for cardiac arrest resuscitation when direct venous access is "unsuccessful or not feasible" [10, 11]. Unfortunately, existing studies are unable to provide an unbiased view on relative outcomes according to vascular access type. In one large systematic review of IO versus PIV drug administration during cardiac arrest including six observational studies and two randomized controlled trials, investigators found that two of the observation studies did not adjust for covariates, establishing a critical risk of bias to confounding [12]. The other four observational studies used different defined exposures: "IO and IV attempt," "successful IV and IO access," and "successful initial IV and IO access." These variable definitions allow for an inconsistent number of PIV attempts before IO access was attempted, introducing a **resuscitation time bias** [13]. A longer duration of resuscitation during cardiac arrest is associated with worse outcomes. If IO attempts are limited to failed PIV attempts, then patients receiving IO are more likely to have a longer duration of cardiac arrest compared to those who successfully received PIV resuscitation. Therefore, it is inappropriate to conclude that IO is inferior to PIV therapy based upon evidence from such observational studies. Additionally, if access route strategy is based (even in part) upon the judgment of the healthcare provider, then the IO group is likely to have different patient characteristics than the PIV group, which could influence patient outcomes. Any lack of randomization in a comparative study involving IO and PIV access invariably introduces uncontrolled sources of bias against the use of IO infusion.

Recognizing the lack of adequate information and appropriate guidance for route of emergent vascular access, many algorithms for VAD selection have been proposed. These algorithms are based upon a variety of elements that influence appropriate device selection, including the patient's presenting medical condition, injury pattern, medical comorbidities, surgical history, patient mental status and level of cooperation with the provider, anticipated need for fluid and/or medication infusion during stabilization and subsequent hospitalization, environmental factors, device limitations, anticipated device dwell time, availability and prior training of care providers, availability of adjunct technology (e.g., ultrasound, vein finders), and presence of preexisting venous access devices (e.g., ports, fistulae, tunneled catheters). An example of one such algorithm is provided in Fig. 11.3. As this algorithm illustrates, VAD selection is a complex medical decision that incorporates a wide range of considerations that may be unique to the care environment, care provider, and patient receiving vascular access device placement.

While it is desirable for care providers to have some form of guidance when selecting a VAD for their patient, the provider's healthcare institution or professional guidelines may offer little help. In the absence of institutional guidance, providers should develop their own explicit or implicit algorithm that is informed by their own personal experience, training, and beliefs. While such algorithms do permit a certain degree of cognitive off-loading, especially under austere or chaotic conditions, providers should recognize that VAD selection is very much an art as well as a science. Optimally, providers will apply a sound understanding of the evidence provided in the medical literature (as limited as it is), as well as their own creative problem-solving skills and technical prowess to the task.

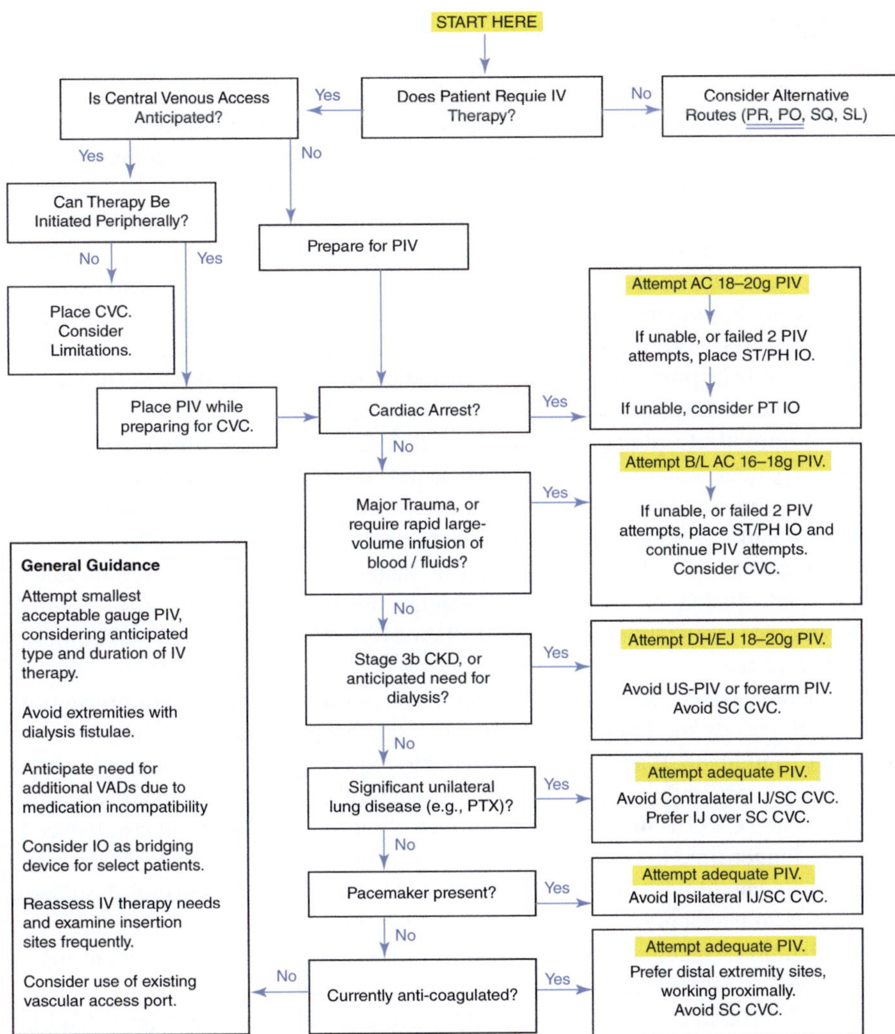

Fig. 11.3 Example of a VAD placement algorithm for adult patients [14]. Notes: *AC* antecubital; *B/L* bilateral CKD chronic kidney disease; *CVC* central venous catheter; *DH* dorsal hand; *EJ* external jugular; *IJ* internal jugular; *IO* intraosseous; *PIV* peripheral intravenous; *PO* per oral; *PR* per rectum; *PTX* pneumothorax; *SC* subclavian; *SL* sublingual; *SQ* subcutaneous; *ST* sternal; *US-PIV* ultrasound-guided peripheral intravenous

A Bridge to Definitive Access

As mentioned above, many institutions and professional societies have offered recommendations on the forms of vascular access that are most appropriate under a variety of therapeutic circumstances. Generally speaking, these guidelines usually endorse specific forms of definitive vascular access according to the patient's broadly categorized therapeutic needs. These needs are usually very simply defined as the type of medications and fluids to be infused and the period of time over which those infusions will be required. Unfortunately, it is often difficult or impossible to accurately predict the medications that a patient will need throughout the course of their medical care, and the needed duration of therapy may be similarly unpredictable. Thus, **it is important to think of vascular access as a multi-staged process that may evolve throughout the patient's care episode**.

In the **immediate phase**, providers are first faced with the binary decision of whether a patient requires venous access or not. If so, the decision is usually quite simple, with most medications and other interventions indicated for patient stabilization compatible with PIV or IO infusion. In some cases, of course, CVC insertion may be required for safe administration of medications such as with continuous vasopressor infusion or when central venous pressures are required to confirm hemodynamic stabilization. However, a PIV or IO catheter will often suffice in the immediate phase.

A patient's subsequent vascular access needs during the **short-term phase** (i.e., in-hospital period) and **long-term phase** (i.e., posthospital discharge) may be more difficult to anticipate. If a patient is expected to require prolonged vasopressor infusion or long-term antibiotic therapy, it may be tempting for the provider to consider placement of a CVC as initial therapy. Unfortunately, CVC placement requires considerably longer time to be achieved than PIV or IO cannulation when done safely under sterile conditions; thus, excessive focus on a patient's anticipated short-term and long-term needs may lead to delays in achieving the patient's immediate need for stabilization. Examples of immediate, short-term, and long-term patient needs that may be served with IO infusion are provided in Table 11.1.

The 2015 Michigan Appropriateness Guide for Intravenous Catheters (MAGIC) guidelines provide recommendations on appropriate use of various intravenous catheter types, including indications for insertion and duration of their use [15]. These guidelines are generally consistent with recommendations by other groups that peripheral IV catheters should be used when the duration of medication therapy is short (i.e., ≤ 5 days), but ultrasound-guided peripheral IV (US-PIV) or central venous catheters should be used for prolonged therapy (Table 11.2).

While the MAGIC guidelines do not specifically address the use of IO catheters, many providers consider IO infusion to be equivalent to PIV infusion during the stabilization of critically ill patients. However, many institutions have policies and guidelines requiring that the **dwell time** (i.e., how long a catheter may be left in place) for IO catheters be limited to 1–2 days, necessitating the placement of additional vascular access devices (e.g., PIV or CVC) to maintain vascular access during subsequent care. Some institutions may even require that IO catheters be removed

Table 11.1 Examples of immediate, short-term, and long-term vascular access needs [14]

Immediate needs (stabilization)	Short-term needs (hospitalization)	Long-term needs (post-hospitalization)
Intubation (RSI)	Continuous infusions	Central vein preservation
Vasopressors	Vasopressors	Minimal risk of CRBSI
Fluids (bolus)	Fluids (maintenance)	Minimal risk of CRT
Antibiotics	Antibiotics (inpatient)	Antibiotics (long term)
Hyperosmolar agents	"As-needed" medications	
Anticoagulation	Anticoagulation	
ACLS medications/CPR	Parenteral nutrition	
Blood sampling	Blood sampling	
Hemodynamic monitoring	Hemodynamic monitoring	
Intravenous contrast	Intravenous contrast	
Patient preference	Patient comfort	
Interventional procedures	Low risk of line failure	
Low risk of complications	Low risk of complications	

Notes: *RSI* rapid sequence induction; *CRBSI* catheter-related bloodstream infection; *CRT* catheter-related thrombosis; *ACLS* advanced cardiac life support; *CPR* cardiopulmonary resuscitation

Table 11.2 MAGIC recommendations for VAD selection according to the duration of infusion [13, 14]

Duration of infusion	Preferred device	Considerations
≤5 days	PIV or US-PIV	
6–14 days (non-critically ill)	US-PIV	US-PIV is preferred to PIV. Midline catheter is preferred to PICC
6–14 days (critically ill)	Non-tunneled CVC	If hemodynamic monitoring is needed for 6–14 days
15–30 days	PICC	PICC preferred to midline catheter, tunneled CVC, or port
≥30 days	Tunneled catheter or port	

when the patient leaves the emergency department or as soon as possible after admission to the hospital or operating room, despite evidence that dwell times for IO catheters up to 48-h induration appear to be safe [16]. This may lead some providers to avoid placement of an IO catheter, even when clinical circumstances suggest that IO infusion is indicated, since an alternative form of vascular access will ultimately be required.

The fallacy that delayed PIV or CVC placement is somehow more efficient than immediate placement of an IO catheter can be easily dispelled if providers think of IO devices as a "**bridge**" from "no access" to definitive vascular access. In many ways, IO catheters are the optimal bridging device, with large fluid volumes able to be quickly and reliably infused to increase intravenous filling and enlarge target veins for subsequent PIV or CVC attempts. Refusal to consider "filling the tank" via IO infusion to facilitate subsequent direct venous cannulation should be considered a failure on the part of the emergency care provider to consider means by which they can optimize future vascular access attempts.

Selection of an Intraosseous Access Device

Once the decision has been made to place an IO catheter, providers should consider the specific advantages and limitations for each device and deployment site. Although many different IO access devices are commercially available, certain device characteristics may be helpful in deciding which IO catheter to use. These characteristics include:

- Degree of manual control with insertion (manual > semiautomatic > automatic)
- Force required to achieve adequate insertion
- Length and gauge of available cannulae
- Anatomic sites compatible with the selected device
- Known incidence of complications and device failures
- Provider familiarity and level of comfort with device use
- Availability of the selected device to the care provider

The **degree of manual control** among modern devices varies according to the mechanisms for insertion force available by device. Manually inserted IO devices have been largely phased out of production, but commercially available options at present include the Cook needle with Dieckmann™ modification (Cook Medical), the TALON® (Teleflex, Inc.), the FAST-1® (Teleflex, Inc.), and the SAM IO® system (SAM Medical). The Cook needle is available in 14-gauge, 16-gauge, and 18-gauge sizes with lengths from 25 to 40 mm. The TALON® comes in only one size (15 gauge, 38.5 mm length), as does the FAST-1®. Of course, manual IO catheters offer the greatest possible control over the insertion process, but can be challenging to place in dense, adult bones. Sternal insertion requires the least force (approximately 8.5 kg) as the bone is less dense, but other sites may require considerably more force to achieve insertion [16]. Semiautomatic devices such as the EZ-IO® (Teleflex, Inc.) system allow provider control with augmented insertion force due to the use of a mechanical, battery-operated rotary driver. Automatic devices such as the BIG® catheter (Safeguard Medical) offer the benefit of augmented insertion force but do not allow provider control over the force being used for insertion as they are injected into the bone by a tension-loaded spring.

Providers may be concerned about the risk of injury to the target bone or adjacent structures during IO catheter insertion. Pediatric bones are not as firm as adult bones, and excessive force during pediatric IO catheter insertions may increase the risk of target bone fracture during insertion. Excessive force or depth of insertion can also increase the risk of complications when IO devices are placed near vulnerable structures, such as arteries, veins, nerves, and joint capsules. For this reason, **IO insertion at the sternum, clavicle, radius, or ulna may be most safely achieved with device characterized by a high degree of provider control during insertion** (e.g., manual or semiautomatic devices), rather than automatic IO devices. Automatic devices (e.g., BIG®) may be preferred for target sites that are low risk for fracture or iatrogenic injury to adjacent structures, such as the proximal humerus, distal femur, proximal tibia, or distal tibia in adults.

The length and gauge of IO devices should also be considered when making decisions about IO catheter insertion. Of course, modern IO devices are generally 14 or 15 gauge in diameter, and the effects of catheter length may be clinically negligible in regard to infusion rate. That said, narrower and longer catheters likely have lower infusion flow rates under constant infusion pressure. In general, **providers should prefer shorter and larger diameter catheters when available**, especially if high-volume fluid infusion is required.

Available IO infusion sites may differ by patient, but **IO infusion sites closest to the central circulation (e.g., sternum, clavicle, proximal humerus) should be preferred when high-volume infusion is needed**. More distal sites (e.g., proximal tibia, distal tibia, distal radius, distal ulna) should be considered when proximal sites are not available or when high-volume infusion is not required. Choosing the ideal site for IO access depends on the patient's age, type of IO device, and contraindications (e.g., underlying fracture or overlying cellulitis). The ideal site will contain a large medullary cavity, thin cortical bone, a flat surface, and anatomic landmarks for a safe and quick cannulation.

The medullary cavity is highly vascularized and serves as a non-collapsible venous system even in the presence of shock. The **central sinus**, running through the diaphysis of long bones, is a distensible system that can expand to accommodate a fivefold increase in volume [17]. Blood from within the intraosseous space travels through a system of canals within the bone before joining the local vasculature. **Haversian canals** are bony tubes deep within the bone that run parallel to the long axis of the bone. These Haversian canals connect with smaller **Volkmann canals** running perpendicular to the long axis to allow blood to exit the bone. Haversian canals are found only in compact bone, while Volkmann canals are found in both compact and spongy bones. **Nutrient veins** exit the bone to join with **periosteal veins** draining the periosteum. Nutrient and emissary veins coalesce to form the larger named veins of the extremity [17, 18]. In the case of the proximal humerus, the **axillary vein** is the primary vessel carrying blood and infusates into the central circulation, while the proximal tibia is drained by the **popliteal vein**, and the distal tibia is drained by the **saphenous vein**. It is important to consider the crucial role of this venous network in facilitating IO infusion. Although the central sinus may be able to accommodate large volumes of infusate and expand with increased pressure, the smaller draining vessels may serve as a bottleneck, limiting flow. These smaller vessels may also be more prone to rupture or occlusion than the larger veins of the extremity.

Upon washout of the medullary cavity contents, bone spicules remain. These spicules provide structural reinforcement to the bone. However, during IO fluid resuscitation, bony spicules may impede the flow of fluids and high-volume medications. The mean blood pressure within the intraosseous space is roughly one-third of the systemic blood pressure [19], which is significantly higher than the usual pressure within the venous circuit (e.g., 0–6 mmHg in central veins and 8–10 mmHg in named peripheral veins) [20, 21]. Thus, even in the hypotensive patient, intrinsic intramedullary pressure can limit the forward flow of fluids. A pressure bag placed around the fluid bag may help to achieve needed flow rates by overcoming this intrinsic IO pressure [22].

Conclusion

The first decision to be made when considering the use of IO cannulation is whether the patient requires venous access at all. Once this determination has been made, the provider should assess whether PIV access may be readily achieved. In those cases in which PIV access is deemed to be impossible or likely to be delayed, providers should decide whether IO access is appropriate. If IO access is required, providers will need to determine whether they have the proper equipment to achieve IO cannulation and which target bones are accessible. Provider comfort with IO cannulation is an essential component of the decision to attempt IO access, and providers should be aware of which IO access devices are available to them and whether they are adequately trained to attempt IO placement. Various IO vascular access devices are available to most providers, including manual, semiautomatic, and automatic devices. Providers should consider which devices they have access to and whether they are adequately trained on IO catheter placement. Intraosseous devices should be used for cases in which direct venous access is deemed to be impossible or associated with unacceptable delays in care. While providers must consider short-term (i.e., during the hospitalization) and long-term (i.e., post-hospitalization) needs for the patient, immediate (i.e., stabilization) needs must be prioritized above these considerations, with an understanding that additional VAD placement may be required after IO access has facilitated immediate vascular access needs. The risks of IO catheter placement must be weighed against the benefits of IO infusion therapy, including the need for immediate infusion.

Key Concepts
- Intraosseous vascular access should be considered when immediate venous access is required, but direct venous access (i.e., peripheral or central venous access) is deemed impossible or associated with unacceptable delays in therapy.
- Providers should consider environmental, patient-specific, provider-specific, and device-specific factors that may contribute to difficult vascular access when assessing the need for IO access.
- When deciding upon optimal venous access for a patient, providers should consider immediate (i.e., stabilization) needs as well as short-term (i.e., during hospitalization) and long-term (i.e., post-hospitalization) needs for venous infusion of medications and fluids.
- Studies comparing IO to PIV infusion of medications should be designed in a randomized fashion, in order to reduce the risk of bias as it relates to selection of vascular access device. Studies comparing IO to PIV infusion of medications and fluids are largely biased against IO infusion due to resuscitation time bias and other factors that appear to suggest that IO infusion is associated with less favorable outcomes than PIV infusion.
- Intraosseous access devices differ in regard to catheter length, appropriate insertion site, and other factors that may influence clinical outcomes. Device-specific factors should be considered when comparing clinical outcomes associated with specific IO devices.

References

1. Hallas P, Brabrand M, Folkestad L. Reasons for not using intraosseous access in critical illness. Emerg Med J. 2012;29(6):506–7. https://doi.org/10.1136/emj.2010.094011. Epub 2010 Oct 18.
2. Bloch SA, Bloch AJ, Silva P. Adult intraosseous use in academic EDs and simulated comparison of emergent vascular access techniques. Am J Emerg Med. 2013;31(3):622–4. https://doi.org/10.1016/j.ajem.2012.11.021. Epub 2013 Feb 4.
3. Cheung WJ, Rosenberg H, Vaillancourt C. Barriers and facilitators to intraosseous access in adult resuscitations when peripheral intravenous access is not achievable. Acad Emerg Med. 2014;21(3):250–6. https://doi.org/10.1111/acem.12329.
4. Eichenlaub JM, Eichenlaub CT, Shuck JM, Paxton JH. Chapter 3. Landmark-based peripheral intravenous catheters. In: Paxton JH, editor. Emergent vascular access: a guide for healthcare professionals. Basel, Switzerland: Springer Nature; 2021. p. 23–53.
5. Paxton JH, Szydlowski B, Coddington CG. Chapter 10. Difficult vascular access. In: Paxton JH, editor. Emergent vascular access: a guide for healthcare professionals. Basel, Switzerland: Springer Nature; 2021. p. 217–48.
6. Rodríguez-Calero MA, Blanco-Mavillard I, Morales-Asencio JM, et al. Defining risk factors associated with difficult peripheral venous cannulation: a systematic review and meta-analysis. Heart Lung. 2020;49(3):273–86. https://doi.org/10.1016/j.hrtlng.2020.01.009. Epub 2020 Feb 11.
7. Leidel BA, Kirchhoff C, Braunstein V, et al. Comparison of two intraosseous access devices in adult patients under resuscitation in the emergency department: a prospective, randomized study. Resuscitation. 2010;81(8):994–9. https://doi.org/10.1016/j.resuscitation.2010.03.038.
8. Fields JM, Piela NE, Au AK, Ku BS. Risk factors associated with difficult venous access in adult ED patients. Am J Emerg Med. 2014;32(10):1179–82. https://doi.org/10.1016/j.ajem.2014.07.008. Epub 2014 Jul 30.
9. Sebbane M, Claret PG, Lefebvre S, et al. Predicting peripheral venous access difficulty in the emergency department using body mass index and a clinical evaluation of venous accessibility. J Emerg Med. 2013;44(2):299–305. https://doi.org/10.1016/j.jemermed.2012.07.051. Epub 2012 Sep 13.
10. Nolan JP, Maconochie I, Soar J, et al. Executive summary: 2020 international consensus on cardiopulmonary resuscitation and emergency cardiovascular care science with treatment recommendations. Circulation. 2020;142(16_suppl_1):S2–S27. https://doi.org/10.1161/CIR.0000000000000890. Epub 2020 Oct 21.
11. Soar J, Böttiger BW, Carli P, et al. European Resuscitation Council guidelines 2021: adult advanced life support. Resuscitation. 2021;161:115–51. https://doi.org/10.1016/j.resuscitation.2021.02.010. Epub 2021 Mar 24. Erratum in: Resuscitation. 2021;167:105–106.
12. Granfeldt A, Avis SR, Lind PC, et al. Intravenous vs. intraosseous administration of drugs during cardiac arrest: a systematic review. Resuscitation. 2020;149:150–7. https://doi.org/10.1016/j.resuscitation.2020.02.025. Epub 2020 Mar 3.
13. Andersen LW, Grossestreuer AV, Donnino MW. "Resuscitation time bias"—a unique challenge for observational cardiac arrest research. Resuscitation. 2018;125:79–82. https://doi.org/10.1016/j.resuscitation.2018.02.006. Epub 2018 Feb 6.
14. Paxton JH, Lemieux A. Chapter 11. Decision-making for emergent vascular access. In: Paxton JH, editor. Emergent vascular access: a guide for healthcare professionals. Basel, Switzerland: Springer Nature; 2021. p. 249–71.
15. Chopra V, Flanders SA, Saint S, et al. The Michigan appropriateness guide for intravenous catheters (MAGIC): results from a multispecialty panel using the RAND/UCLA appropriateness method. Ann Intern Med. 2015;163:S1–S39.
16. Philbeck TE, Puga TA, Montez DF, et al. Intraosseous vascular access using the EZ-IO can be safely maintained in the adult proximal humerus and proximal tibia for up to 48 h: report of a

clinical study. J Vasc Access. 2022;23(3):339–47. https://doi.org/10.1177/1129729821992667. Epub 2021 Feb 5.

17. Laroche M. Intraosseous circulation from physiology to disease. Joint Bone Spine. 2002;69(3):262–9. https://doi.org/10.1016/s1297-319x(02)00391-3.

18. Johnson DL, Findlay J, Macnab AJ, Susak L. Cadaver testing to validate design criteria of an adult intraosseous infusion system. Mil Med. 2005;170(3):251–7. https://doi.org/10.7205/milmed.170.3.251.

19. Tøndevold E, Eriksen J, Jansen E. Observations on long bone medullary pressures in relation to arterial PO2, PCO2 and pH in the anaesthetized dog. Acta Orthop Scand. 1979;50(6 Pt 1):645–51. https://doi.org/10.3109/17453677908991287.

20. Debrunner F, Bühler F. "Normal central venous pressure," significance of reference point and normal range. BMJ. 1969;3:148–50. https://doi.org/10.1136/bmj.3.5663.148.

21. Levick JR. An introduction to cardiovascular physiology. London: Hodder Arnold; 2010.

22. LaSpada J, Kissoon N, Melker R, et al. Extravasation rates and complications of intraosseous needles during gravity and pressure infusion. Crit Care Med. 1995;23(12):2023–8. https://doi.org/10.1097/00003246-199512000-00011.

The Future of Intraosseous Vascular Access

12

James H. Paxton

Introduction

Modern clinicians can scarcely imagine what it must have been like to practice medicine a century ago, when the pioneers of intraosseous (IO) infusion were just beginning to explore the potential utility of this technique. In those days, peripheral intravenous (PIV) catheters were reusable and made of heavy steel, the central veins were considered to be off-limits for cannulation, and antibiotics were not yet widely available. At the time, medical care providers were desperate for emergent vascular access techniques, and the IO route was interpreted by many in the medical community to be a safer and more reliable means by which fluids and medications could be provided to critically ill patients. Fast-forward nearly a century later, and much has changed in the realm of peripheral and central venous access. Peripheral IV lines made of disposable plastic materials are the standard of care, and the placement of central venous catheter (CVC) devices is considered to be commonplace; infections associated with vascular access devices (VADs), once common, are now considered to be "never events" within the medical community.

By contrast, IO devices are still made of surgical steel, often still inserted at the same anatomic sites utilized nearly a century ago, and remain relatively underutilized in the management of most medical conditions. One wonders what clinicians will think in a hundred years about the lack of progress that we have made in understanding the utility of the IO technique over the last century. While the medical community appears to have embraced and refined the science of direct venous access to a fine point, IO access remains relatively undeveloped and far less studied. Most analyses of IO infusion data are secondary reports of studies conducted for other reasons, with little attention paid to the primary use of this approach in clinical

J. H. Paxton (✉)
Department of Emergency Medicine, Wayne State University School of Medicine, Detroit, MI, USA
e-mail: james.paxton@wayne.edu

© The Author(s), under exclusive license to Springer Nature Switzerland AG 2024
J. H. Paxton (ed.), *Intraosseous Vascular Access*,
https://doi.org/10.1007/978-3-031-61201-5_12

301

practice. Suboptimal outcomes are accepted to be inherent to the IO technique, with a clear preference in published reports to the use of intravenous access techniques. Many modern providers still consider IO infusion to be a second-line choice (at best), with inadequate effort made to advance the field outside of industry-funded studies designed to show equivalency to the gold standard of PIV infusion. Few providers have suggested, let alone scientifically evaluated, the premise that IO infusion may one day prove to be superior to PIV access in the treatment of emergent medical conditions.

Much about the IO route remains cloaked in mystery and tradition, with conflicting evidence from the last century of medical literature left in place, undisturbed, as if it represents some inviolable shroud that cannot be lifted for fear of the controversy that would ensue. The reality is that we do not know whether IO infusion is truly equivalent to PIV or other direct venous access methods. But future generations will undoubtedly question the truth of this construct, calling for better designed trials to confirm or refute the equivalency paradox. This chapter describes many of the areas in which IO device development and study are likely to change practice for future clinicians. Now that direct venous access methods appear to have been fully explored in the medical literature, the time may be right for improved attention to IO infusion methods to advance the field. In this chapter, challenges to prevailing doctrine are described that the author expects will eventually lead to important breakthroughs in the study of IO infusion techniques.

Equivalency to PIV Infusion

The assumption of **bioequivalency** between IO and PIV infusion has been implicit in the clinical use of IO technology since its inception more than 80 years ago. Even when studied in animal models, equivalency is generally assessed on the basis of a clinical response: That is, does IO infusion generate the same clinical response from the subject as PIV infusion? Strictly speaking, it never does. Over the last century, the scientific community has accumulated vast knowledge from preclinical studies on the relative efficacy of IO infusion for fluids and medications, yet clinical studies comparing PIV to IO infusion have produced inconsistent results. This has led to an **equivalency paradox**, in which clinicians are asked to utilize the IO approach as if it is equivalent to PIV infusion despite popular evidence that it is not. This is not to say that IO infusion is inherently inferior to direct venous infusion; rather, we do not really understand how it is different. If one considers the bone marrow space to be a simple conduit for substances arriving, unchanged and unfiltered, into the venous circulation, the equivalency proposal seems to be sound. But bones are not simply tubes or conduits. They house a complex network of physiological processes that may (and should) be expected to interfere or otherwise alter how substances are transmitted into the bloodstream. Unfortunately, we have not yet scratched the surface of understanding how the circulatory system of the bone interacts with the fluids and medications that clinicians infuse into it.

Modern clinicians are just beginning to recognize that all bones used for IO infusion are not the same. Of course, we know that some bones have more red marrow or yellow marrow than others. We have also established that different bones have different reservoir volumes and different degrees of connectivity with the local and central circulation. But even these basic facts about bony anatomy are not generally considered when utilizing IO infusion in the clinical realm. As an example, let us consider the use of distal IO infusion sites (e.g., proximal tibia, distal tibia) for cardiac arrest (CA) resuscitation. It has been well established in both the CA and trauma resuscitation literature that the location of venous access matters [1, 2]. In fact, central venous access via the internal jugular or subclavian vein has been shown to deliver higher peak concentrations of drug and more rapid circulation times than PIV infusion in the CA model, although the challenges of safely and rapidly establishing central venous access have led professional guidelines to promote PIV access over CVC access for initial access attempts [1, 3–6]. At least one study comparing subclavian CVC to antecubital PIV infusion of Cardio-Green dye during active CPR chest compressions in human subjects showed a peak concentration of dye (2.4 mcg/mL) at the first sampling time (30 s post-infusion) that was six times higher than the greatest concentration ever achieved with PIV infusion (0.4 mcg/mL) during the 5 min following infusion [4]. The results of this study suggest that supradiaphragmatic CVC infusion of resuscitative medications for CA dramatically outperforms upper extremity PIV infusion, yet PIV infusion is still recommended.

It has also been well established that blood flow to structures below the diaphragm, including the intra-abdominal organs, is profoundly compromised during cardiopulmonary resuscitation (CPR) [7]. This suggests that resuscitative vascular access sites above the diaphragm should be preferred in such low-flow states [7]. Current ACLS and ATLS guidelines recommend that PIV access be established in the antecubital fossae of the upper extremity, and not in the lower extremities, presumably for this reason [1, 2]. It is clear from such recommendations that PIV access attempts at the upper extremities are preferred to lower extremity targets, yet modern scientists seem content to compare upper extremity PIV infusion with lower extremity (e.g., proximal tibia) IO infusions. Why would this be true? Clinicians would never select a lower extremity PIV infusion for CA or trauma resuscitation, but the vast majority of comparative data on IO infusion in CA utilizes a lower extremity IO site. This corollary of the equivalency paradox is especially enigmatic, in that supradiaphragmatic IO access sites (e.g., sternum, proximal humerus) have been described but are not well represented in the CA literature. Perhaps, there is an (obviously inaccurate) assumption that all IO sites are equivalent. But why would they be considered equivalent, when analogous PIV insertion sites are not viewed in the same light? Future CA investigators will realize that supradiaphragmatic IO sites are preferred for hypotensive patients and will begin to consider proximal humeral and sternal IO sites to be inherently different than subdiaphragmatic sites in regard to their resuscitative capabilities. But this paradigm shift has not yet happened.

Pharmacokinetic studies will undoubtedly continue to offer insight into the difference between various PIV and IO insertion sites, and existing studies have already begun to demonstrate this distinction. For example, the **Tmax** (i.e., time to peak drug concentration) and **Cmax** (i.e., highest serum concentration of drug) of amiodarone have been shown to be similar between IO and PIV infusion in a hypovolemic porcine model of cardiac arrest at the proximal humerus (PHIO), proximal tibia (PTIO), and sternum (STIO) infusion sites [8–10]. But other groups have found a significant lag in medication uptake with PTIO infusion of amiodarone when compared to STIO infusion, presumably due to the depot effect of this highly lipophilic medication [11, 12]. Other medications, such as ceftriaxone (but not ampicillin or cefotaxime), also appear to be bound by proteins in the marrow space with PTIO infusion demonstrating lower concentrations than those seen with upper extremity PIV infusion [13]. While some drugs such as phenytoin appear to have equivalent uptake between PTIO and PIV routes [14], epinephrine infusion in a porcine model of cardiac arrest appears to achieve a higher concentration at 30-s post-infusion with PHIO infusion than with peripheral intravenous (PIV) infusion although other parameters appear to be similar [15].

These preclinical studies routinely suggest that different medications behave differently within the IO space when compared to PIV infusion, especially in regard to protein and fat binding. Unfortunately, very few medications have been studied to determine whether their infusion via the IO space yields different bioavailability than PIV infusion. To date, the only IO pharmacokinetic study conducted in live human subjects was published in 2008, describing the experience of 22 adult cancer patients who received both PIV and IO infusion of a 5 mg dose of morphine sulfate [16]. The authors concluded that the Cmax and Tmax of these two routes were similar, but the volume of distribution (Vd) in the central compartment was significantly different ($p = 0.0247$), suggesting a "minor deposition effect" within the bone marrow space [16]. Considering the low lipophilicity of morphine, it seems likely that other medications with a higher degree of affinity for lipid binding would have a greater depot effect. Findings such as this will open the door for future studies in human subjects to determine (at least) the magnitude of marrow deposition with IO infusion, although no subsequent human trials have capitalized on this finding to date. Future investigators will undoubtedly exploit this gap in our understanding of how different medications interact with marrow contents to produce differing results when compared to direct venous infusion.

Randomized Controlled Trials

Randomized controlled trials (RCTs) are generally considered to be the gold standard for research studies, although very few RCTs have been designed to directly compare IO to PIV infusion for any indication. The most obvious patient population to be targeted for an RCT comparing IO to PIV infusion is the CA population, as IO catheters are commonly used for this indication. However, no RCT to date has directly compared the clinical outcomes associated with IO and PIV medication infusion in the management of CA [17]. Despite the abundance of opinion on the matter, there appears to be little interest in conducting an RCT for IO and PIV infusion in the treatment of CA in the United States, although many other countries have recently initiated such studies. In Taiwan, the "Venous Injection Compared to IntraOsseous Injection During Resuscitation of Patients With Out-of-hospital

Cardiac Arrest (VICTOR)" trial (Clinical Trials ID # NCT04135547) is nearing completion, which may offer some insight into the potential advantages of IO infusion for OHCA when compared to traditional PIV catheter-based resuscitation. This study is intended to explore clinically important outcomes following OHCA according to the type of venous access achieved by prehospital providers. Another ongoing Chinese study (Clinical Trials ID # NCT04130984) is also looking at the proximal tibial IO insertion site as it relates to clinical outcomes in OHCA patients according to the type of resuscitative line. If such RCTs are eventually to be reported, it appears likely that they will come from the Asian medical literature, as this subject appears to be a higher research priority in that region than in other areas.

Infusion Pressures

It has been well established that intramedullary pressures are higher than the ambient pressure within venous channels, with the average IO pressure being approximately one-third of a patient's systolic blood pressure. Thus, **pressurized infusion with the use of a pressure bag, infusion pump, syringe, or other pressure device is essential to achieving adequate flow rates with IO infusion**. While most PIV or central venous catheter (CVC) lines can achieve acceptable flow rates using gravity infusion of fluids alone, this is not true for IO lines. High-volume fluid infusion through an IO catheter requires pressurized infusion, but the optimal amount of pressure to be applied with IO infusion remains unknown. Syringes can generate significantly more pressure than other methods, but syringe infusion is very labor intensive and requires continuous effort on the part of medical providers to achieve forward flow.

Future research will likely focus on the amount of infusion line pressure needed to achieve adequate fluid flow rates with IO infusion, including investigation into more effective methods of applying infusion pressure during IO fluid resuscitation. Novel methods of augmenting flow through IO lines include the use of syringe-like technology, such as the LifeFlow™ device (Research Triangle Park, North Carolina, USA), which uses a manually driven hand pump to deliver high volumes of resuscitative fluids into the patient with greater infusion pressures than are generally achievable with fully automated devices such as infusion pumps. The use of high-pressure infusion devices such as the LifeFlow™ device may allow IO infusion to achieve flow rates comparable (or superior) to intravenous infusion. However, greater IO infusion pressures may reasonably be expected to increase the risk of infiltration and extravasation if infusion pressure exceeds the capacitance of the venous drainage channels to remove infusates from the medullary cavity once deposited. When infusion pressure exceeds the ability of the venous drainage system to empty the medullary space, excessive IO pressure will likely increase the risk of vein rupture or retrograde flow around the IO cannula into the soft tissues. **It is likely that excessive IO infusion pressures will increase the risk of extravasation, although this pressure-infusion relationship has not yet been fully explored**. Measurement of IO infusion pressures using readily available pressure transducers attached to the IO infusion circuit may allow correlation between infusion pressures and incidence of infiltration and extravasation events, although this relationship has not yet been explored in the medical literature.

Local Effects

The potential effects of IO infusion on bony metabolism and the regulation of local vasculature remain poorly understood, and further study into these local effects may yield a better understanding of complications seen with IO infusion. Soft tissue destruction adjacent or distal to an IO infusion site has been reported, presumably due to extravasation of vasopressors or hypertonic solutions into the region with resultant vasoconstriction and avascular necrosis. But these complications are not commonly seen, despite many preclinical animal studies and human subject clinical case reports of vasopressor infusion via the IO route. This suggests that certain characteristics of the patient or insertion site may be at least partially responsible for these potentially life-threatening complications. Yet, prospective studies involving IO vasopressor infusion, such as that seen commonly with cardiac arrest resuscitation, remain lacking in the medical literature. It is likely that future investigators will choose to more carefully monitor IO insertion sites in post-cardiac arrest patients (and others who routinely receive IO infusion) in search of better insight into how these deleterious local effects may be manifested and mitigated.

Epinephrine infusion via the IO route appears to induce local vascular vasoconstriction and increase bony vascular resistance, although this effect is not seen with vasopressin in the porcine model [18]. This suggests that **different vasopressor medications may have differing effects on blood flow regulation within the bone**, which could have significant implications for the use of specific vasopressors when IO infusion is required for cardiac arrest resuscitation. Although vasopressin was removed from the Advanced Cardiac Life Support (ACLS) guidelines cardiac arrest algorithm in 2015 [19], it seems possible that IO vasopressin could offer a better clinical profile than IO epinephrine, at least in regard to potential reduced efficacy for subsequent medication doses. A randomized controlled trial (or at least a well-designed clinical study) comparing IO vasopressin to IO epinephrine for cardiac arrest management might reveal differences in the clinical response to subsequent IO infusion of these vasopressors and other medications given later in the resuscitative event.

Standardization of Complications Reporting

To date, most reports of outcomes related to IO infusion have been described in terms of **provider-centered outcomes** such as time to placement, first-attempt deployment success rate, and ease of use. While such outcomes are understandable in the earliest phases of device adoption, evaluation of IO infusion devices must eventually progress beyond such provider-centered outcomes to address

patient-centered outcomes such as pain with placement and infusion, long-term complications, survival, and other outcomes that are of importance to patients. The likelihood of first-attempt success is undoubtedly higher with IO than with PIV access attempts, although the number of PIV attempts required to achieve adequate PIV access is not usually reported in clinical studies. It is not uncommon for clinicians to require multiple attempts at PIV placement before they achieve reliable PIV access, but this is seldom reported.

Complications of IO infusion are usually not reported according to any standardized format. In fact, what constitutes a "complication" of IO device deployment has never been standardized. Reports of complications attributed to IO cannulation among early adopters in the 1940s and 1950s included primarily infectious complications such as osteomyelitis and insertion site abscess, which are rarely seen. This has led to a very favorable complication profile for IO access, with early reports generally in agreement that the rate of "serious" complications following IO cannulation is less than 1% [20]. But **these traditional definitions of serious complications attributable to IO cannulation may not reflect the actual patient experience**. A modern perspective suggests that other noninfectious complications (e.g., soft tissue necrosis, extravasation, pain) may deserve additional attention. In fact, recent reviews of IO complications have suggested that the actual rate of complications from IO access may be much higher when also considering noninfectious complications [21, 22]. Unfortunately, inconsistent reporting of complications makes it impossible to perform a proper meta-analysis of the existing data to determine whether the conventional assumption of safety with IO infusion is deserved.

Device-Specific Differences

The modern industry standard for IO catheter length appears to be 15 mm for infants and small children, 25 mm for older children and adult proximal tibial insertions, and 45 mm for proximal humerus and obese adult distal femur/proximal tibial insertions. But these catheter length recommendations are based entirely upon preclinical studies and manufacturer recommendations and are not informed by clinical trials. In fact, very few studies have attempted to determine the optimal catheter length at any site for any human subjects. The internal diameter of modern IO catheters appears to be almost universally 15 gauge (1.8 mm), but selection of this conventional gauge is completely uninformed by any clinical data.

Future studies on the optimal depth of catheter insertion (i.e., catheter length) and gauge are needed to optimize clinical use of these devices. We know from **Poiseuille's law** that the rate of a liquid's flow (V) through a tube of a given length (L) and radius (r) under a pressure difference (p) is predicted by the equation, $V = (\pi\,pr^4/8\eta L)$, where η is the viscosity of the fluid. Given this relationship, it is predicted that larger gauge cannulae with shorter lengths should permit higher flow rates for any fluid. The usual internal diameter of IV tubing is 3–4 mm [23], which suggests that the bottleneck for IO infusion is the IO cannula, not the IV tubing setup. After all, the internal diameter of an IO cannula (1.8 mm) is often less than one-half of the internal diameter of the infusion tubing that is attached to it. Thus, **it seems likely that shorter, larger gauge IO cannulae should be able to deliver higher infusion rates with standard IV tubing**, assuming that all other factors are equal. Unfortunately, no major manufacturers of IO devices have chosen to introduce a larger gauge IO cannula into the market. Once manufacturers and IO device investigators recognize this bottleneck, it seems likely that larger gauge cannulae will be available, with greater attempts at guidance for minimal cannula length according to site- and patient-specific anthropomorphic soft tissue depth.

It is likely that patient sex, body mass index, and other patient-specific factors influence the amount of soft tissue overlying common IO catheter insertion sites. Unpublished data from our group suggest that female sex may be a risk factor for increased soft tissue depth at the PTIO insertion site, and other sex-specific differences may also exist. Future research will undoubtedly provide guidance for providers in selection of appropriate IO cannulae at specific insertion sites, with consideration for sex, comorbidities, and other determinants of soft tissue depth.

At present, clinicians and investigators appear to have adopted an unsettling tendency to assume that all IO devices are equivalent in regard to their placement success rates, flow rates, and risk of complications. This fallacy is understandable, as such distinctions between devices are unique within the vascular access community. Providers are not accustomed to distinguishing between different PIV or central venous catheter (CVC) devices in regard to their flow rates, complications, or other clinically relevant attributes. However, **the assumption that all IO devices are equivalent is both unfounded and potentially deleterious to patient care**. Different devices may be more or less appropriate for different sites and may have different indications with different complication profiles. Future research will focus upon how different IO infusion devices perform clinically, including reporting of complications according to the IO infusion device used, rather than a biased assumption that all IO catheters are the same. It is likely that future reports on IO infusion complications will eventually begin to include the rates of complications observed for specific devices and anatomic site selected for infusion. This may allow providers to make a more accurate assessment of the risks and benefits of IO infusion for a specific device or site, rather than assuming that all IO infusions are equally efficacious and safe.

Preloaded IO Infusion Devices

At present, IO infusion devices are never preloaded with medications for immediate injection. However, the use of IO devices to treat certain conditions such as cardiac arrest or life-threatening allergic reactions may seem to lend itself to the use of preloaded epinephrine cartridges (for example), especially when devices are to be deployed in austere environments. Preloading devices with an effective local anesthetic (e.g., lidocaine) might also save time when devices are to be deployed in sensate patients. The obvious challenge here is the development of pharmaceutical compounds with a longer shelf life, as the potential value of preloaded IO devices would seem to hinge on the stability of the preloaded medication over time. At present, such innovations may be infeasible due to storage limitations inherent to the drugs themselves. However, future developments in this field could liberate this approach to care.

Novel Devices

Review of recent trends in the development and release of novel IO infusion devices reveals certain trends. In general, cannula design remains similar between the traditional manual IO devices and more modern devices, notwithstanding changes to the connector hub linking the cannula to the infusion tubing. The basic design of an IO catheter is a straight stainless steel tube with a constant internal diameter (15 gauge, approximately 1.8 mm) and a beveled tip. In most cases, a removable stylet is inserted inside of the cannula, which is in turn attached to the handle or some adapter permitting interface with a mechanical driver. Of course, some notable modifications have been introduced by necessity. For example, the FAST1™ (and other derivative products based upon that device design) includes a ring of stabilizer needles around the cannula that facilitate a perpendicular angle of insertion and help the user to gauge depth of insertion at the sternum (Fig. 12.1). These modifications

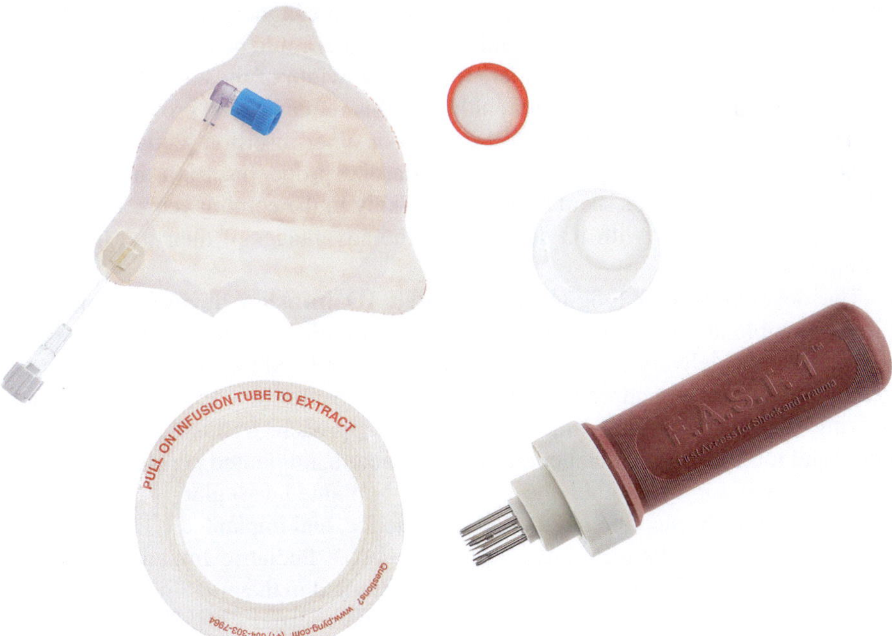

Fig. 12.1 The FAST1® intraosseous system. (*Image courtesy of Teleflex Incorporated. © 2023 Teleflex Incorporated. All rights reserved*)

are needed because of the shallow position of the target sternum and the narrow space within the flat cancellous bone to be accessed. Overpenetration is a major concern at the sternal site, so this modification has enabled this device to position itself as a preferred device at this anatomic site. The FAST1™ also features a much shorter steel cannula prefabricated with an attached flexible infusion tube, allowing a low profile relative to the skin surface that may reduce the risk of post-placement levering and dislodgement. But this novel design has also led to some early challenges, including multiple cases of retained catheter tip after extraction attempts, likely due to difficulties in properly using the catheter extraction tool [24–27]. More recent versions of the device do not require an extraction tool for device removal and have not yielded any further reports of retained catheter tip. This example of how novel devices can lead to unanticipated challenges may be one reason that modern IO devices have not deviated far from the standard design for IO cannulae.

Despite the potential challenges associated with novel IO device designs, it is likely that truly unique modifications to the existing design model will be introduced in the future. For example, **radiopaque materials other than stainless steel** could be considered that may be less prone to bending with excessive torque without shattering. Concerns about infectious complications may eventually lead to **antibacterial coatings or impregnated materials** that could mitigate this risk with prolonged infusion times. Some progress on antibacterial coatings for intraosseous implants has already been made [28]. Similarly, the incorporation of **heparin or other anticoagulants** into an IO device might reduce the risk of catheter clotting or help with the clearance of marrow contents to facilitate higher infusion rates. **Wider cannula** (i.e., beyond the 15 gauge industry standard) could be expected to improve infusion rates as well, if one considers the narrow width of the cannula to be a significant bottleneck for fluid infusion, although this remains to be proven. The use of a **target patch** (as with the FAST1™ device) or other insertion guidance tools for new or existing devices may also help to standardize proper insertion site. These and other novel modifications seem feasible and likely in the coming years as providers become more familiar with IO devices and the advantages of their use in a wider patient population.

The development of long-term **implanted IO infusion devices** seems to be highly feasible and may offer an alternative to traditional methods. Subcutaneous implanted drug delivery devices are already being utilized for the infusion of analgesic medications for chronic pain patients and insulin among diabetic patients, proving the potential value and safety of this approach. Synthetic arteriovenous grafts and long-term tunneled hemodialysis catheters, implanted ports connecting to a central vein for chemotherapy, and other implanted vascular access aids are already commonly encountered in medical practice, and implanted IO devices are a likely extension of this technique. The Osteoport™ Pediatric Implant (LifeQuest Medical, San Antonio) was a promising device studied in the preclinical goat model 30 years ago but was never subsequently commercialized [29]. This device was patented in several countries for use with chemotherapy infusion, but never reached clinical trials. More recently developed devices could reinvigorate this approach.

One such device, the PortIO™ Intraosseous Infusion System (PAVmed Inc., Columbia), is currently being studied in a human clinical trial expected to enroll 40 patients with chronic kidney disease requiring non-emergent delivery of fluids and medications [30]. Although this device is currently being studied for a dwell time of up to 60 days, the investigators plan to assess complications at 30 days post-explant to determine whether such devices have any long-term effects on the bone and surrounding tissues [30]. Studies like this could offer patients with long-term vascular access needs an alternative means of infusing medication and fluids that allows for the preservation of veins for other purposes such as dialysis maintenance therapy.

Novel Infusion Sites

Although the proximal humerus and proximal tibia are the most commonly used IO infusion sites, the sternum, distal femur, and distal tibia are also commonly reported in the medical literature [22]. Current evidence suggests that **intrinsic flow rates are highest at the more central and proximal sites** (i.e., proximal humerus, sternum) with resistance to flow gradually increasing at bony targets more distant from the central circulation. The distal femur has been a standard target bone for pediatric resuscitation for many years due to its greater proximity to the heart and improved flow rates relative to the proximal tibia, but this site is also gaining traction in the adult prehospital population [31]. Specialty devices including the FAST1™, along with the occasional use of manual catheters, allow for infusion at the sternum, which likely has the best flow rate of all IO devices when properly inserted. Meanwhile, traditional sites such as the distal tibia (i.e., internal malleolus) and distal fibula (i.e., external malleolus) have been largely neglected in favor of more proximal targets [32].

Newer target bones for IO infusion have been gradually appearing on the scene and may offer unique advantages over traditional access sites. The calcaneus has been studied in a cadaver model [35, 36], but clinical use appears to be limited to a single case report [35]. The iliac crest and clavicle have been studied [36] in older reports, but these sites have been underutilized to date by emergency care providers. The distal radius and ulna have been suggested [33, 37, 38]. It is likely that increased use of these nontraditional IO insertion sites will expand the list of available IO infusion sites for future clinicians without significantly increasing the risks associated with this infusion technique.

Dwell Time

Dwell time is the length of time that a properly placed, functional venous access device can be left in situ for clinical use. The optimal dwell time for a PIV catheter remains controversial, with the US Centers for Disease Control and Prevention (CDC) recommending routine replacement of PIV catheters every 72–96 h [37], although multiple studies suggest that PIV catheters can be safely maintained until replacement is clinically indicated due to catheter malfunction, infiltration, blockage, phlebitis, or evidence of infection [40]. While a great deal of time and effort have been dedicated to studying the safety of extended dwell times with PIV catheters, **very little has been done to advance our understanding of the safety of extended IO dwell times** [41]. Following their initial approval of the IO route, the United States Food and Drug Administration (FDA) established a 24-h safe dwell time recommendation for IO cannulae, which was extended in November 2018 to 48 h when alternative intravenous access is not available or reliably established [41]. Although the European Union has advanced the dwell time for IO catheters to 72 h, the Canadian government (and many American institutions) still endorses a 24-h dwell time limit for IO catheters [41, 42]. In clinical practice, many providers remove functional IO catheters as soon as direct venous access has been established. As a result of these short dwell times, little clinical evidence is available to inform providers about the safety (or risks) of extended IO dwell times greater than 48 h.

Philbeck and colleagues studied 121 healthy volunteers who were randomized to receive a total of 61 proximal humerus and 66 proximal tibia IO insertions with a 48-h dwell time [41]. While 79 (65.3%) subjects reported pain at the insertion site, other complications were rare, including four cases (3.3%) of insertion site swelling, two cases (1.7%) of fluid infiltration, and one case (0.8%) of fluid leakage. The insertion site was examined at 48 h post-placement, and marrow cultures were taken from the catheter just prior to removal. The insertion site was re-examined at 30 days post-removal, at which time X-rays were taken to identify signs of bony injury or infection. No evidence of infection (e.g., positive marrow culture, radiographic evidence of osteomyelitis) was found.

One of the few reports of extended IO dwell times beyond 48 h was published in 1977 by Dr. Manuel Valdes from the Institute of Tropical Diseases (Mexico City, Mexico) [32]. In this case series, 15 adult patients were treated clinically with IO infusion at the distal tibia (12 cases) or distal fibula (three cases). The average volume of IO fluid infusion for these patients was 4 L (SD ± 10.05, median 7.4) over a mean period of 5.4 days (SD ± 7.7, median 3.4 days). At least one patient experienced an IO dwell time of 30 days, and there were no "gross complications," with only "moderate fluid infiltration" in a few patients [32].

Unfortunately, without high-quality data on patient outcomes after extended dwell times, it is impossible to predict the true rate of complications associated with long-term continuous use of these devices. Many studies like the Philbeck study have obtained plain films of the target bones weeks or months after a limited infusion and have shown no discernible evidence of infection or bone injury. But this does not prove the safety of extended dwell times beyond the clinically utilized time periods. Unfortunately, this paucity of data is not likely to be improved by American investigators due to time-restrictive use of these devices, although some evidence on long-term complications may be expected from European investigators or others who practice in countries where dwell times >48 h are routinely employed.

Pain Control

The most important limitation to widespread use of the IO route for infusion of medications and fluids is pain with infusion. If clinicians are to ever expand the use of this technique beyond insensate patients (e.g., cardiac or respiratory arrest), this common complication of IO infusion will need to be more effectively managed. Current guidelines suggest the use of 40 mg IO preservative-free lidocaine as an initial bolus, followed by additional doses as needed. But this regimen is not universally effective at treating pain caused by stretch receptors in the intramedullary space. Future research will undoubtedly focus upon alternative means of controlling IO infusion pain, which could include distraction techniques, use of alternative local anesthetics, and regional nerve blocks. None of these approaches have been well described in the existing medical literature for this indication, but all seem to be viable means of reducing the discomfort associated with IO infusion. Buffered lidocaine-containing sodium bicarbonate solution has been suggested, but has not been adequately studied. Whatever the solution, future clinicians will find that adequate pain control with IO infusion is essential to making this approach palatable to the majority of sensate patients.

Intraosseous Pressure Monitoring

Critically ill patients often present with hemodynamic instability, requiring aggressive blood pressure monitoring. Although serial blood pressure measurement with a sphygmomanometer (i.e., blood pressure cuff) can be performed noninvasively in selected cases, blood pressure measurements obtained with such devices are very labor intensive and can be unreliable in the setting of hypotension. Consequently, patients with exceedingly low systemic blood pressures may require placement of an invasive intra-arterial catheter, which can be attached to a pressure transducer to allow for continuous blood pressure monitoring. These arterial lines are most commonly placed peripherally at the radial artery or centrally at the femoral artery [43]. Although complications of arterial line placement are rare, they can include air embolism (0.2%), pseudoaneurysm formation (0.3%), local soft tissue infection (0.8%), and even thrombosis or compartment syndrome leading to permanent ischemic damage to the extremity (0.2%) [43]. Although ultrasound guidance can be used to expedite the process, published reports suggest that radial arterial line placement by landmark method takes about 5 min, requires an average of 2.2 attempts to achieve success, and requires attempts at a second location in about 60% of cases [44].

Recent studies have shown that IO pressure can be successfully measured using commonly available arterial line monitoring equipment attached to a standard IO catheter [45], and continuous blood pressure monitoring has already been performed in both healthy [46] and critically ill human subjects [47]. Intraosseous pressure measurements appear to vary widely between subjects, with tibial IO pressures approximating 52% (± 32%) of external cuff pressure and proximal humeral IO pressures approximating 26.5 ± 15.2% of cuff measurements [46]. One small study of ten critical care patients found that the measured IO pressure readings were generally 35–40% range of the blood pressure readings obtained via external blood pressure cuff, although this study did not report anatomic location of the IO devices used [47]. Additional study is needed to identify factors that could alter intrinsic IO pressures at different insertion sites or with different medical conditions, as well as the effects of drugs and other interventions on the accuracy of IO pressure as an indirect indicator of systemic blood pressure.

Conclusion

The future of intraosseous infusion will be guided by the need to improve patient care inasmuch as that need is recognized by future clinicians. It has been said that necessity is the mother of invention, but clinician-investigators must first recognize the need to improve current management strategies in order to achieve future innovation. Complacency with existing IO infusion methods will never adequately advance the field. Fortunately, clinicians are beginning to recognize that the current limitations of the field are not absolute and that better devices and means by which to utilize them are within our grasp if we choose to seek them out. Rather than relying upon historical evidence to inform their vascular access decisions, future investigators will seek out better data pertaining to individual device performance and the intrinsic differences that do exist relating to IO site selection and how different medications behave within the IO space. Pharmacokinetic studies of IO medication infusion are currently lacking, but will necessarily inform how dosing will be adjusted for IO infusion in the future. Our understanding of complications attributed to IO infusion will be enhanced by improved awareness of the cascade of physiologic events that is triggered by the introduction of substances into the intramedullary space. In the future, we will recognize that all IO devices and IO medications are not the same. Armed with this knowledge, we will begin the real work of advancing the field of IO infusion techniques to realize the true potential of this lifesaving approach to indirect vascular access.

Key Concepts
- Although current IO infusion devices are exclusively made of surgical stainless steel, future devices will be composed of other physiologically inert substances that will be less susceptible to inadvertent bending or occlusion. This may include substances intended to reduce the risk of cannula thrombosis or otherwise promote improved flow through the device.
- Future studies of IO infusion will likely better distinguish between different IO insertion sites, as well as different IO devices, allowing investigators to better delineate the clinical profiles of specific IO devices at specific sites.

- Future pharmacokinetic studies will likely explore the medication-specific characteristics of substances infused via the IO route. This will facilitate a better understanding of how drug delivery can be optimized during IO infusion.
- Future randomized controlled studies will likely provide additional evidence on how IO infusion differs from PIV infusion.
- Current evidence on the safety of extended dwell times for IO catheters is lacking, primarily due to the lack of extended dwell times (>48 h) for clinical use. Clinical data following extended dwell times will eventually be acquired to assess the true safety of extended IO infusion periods.

References

1. Panchal AR, Bartos JA, Cabañas JG, et al. Adult basic and advanced life support writing group. Part 3: adult basic and advanced life support: 2020 American Heart Association guidelines for cardiopulmonary resuscitation and emergency cardiovascular care. Circulation. 2020;142(16_suppl_2):S366–468. https://doi.org/10.1161/CIR.0000000000000916. Epub 2020 Oct 21.
2. Vishwanathan K, Chhajwani S, Gupta A, Vaishya R. Evaluation and management of haemorrhagic shock in polytrauma: clinical practice guidelines. J Clin Orthop Trauma. 2020;13:106–15. https://doi.org/10.1016/j.jcot.2020.12.003.
3. Barsan WG, Levy RC, Weir H. Lidocaine levels during CPR: differences after peripheral venous, central venous, and intracardiac injections. Ann Emerg Med. 1981;10:73–8. https://doi.org/10.1016/s0196-0644(81)80339-3.
4. Kuhn GJ, White BC, Swetnam RE, et al. Peripheral vs central circulation times during CPR: a pilot study. Ann Emerg Med. 1981;10:417–9. https://doi.org/10.1016/s0196-0644(81)80308-3.
5. Talit U, Braun S, Halkin H, et al. Pharmacokinetic differences between peripheral and central drug administration during cardiopulmonary resuscitation. J Am Coll Cardiol. 1985;6(5):1073–7. https://doi.org/10.1016/s0735-1097(85)80311-9.
6. Emerman CL, Pinchak AC, Hancock D, Hagen JF. Effect of injection site on circulation times during cardiac arrest. Crit Care Med. 1988;16:1138–41. https://doi.org/10.1097/00003246-198811000-00011.
7. Voorhees WD, Babbs CF, Tacker WA Jr. Regional blood flow during cardiopulmonary resuscitation in dogs. Crit Care Med. 1980;8(3):134–6. https://doi.org/10.1097/00003246-198003000-00008.
8. Holloway CM, Jurina CS, Orszag CJ, et al. Effects of humerus intraosseous versus intravenous amiodarone administration in a hypovolemic porcine model. Am J Disaster Med. 2016;11(4):261–9. https://doi.org/10.5055/ajdm.2016.0248.
9. Hampton K, Wang E, Argame JI, et al. The effects of tibial intraosseous versus intravenous amiodarone administration in a hypovolemic cardiac arrest porcine model. Am J Disaster Med. 2016;11(4):253–60. https://doi.org/10.5055/ajdm.2016.0247.
10. Smith S, Borgkvist B, Kist T, et al. The effects of sternal intraosseous and intravenous administration of amiodarone in a hypovolemic swine cardiac arrest model. Am J Disaster Med. 2016;11(4):271–7. https://doi.org/10.5055/ajdm.2016.0249.
11. Adams TS, Blouin D, Johnson D. Effects of tibial and humerus intraosseous and intravenous vasopressin in porcine cardiac arrest model. Am J Disaster Med. 2016;11(3):211–8. https://doi.org/10.5055/ajdm.2016.0241.
12. O'Sullivan M, Martinez A, Long A, Johnson M, Blouin D, Johnson AD, Burgert JM. Comparison of the effects of sternal and tibial intraosseous administered resuscitative drugs on return of spontaneous circulation in a swine model of cardiac arrest. Am J Disaster Med. 2016;11(3):175–82. https://doi.org/10.5055/ajdm.2016.0237.

13. Pollack CV Jr, Pender ES, Woodall BN, Parks BR. Intraosseous administration of antibiotics: same-dose comparison with intravenous administration in the weanling pig. Ann Emerg Med. 1991;20(7):772–6. https://doi.org/10.1016/s0196-0644(05)80840-6.

14. Vinsel PJ, Moore GP, O'Hair KC. Comparison of intraosseous versus intravenous loading of phenytoin in pigs and effect on bone marrow. Am J Emerg Med. 1990;8(3):181–3. https://doi.org/10.1016/0735-6757(90)90317-s.

15. Johnson D, Garcia-Blanco J, Burgert J, et al. Effects of humeral intraosseous versus intravenous epinephrine on pharmacokinetics and return of spontaneous circulation in a porcine cardiac arrest model: a randomized control trial. Ann Med Surg (Lond). 2015;4(3):306–10. https://doi.org/10.1016/j.amsu.2015.08.005.

16. Von Hoff DD, Kuhn JG, Burris HA 3rd, Miller LJ. Does intraosseous equal intravenous? A pharmacokinetic study. Am J Emerg Med. 2008;26(1):31–8. https://doi.org/10.1016/j.ajem.2007.03.024.

17. Hooper A, Nolan JP, Rees N, et al. Drug routes in out-of-hospital cardiac arrest: a summary of current evidence. Resuscitation. 2022;181:70–8. https://doi.org/10.1016/j.resuscitation.2022.10.015. Epub 2022 Oct 26.

18. Voelckel WG, Lurie KG, McKnite S, et al. Comparison of epinephrine with vasopressin on bone marrow blood flow in an animal model of hypovolemic shock and subsequent cardiac arrest. Crit Care Med. 2001;29(8):1587–92. https://doi.org/10.1097/00003246-200108000-00015.

19. Moskowitz A, Ross CE, Andersen LW, et al. Trends over time in drug administration during adult in-hospital cardiac arrest. Crit Care Med. 2019;47(2):194–200. https://doi.org/10.1097/CCM.0000000000003506.

20. Rosetti VA, Thompson BM, Miller J, et al. Intraosseous infusion: an alternative route of pediatric intravascular access. Ann Emerg Med. 1985;14(9):885–8. https://doi.org/10.1016/s0196-0644(85)80639-9.

21. Bouhamdan J, Polsinelli G, Akers KG, et al. A systematic review of complications from pediatric intraosseous cannulation. Curr Emerg Hosp Med Rep. 2022;10:116–24. https://doi.org/10.1007/s40138-022-00256-x.

22. Palazzolo A, Akers KG, Paxton JH. Complications of intraosseous catheterization in adult patients: a review of the literature. Curr Emerg Hosp Med Rep. 2023;11:35–48. https://doi.org/10.1007/s40138-023-00261-8.

23. Cross GD. Evaluation of 3-mm diameter intravenous tubing for the rapid infusion of fluids. Arch Emerg Med. 1987;4(3):173–7. https://doi.org/10.1136/emj.4.3.173.

24. Johnson DL, Findlay J, Macnab AJ, Susak L. Cadaver testing to validate design criteria of an adult intraosseous infusion system. Mil Med. 2005;170(3):251–7. https://doi.org/10.7205/milmed.170.3.251.

25. Fenton P, Bali N, Sargeant I, Jeffrey SL. A complication of the use of an intra-osseous needle. J R Army Med Corps. 2009;155(2):110–1. https://doi.org/10.1136/jramc-155-02-06.

26. Byars DV, Tsuchitani SN, Erwin E, et al. Evaluation of success rate and access time for an adult sternal intraosseous device deployed in the prehospital setting. Prehosp Disaster Med. 2011;26(2):127–9. https://doi.org/10.1017/S1049023X11000057.

27. Hodgetts JM, Johnston A, Kendrew J. Long-term follow-up of two patients with retained intraosseous sternal needles. J R Army Med Corps. 2017;163(3):221–2. https://doi.org/10.1136/jramc-2016-000699. Epub 2017 Mar 1.

28. Bai X, Yu J, Xiao J, Wang Y, Li Z, Wang H. Antibacterial intraosseous implant surface coating that responds to changes in the bacterial microenvironment. Front Bioeng Biotechnol. 2023;10:1016001. https://doi.org/10.3389/fbioe.2022.1016001.

29. Welch RD, Waldron MJ, Hulse DA, Johnston CE 2nd, Hargis BM. Intraosseous infusion using the osteoport implant in the caprine tibia. J Orthop Res. 1992;10(6):789–99. https://doi.org/10.1002/jor.1100100607.

30. ClinicalTrials.gov. PR-0164 first in human clinical trial of the PAVmed PortIO intraosseous infusion system. ClinicalTrials.gov Identifier: NCT06037265. 2023. https://classic.clinicaltrials.gov/ct2/show/NCT06037265. Accessed 13 Dec 2023.

31. Rayas EG, Winckler C, Bolleter S, et al. Distal femur versus humeral or tibial IO access in adult out of hospital cardiac resuscitation. Resuscitation. 2022;170:11–6. https://doi.org/10.1016/j.resuscitation.2021.10.041. Epub 2021 Nov 5

32. Valdes MM. Intraosseous fluid administration in emergencies. Lancet. 1977;1(8024):1235–6. https://doi.org/10.1016/s0140-6736(77)92441-2.

33. McCarthy G, O'Donnell C, O'Brien M. Successful intraosseous infusion in the critically ill patient does not require a medullary cavity. Resuscitation. 2003;56(2):183–6. https://doi.org/10.1016/s0300-9572(02)00348-9.

34. Clem M, Tierney P. Intraosseous infusions via the calcaneus. Resuscitation. 2004;62(1):107–12. https://doi.org/10.1016/j.resuscitation.2004.02.012.

35. McCarthy G, Buss P. The calcaneum as a site for intraosseous infusion. J Accid Emerg Med. 1998;15(6):421. https://doi.org/10.1136/emj.15.6.421.

36. Iwama H, Katsumi A, Shinohara K, et al. Clavicular approach to intraosseous infusion in adults. Fukushima J Med Sci. 1994;40(1):1–8.

37. Waisman M, Roffman M, Bursztein S, Heifetz M. Intraosseous regional anesthesia as an alternative to intravenous regional anesthesia. J Trauma. 1995;39(6):1153–6. https://doi.org/10.1097/00005373-199512000-00025.

38. Waisman M, Waisman D. Bone marrow infusion in adults. J Trauma. 1997;42(2):288–93. https://doi.org/10.1097/00005373-199702000-00019.

39. Centers for Disease Control and Prevention (CDC). Guidelines for the prevention of intravascular catheter-related infections. 2011. https://www.cdc.gov/infectioncontrol/guidelines/bsi/recommendations.html. Accessed 14 Nov 2023.

40. Webster J, Osborne S, Rickard CM, Marsh N. Clinically-indicated replacement versus routine replacement of peripheral venous catheters. Cochrane Database Syst Rev. 2019;1(1):CD007798. https://doi.org/10.1002/14651858.CD007798.pub5.

41. Philbeck TE, Puga TA, Montez DF, et al. Intraosseous vascular access using the EZ-IO can be safely maintained in the adult proximal humerus and proximal tibia for up to 48 h: report of a clinical study. J Vasc Access. 2022;23(3):339–47. https://doi.org/10.1177/1129729821992667. Epub 2021 Feb 5.

42. Government of Canada. Active device name search results. From Health Canada. Licence No.: 78909. Licence name: EZ-IO Intraosseous Infusion System—Needle Sets. https://www.canada.ca/en/health-canada/services/drugs-health-products/medical-devices.html. Accessed 13 Nov 2023.

43. Scheer B, Perel A, Pfeiffer UJ. Clinical review: complications and risk factors of peripheral arterial catheters used for haemodynamic monitoring in anaesthesia and intensive care medicine. Crit Care. 2002;6(3):199–204. https://doi.org/10.1186/cc1489. Epub 2002 Apr 18.

44. Shiver S, Blaivas M, Lyon M. A prospective comparison of ultrasound-guided and blindly placed radial arterial catheters. Acad Emerg Med. 2006;13(12):1275–9. https://doi.org/10.1197/j.aem.2006.07.015. Epub 2006 Nov 1.

45. Chang CY, Yeh KJ, Roller LA, Torriani M. A measuring technique for intra-osseous pressure. Skeletal Radiol. 2021;50(7):1461–4. https://doi.org/10.1007/s00256-020-03671-x. Epub 2020 Nov 13.

46. Salzman JG, Loken NM, Wewerka SS, Burnett AM, Zagar AE, Griffith KR, Bliss PL, Peterson BK, Ward CJ, Frascone RJ. Intraosseous pressure monitoring in healthy volunteers. Prehosp Emerg Care. 2017;21(5):567–74. https://doi.org/10.1080/10903127.2017.1302529. Epub 2017 Apr 18.

47. Frascone RJ, Salzman JG, Ernest EV, Burnett AM. Use of an intraosseous device for invasive pressure monitoring in the ED. Am J Emerg Med. 2014;32(6):692.e3–4. https://doi.org/10.1016/j.ajem.2013.12.029. Epub 2013 Dec 18.

Index

A

Absolute contraindications, 77, 78
Acid-base disturbances, 256–258
Acidosis, 256
Action potentials, 251
Acute failure of the peripheral circulation, 5
Acute hypotension, 70
Adductor longus muscle, 269
Advanced Cardiac Life Support
      (ACLS), 67, 306
Air emboli, 233
Air Release System (ARS) pneumothorax
      decompression device, 31
Alkalosis, 257
Alteplase, 194
Amide-type local anesthetic (LA) agent, 259
Amiodarone, 70, 177
Amiodarone, Lidocaine or Placebo Study
      (ALPS), 177
Analgesics, 185, 186
Anascorp®, 190
Angle of Louis, 94
Antecubital fossa, 290
Anterior superior iliac spine (ASIS), 107
Antibacterial coatings, 310
Antibiotics, 197
Antidote infusion, 187
Antiseptic methods, 9
Anxiolysis, 274, 276, 277
Arinkin, Mikhael Innokent'evich, 3
Aspiration failure, 219
Atracurium, 198
Atropine, 72, 178, 188
Automatic intraosseous devices, 131
    Bone Injection Gun (B.I.G.), 132–134
    future directions, 144
    New Intraosseous (NIO™), 134–137
Awake and conscious patients, 80
Axillary block, 271
Axillary nerve, 271
Axons, 250

B

Bailey, Henry Hamilton, 9
Bailey's winged catheter design, 118
Basilic vein, 288, 289
BD™ Intraosseous Powered Driver, 33, 34, 126
BD™ Intraosseous Vascular Access System,
      143, 144
Becton-Dickinson needle, 15
Benzodiazepines, 72
Berg, Robert A., 15, 16
Bethell, Frank H., 12
Biceps femoris tendon, 268
BIG® device, 132–134
Bioavailability, 51, 52, 170, 171
Bioequivalency, 302
Bisphosphonates, 196
Bleeding risks, 80
Body mass index (BMI), 104
Bolleter, Scotty, 25, 29, 31
Bone anatomy, 43–46
Bone, factors influencing vascular supply
      to, 47–49
Bone fragility, 218
Bone Injection Gun® (BIG), 22, 23,
      61, 132–134
Bone marrow, 1, 2, 252, 256
Bougie aided cricothyroidotomy (BAC) kit, 31
Brachial plexus, 265, 271–274
Brachiocephalic vein, 52
Buffered lidocaine, 261
Bupivacaine, 263

J. H. Paxton (ed.), *Intraosseous Vascular Access*,
https://doi.org/10.1007/978-3-031-61201-5

C
Calcaneal tuberosity, 107
Calcaneus, 106, 107
Calcium, 178, 251
Cannulation of medullary cavity, 180
Cardiac arrest, 67–69, 171–179
Cardiopulmonary emergencies, 67–70
Cardiopulmonary resuscitation (CPR), 96, 173, 232, 303
Cardiovascular collapse : central nervous system (CC:CNS) ratio, 264
Cefazolin, 197
Central sinus, 297
Central venous catheter (CVC), 14, 43, 62, 63, 66, 287, 290
Centruroides immune F(ab')$_2$ (Anascorp®), 190
Cephalic vein, 288, 289
C-fibers, 253
Clavicle, 105, 106, 296
Clinchy, Richard, 35
Coller, Frederick A., 12
Compartment syndrome (CS), 217, 224, 235, 238
Complications of intraosseous access, 215
  delayed
    compartment syndrome (CS), 235, 238
    infectious complications, 229–232
    pulmonary fat embolism (PFE), 232, 233
    rates of, 238–240
    soft tissue ischemia / necrosis, 233
  early (placement)
    dermal injury, 225, 226
    device malfunction, 218–221
    immediate dislodgement/extravasation, 221–223, 225
    inability to cannulate, 217, 218
    pain, 228, 229
    sternal perforation, 227, 228
  major, 215
  minor, 215
  moderate, 215
  pediatric and adult patients, 216, 217
Cook manual IO needle with Dieckmann™ modification, 20, 122
Cortex, 44, 252
COVID-19, 137

D
Davila, Nick, 25
Decision-making
  general approach to vascular access, 288–293
    immediate phase, 294, 295
    long-term phase, 294, 295
    MAGIC guidelines, 294, 295
    selection of an intraosseous access device, 296, 297
    short-term phase, 294, 295
Degree of manual control, 296
Dendrites, 250
Depolarization, 251
Depot effect, 11, 52, 53, 66, 171
Depth of target bone, 154
Dermal injury, 225, 226
Device malfunction, 215, 218–221
Device-specific causes, 291
Dextran-containing solutions, 181
Dextrose, 187
Diaphysis, 43, 93, 252
Diazepam, 191
Direct venous cannulation, 93
Direct venous infusion, 150
Dislodgement, definition of, 223
Distal femur, 99–101
Distal tibia, 101, 102
Distraction techniques, 264–266
Doan, Charles A., 2, 4
Dobutamine, 184
Dopamine, 184
Dorsal venous network, 288
Drinker, Cecil Kent, 1, 2
Dwell time, 294, 311, 312
Dysrhythmias, medication for, 172–179

E
Egress, 150
Eisbrenner, Eric, 25, 27
Electromyographic (EMG) data, 199
Ellison, Joseph Bramhall, 9
Endosteum, 44
Endothelial nitric oxide synthase (eNOS), 48
End-tidal carbon dioxide (ETCO$_2$), 179
Epinephrine, 67, 173, 174, 176, 267
Epiphyseal growth plate, 98, 217
Epiphysis, 43, 252
Equivalency paradox, 302
Equivalency to PIV Infusion, 302–304
Ester-type LAs, 259
Estrogen, 49
Etomidate, 198
Excessive soft tissue depth, 217
External jugular (EJ) vein, 289
Extravasation, 155, 221–223, 225, 234
Extrinsic factors, 149
EZ-IO® Intraosseous Vascular Access System, 27, 28, 30, 60, 134, 135, 138–142, 219

F
FAST-Responder®, 124, 125
Fat and bone marrow emboli, 17
Fat embolism, 155
Femoral nerve block, 265, 268–274
Femoral triangle, 269
Fentanyl, 198
Filtration coefficient, 50
First Access for Shock and Trauma (FAST-1®)
       intraosseous infusion system, 22,
       123, 124, 309
First-line therapy, 75
Flow rates
    future directions, 163
    infusion pressures, 155
    infusion site selection, 153, 154
    infusion tract, 156
    patient-related factors, 151–153
    pressurized infusion
       risk of, 155, 156
       techniques for, 154, 155
    subject, 157–160
    troubleshooting
       catheter insertion, 161
       marrow aspiration, 161
       obstacles to flow, 162, 163
Fluid dynamics, 150, 151
Fluid flux, 50
Fluid resuscitation, 71
Fojtik, Shawn, 34
Future of intraosseous vascular access, 301, 302
    device-specific differences, 307
    dwell time, 311, 312
    equivalency to PIV infusion, 302–304
    infusion pressures, 305
    intraosseous pressure monitoring, 313, 314
    local effects, 306
    novel devices, 309–311
    novel infusion sites, 311
    pain control, 313
    RCTs, 304, 305
    standardization of complications reporting,
       306, 307

G
Gadolinium contrast agents, 74
Ghedini, Giovanni, 4
Gimson, Janet Dinah, 10
Gimson needle, 11, 119
Greater saphenous vein, 101

H
Haversian canals, 44, 45, 297
Heinild, Svend, 13
Hematologic emergencies, 194, 195
Henderson-Hasselbalch equation, 259
Henning, Norbert, 7
Heparin, 310
Hub connector, 115
Humeral IO infusion, 51
Hyaluronic acid, 234
Hydrophilic opioid, 186
Hydrostatic pressure, 50
Hydroxocobalamin, 73, 188, 189
Hydroxyethyl starch, 182
Hyperglycemia, 187
Hypertonic saline, 181, 192
Hypodermic needle, 15
Hypoglycemia, 5, 187
Hypotension, 65
Hypovolemia, 153, 171
Hypovolemic cardiac arrest swine
       model, 176
Hysteresis, 183

I
Ibandronate, 196
Iliac bone, 107, 108
Immediate dislodgement, 221–223, 225
Immediate phase, 294, 295
Implanted IO infusion devices, 310
Impregnated materials, 310
Improper insertion technique, 215
Inadequate monitoring, 215
Inappropriate infusion pressures, 215
Indirect infusion, 43
Indirect venous access, 150
Infectious complications, 229–232
Infiltration, 233
Infraclavicular block, 271
Infusate, 156
Infusion pressures, 155, 305
Infusion tract, 156
Ingress, 150
Inguinal ligament, 269
Inotropes, 183, 184
Insulin, 187
Internal motors, 131
Internal thoracic vein, 52
Interscalene block, 271
Intramedullary pressure, 256

Intraosseous access site selection
calcaneus, 106, 107
clavicle, 105, 106
distal femur, 99–101
distal tibia, 101, 102
general considerations, 110, 111
iliac bone, 107, 108
proximal humerus, 102–104
proximal tibia, 97–99
radius and ulna, 108
sternum, 94–97
Intraosseous Access System by SAM Medical
(SAM IO), 33, 34, 126, 127
Intraosseous cannulation, history of, 37
Intraosseous capillary system, 3
Intraosseous contrast media, 195, 196
Intraosseous (IO) infusion, 43
bioavailability, 52
cardiopulmonary emergencies, 67–70
contraindications
absolute, 77, 78
relative, 78–80
depot effect, 52, 53
diagnostic studies, 73, 74
indications
for age and health status, 75
for awake patients, 74
for older patients and patients with
chronic medical conditions, 77
for pediatric patients, 75–77
IOP and flow, 49, 51
neurohormonal regulation, 46
neurologic and toxicologic
emergencies, 72, 73
shock and circulatory emergencies, 70
traumatic emergencies, 70, 71
vascular supply to bone, factors
influencing, 47–49
Intraosseous pressure (IOP), 49–51, 152,
313, 314
Intraosseous vascular access, 1–3, 6, 24, 61
BD™ Intraosseous Powered Driver, 34
Bone Injection Gun (BIG®), 22
EZ-IO® infusion system, 27, 28
Gimson needle, 11
hypodermic needle, 15
Jamshidi™ modified Illinois disposable
needle, 19
Klima and Salah needles, 18
Monoject® Illinois Needle, 19
Next Generation Intraosseous (NIO®)
device, 33
Osteoport®, 25
proximal tibia/distal femur, 7

proximal tibial IO catheter, 31
reusable Jamshidi™ needle, 19
Rochester needle, 14
SAM IO® Intraosseous system, 34
success rates and speed of, 64–67
Sussmane-Raszynski needle, 20
TALON™ device, 32
Turkel Trephine Instrument, 13, 14
Vidacare™ LLC, 25
VidaPen® device, 27
winged catheter design, 10
Witts needle, 9
Intravascular volume status, 175
Intrinsic factors, 149
Ischemic osteonecrosis, 196
Isoproterenol, 184

J
Jacobs, Michael W., 21
Jamshidi, Khosrow, 18
Jamshidi™ modified Illinois disposable needle,
19, 121, 122
Josefson, Arnold R., 3
Jugular notch, 96

K
Ketamine, 198
Klima, Rudolph, 18
Klima and Salah needles, 18, 120
Klima-Rosegger needle, 119
Korth, Josef, 7
Kramer, George C., 25
Kuhn, John G., 24

L
Lamprecht, Werner, 7
Lateral side of tibia, 235
Levetiracetam, 72
Levobupivacaine, 263, 264
Lidocaine, 53, 70, 177, 185, 186, 260, 264
Lipid emulsion, 189
Lipophilic cortices, 177
Lipophilic opioids, 186
Local anesthetics, 258, 259, 261, 262
bupivacaine, 263
tetracaine, 262
toxicity, 263, 264
Local anesthetics systemic toxicity (LAST), 264
Long bones of the human body, 43
Long-term phase, 294, 295
Lorazepam, 71, 191

M
Macht, David I., 10
Manual intraosseous devices, 115–119
    Bailey's winged catheter design, 118
    BD™ Intraosseous Powered Driver, 126
    Cook manual IO needle with Dieckmann™
        modification, 122
    FAST-Responder®, 124, 125
    First Access for Shock and Trauma
        (FAST-1®) intraosseous infusion
        system, 123, 124
    general considerations, 127
    Gimson needle, 119
    Intraosseous Access System by SAM
        Medical (SAM IO), 126, 127
    Jamshidi™ modified Illinois disposable
        needle, 121, 122
    Klima and Salah needles, 120
    Original Jamshidi™, 121
    push-pull system, 117
    Reusable Jamshidi™ needle for iliac crest
        biopsy, 120
    Sur-Fast™ needle, 123
    Sussmane-Raszynski™ needle, 122, 123
    TALON™ device, 125
    Turkel Trephine Instrument, 117
Manubrial intraosseous insertion site, 95
Manubriosternal junction, 95
Marrow aspiration, 161
Maximal serum concentration, 174
Mean arterial pressure (MAP), 176
Medial side of the tibia, 235
Median antecubital vein, 289
Medication administration, IO for, 167–169
    antibiotics, 197
    atropine/pralidoxime, 188
    for cardiac arrest / dysrhythmias,
        172–180
    general considerations, 169–172
    hematologic emergencies, 194, 195
    hydroxocobalamin, 188, 189
    hypoglycemia/hyperglycemia, 187
    inotropes, 183, 184
    intraosseous contrast media, 195, 196
    lidocaine/analgesics, 185, 186
    lipid emulsion, 189
    methylene blue, 189
    naloxone, 190
    osteopathy, 196
    poisoning/antidote infusion, 187
    respiratory failure, 198, 199
    scorpion antivenom, 190
    seizures/neurological emergen-
        cies, 191–193
    for shock states, 180–182
    vasopressors, 183, 184
Medullary bone pain, 256
Medullary cavity, 43, 252
Membrane potential, 251
Metaphyseal vessels, 45
Metaphysis, 43, 252
Methylene blue, 73, 189
Michigan Appropriateness Guide for
        Intravenous Catheters (MAGIC)
        guidelines, 294, 295
Midazolam, 191
Miller, Larry, 24, 27
Minimal inhibitory concentration (MIC), 197
Monoject® Illinois Needle, 19, 120, 121
Morphine sulfate, 186
Morrison, Maurice, 11
Müller, Franz, 1
Myelinated nerve conduction, 252
Myelin sheath, 250, 251
Myeloproliferative disorders, 80

N
Naloxone, 73, 190
Near Needle Holder™, 21
Necrosis, 233
Nerve growth factor (NGF), 256
Nerve stimulation, 269
Neurohormonal regulation, 46, 47
Neurological emergencies, 71–73, 191–193
New Intraosseous (NIO™), 134–137
Next-Generation IO (NIO®), 61
NIO Infant®, NIO Pediatric® and NIO Adult®
        devices, 33
Nitric oxide (NO), 47
Nociception, 253
Nodes of Ranvier, 252
Non-collapsible vein, 63
Non-essential organs, 171
Norepinephrine, 46, 183
Nutrient arteries, 45
Nutrient foramina, 45, 256
Nutrient veins, 297

O
Octanol-water partition coefficient, 170
Oncotic pressure, 50
O'Neill, James F., 5
Ong, Marcus Eng Hock, 32
Optimal central venous concentrations, 171
Original Jamshidi™, 121
Orlowski, James P., 17

Osteoclast, 257
Osteogenesis imperfecta, 79, 218
Osteomyelitis, 229, 231–232
Osteopathy, 196
Osteoport®, 24, 310
Osteotomy, 223, 269, 273
Out-of-hospital cardiac arrest (OHCA),
    67, 68, 170

P
Packed red blood cells (pRBCs), 71
Pain, 228, 229, 235, 250, 313
    distraction techniques, 264–266
    femoral nerve block, 268–274
    local anesthetics, 258, 259, 261, 262
        bupivacaine, 263
        tetracaine, 262
        toxicity, 263, 264
    popliteal nerve block, 268–274
    regional nerve blocks to shoulder and tibia,
        265, 267
    skeletal pain
        anatomy of, 250, 252
        pathophysiology of, 253, 255–258
    systemic analgesia and anxiolysis, 274,
        276, 277
Pallor, 235
p-aminobenzoic acid (PABA) metabolite
    formation, 259
Papper, Emanuel M., 7, 8
Paralysis, 235
Paraneural sheath, 268
Paresthesia, 235
Patient-centered outcomes, 307
Patient-specific factors, 215, 291
Paxton, James H., 32
Peabody, Francis Weld, 4
Pediatric Advanced Life Support
    (PALS), 59, 173
Periosteal bone pain, 255, 256
Periosteal veins, 297
Periosteum, 44, 252, 255
Peripheral intravenous (PIV) access, 59, 62,
    64–66, 69, 170, 171, 287,
    290, 302–304
Peripheral nerve blocks, 265
Peripheral nerve sheath, 266
Peripheral vein in the upper extremity, 288
Peripheral venous cutdown, 76
Pernicious anemia, 3
Perpendicular to the cortex of the bone, 98
Persistent loss of function, 62
Pharmacokinetics, 53, 66, 170, 274

Phenobarbital, 192
Phenytoin, 72, 191
Pianese, Giuseppe, 1
Poikilothermia, 235
Poiseuille's Law, 150, 152, 307
Poisoning, 187
Popliteal nerve block, 265, 268–274
Popliteal vein, 297
PortIO™ Intraosseous Infusion System, 311
Posterior distal metaphysis, 109
Potency, 261
Pralidoxime, 188
Pressurized infusion
    risk of, 155, 156
    techniques for, 154, 155
Price, Alison H., 5
Profilnine® SD, 194
Prolonged therapy, 294
Proportionality constant, 186
Prothrombin complex concentrate, 73, 194
Provider-centered outcomes, 306
Provider-specific causes, 291
Proximal humerus, 102–104, 154
Proximal insertion sites, 154
Proximal tibia, 31, 97–99, 154
Pulmonary fat embolism (PFE), 232, 233
Pulselessness, 235
Push-pull infusion system, 6, 117

R
Radial and musculocutaneous nerves, 271
Radiopaque materials, 310
Randomized controlled trials (RCTs), 68,
    304, 305
Rapid sequence intubation (RSI), 198
Raszynski, Andre, 20
Recombinant factor VIIa (rFVIIa), 195
Red marrow, 44, 151, 170, 252
Reflection coefficient, 51
Regional nerve blocks to shoulder and tibia,
    265, 267
Relative contraindications, 78–80
Relative mass, 266
Rendina, Romeo, 8
Respiratory failure, 198, 199
Resuscitation, 155, 287, 292
Return-of-spontaneous-circulation (ROSC),
    67, 69, 174, 177
Reusable Jamshidi™ needle, 19, 120
Rivaroxaban, 194
Robin, Charles-Philippe, 4
Rochester needle, 14
Rocuronium, 53, 198

Rosegger, Hellfried, 18
Rosenberg, Bonnie, 27
Rosenberg, Norman, 26, 27
Rovenstine, Emery A., 8

S
Safety and Efficacy of Intraosseous
Ropivacaine in Lower Extremity
(SORE) study, 185
Saltatory conduction, 252
Saphenous vein, 297
Sartorius muscle, 269
Schamberg, Ira L., 11
Scheinberg, Sam, 34, 35
Sciatic nerve, 268
Scorpion antivenom, 73, 190
Seizures, 191–193
Seldinger, Sven Ivar, 14
Semi-automatic intraosseous devices, 132
BD™ Intraosseous Vascular Access System,
143, 144
EZ-IO® Intraosseous Vascular Access
System, 138–142
future directions, 144
Semimembranosus tendon, 268
Semitendinosus tendon, 268
Septic shock, 70
Septicemia, 80
Serum laboratory tests, 60
Seyfarth, Paul Carly, 3
Shear stress (SS), 48
Shock and circulatory emergencies, 70
Shock states, medication for, 180–182
Short-term phase, 294, 295
Simplified pneumothorax emergency air
release (SPEAR) system, 31
Sinusoids, 45, 50
Site-specific contraindications, 78
Skeletal pain
anatomy of, 250, 252
pathophysiology of, 253, 255–258
Sodium bicarbonate, 73, 179, 180
Sodium-potassium pump, 251
Soft tissue ischemia, 233
Soft tissue necrosis, 60
Soma, 250
Spivey, William H., 17
Starling's equation, 50
Starling forces, 50
Status epilepticus, 71
Sternal Access Vascular Entry (SAVE)
manual, 21
Sternal infusion approach, 6

Sternal perforation, 227, 228
Sternum, 94–97, 153, 296
Sturgis, Cyrus C., 12
Stylet, 115
Subclavian vein, 52
Succinylcholine, 198
Supraclavicular block, 271
Suprasternal notch, 96
Supraventricular tachycardia (SVT), 177
Sur-Fast™ needle, 20, 21, 123
Surgical intervention kit (SIK), 31
Sussmane, Jeffrey B., 20
Sussmane-Raszynski™ needle, 20, 122, 123
Synapse, 250
Systemic analgesia, 274, 276, 277
Systemic vascular resistance (SVR), 290

T
Tactically Advanced Lifesaving Intraosseous
Needle (TALON™) device, 32, 125
Target patch, 310
Technological limitations, 215
Tenecteplase, 194
Tetracaine, 262
T-Handle Jamshidi™ disposable IO cath-
eters, 121
Thermal skin burn, 80
Thiopental, 198
Threshold potential, 251
Tibial nerve, 268
Tibial tuberosity, 97
Time to maximal concentration, 174
Time-to-vascular access, 287
Titkemeyer, Bob, 25
Tocantins, 5, 7, 8
Tranexamic acid (TXA), 182
Transcortical, 220
Traumatic emergencies, 70, 71
Turkel, Heinrich, 12
Turkel Trephine Instrument, 13, 14, 117

U
Ulna, 109, 110, 296
Ultrasound, 269

V
Valdes, Manuel M., 15
Vancomycin, 197
Vascular access devices (VADs), 301
Vascular supply to bone, factors
influencing, 47–49

Vasopressin, 47, 176
Vasopressors, 71, 183, 184
Venous Injection Compared to IntraOsseous
Injection During Resuscitation of
Patients With Out-of-hospital
Cardiac Arrest (VICTOR)
trial, 304–305
Vesicants, 233
Vidacare™ LLC, 25
VidaPen®, 27, 28
Virtual reality (VR), 265
Visual Analog Scale (VAS), 229, 276
Volkmann canals, 297
Voltage-gated sodium channels, 259
Volume of distribution (Vd), 186, 304
Von Hoff, Daniel D., 24
von Kölliker, Rudolf Albert, 4

W
Waisman, Marc, 22
Wider cannula, 310
Wile, Udo J., 11
Witts, Leslie John, 9, 116
Witts lumbar puncture needle, 9, 10, 116
Wolff-Eisner, Alfred, 1

X
Xiphoid process, 94

Y
Yellow marrow, 43, 53, 152, 252